UNIVERSITY OF MEMPHIS LIBRARIES
3 2109 00843 7601

P9-CLC-055

THE FOOD SAFETY INFORMATION HANDBOOK

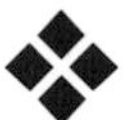

Cynthia A. Roberts

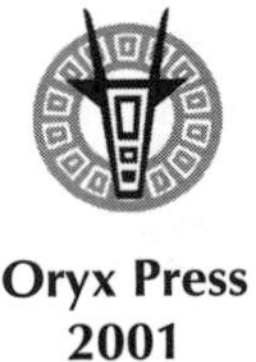

Oryx Press
2001

The rare Arabian Oryx is believed to have inspired the myth of the unicorn. This desert antelope became virtually extinct in the early 1960s. At that time, several groups of international conservationists arranged to have nine animals sent to the Phoenix Zoo to be the nucleus of a captive breeding herd. Today, the Oryx population is over 1,000, and over 500 have been returned to the Middle East.

Library of Congress Cataloging-in-Publication Data

Roberts, Cynthia A.
The food safety information handbook / Cynthia A. Roberts.
p. cm.
Includes bibliographical references and index.
ISBN 1-57356-305-6 (alk. paper)
1. Food adulteration and inspection. 2. Food contamination.
TX531.R57 2001
363.19'26—dc21 2001021435

British Library Cataloguing in Publication Data is available.

Library of Congress Catalog Card Number: 2001021435
ISBN: 1-57356-305-6

First published in 2001

Oryx Press, 88 Post Road West, Westport, CT 06881
An imprint of Greenwood Publishing Group, Inc.
www.oryxpress.com

Printed in the United States of America

The paper used in this book complies with the Permanent Paper Standard issued by the National Information Standards Organization (Z39.48–1984).

10 9 8 7 6 5 4 3 2 1

For Andy, who had to do without

Contents

PREFACE

Food safety is both a solid issue and an enigmatic one. Ask anyone on the street for a definition, and they'll probably answer that it means food that is safe to eat. But breaking this down into its components is a harder task. If one asks important questions such as what is safe food, how safe is safe, how many people get sick from unsafe food, what are the major causes of unsafe food, how can food be made safe, and who's responsibility is food safety, the seemingly solid nature of the discipline dissolves.

While this book cannot pretend to answer questions that even experts in the field are grappling with, it does try to give the reader some possible answers, a broad overview of the subject, and the tools necessary to interpret the quality of the food they eat and the validity of the information to which they are exposed. The audience for the book includes those who eat food, whether they be parents, students, cooks, food industry workers, dietitians, health professionals, educators, or librarians.

The first part of the book offers an introduction and overview to the field of food safety. Chapter 1 begins with food hazards, exposing the reader to information about viruses, pathogenic bacteria, naturally occurring toxins, pesticides, and other dangers. Although humankind has been working to protect the food supply for millennia, pathogens and other forces have been similarly changing throughout the millennia to thwart attempts to make the food supply safe. These factors are examined, followed by a short history of discoveries that have contributed to the current state of scientific knowledge about food safety. Finally, readers are introduced to some of the techniques that have been developed to make food safer, the result of which can be seen in the aisles of grocery stores.

In Chapter 2 the reader is introduced to several hot topics and the issues on each side of the debate over food biotechnology, bovine somatotropin, food irradiation, pesticides, drinking water quality, and restaurant food safety. Chapter 3 provides a chronology of events covered under the umbrella of food safety—inventions, discoveries, foodborne illness outbreaks, legislation, and other events that have shaped our understanding of the safety of food. Chapter 4 traces the evolution of the laws and policies that guide food production in the United States. The reader will follow a chronological path from the earliest laws enacted in the 1600s to modern food safety regulations of the late 1990s. Agencies responsible for regulating food safety at the federal, state, and local levels are examined. Foodborne and waterborne illness statistics make up Chapter 5, which includes what we know, what we don't know, and why we don't know it. Chapter 6 explores options for working in the field of food safety and choices of education and certifications available, along with ideas on where to find scholarships, internships, and fellowship opportunities.

The second part of the book, Chapters 7 through 11, offers food safety resources. These resources cover the whole range of food safety—food allergy, food biotechnology, general food safety, food microbiology, pesticides, food irradiation, water quality and safety, and food preservation. Chapter 7 presents reports on food safety topics from government agencies, nonprofit research institutions, consumer advocacy groups, and academic institutions. This chapter also lists consumer-level brochures. Chapter 8 covers books, from those suitable for children to those for food professionals. Internet and electronic resources are highlighted in Chapter 9, including Web sites, databases, reference tools, and Internet news and discussion groups. Chapter 10 lists food safety educational materials for children; adult consumers; food service workers; providers at child day care centers and other institutions; school food service workers; and volunteers at picnics, church suppers, fairs, and food banks. Chapter 11 lists organizations involved in food safety, including Cooperative Extension Service Offices, Food and Drug Administration public affairs specialists, hotlines, and state agencies and programs. The book closes with a glossary of food safety terms.

ACRONYMS

AMS	Agricultural Marketing Service
APHIS	Animal and Plant Health Inspection Service
ARS	Agricultural Research Service
B.C.E.	Before current era
CDC	Centers for Disease Control and Prevention
CRADA	Cooperative Research and Development Agreement
CSREES	Cooperative State Research, Education, and Extension Service
DHHS	Department of Health and Human Services
EPA U.S.	Environmental Protection Agency
ERS	Economic Research Service
FAO/WHO	Food and Agriculture Organization/World Health Organization
FDA U.S.	Food and Drug Administration
FIFRA	Federal Insecticide, Fungicide, and Rodenticide Act
FQPA	Food Quality Protection Act
FSI	National Food Safety Initiative
FSIS	Food Safety and Inspection Service
GIPSA	Grain Inspection, Packers and Stockyards Administration
GRAS	Generally Recognized as Safe as designated by FDA
HACCP	Hazard Analysis Critical Control Points
JIFSR	Joint Institute for Food Safety Research
NASS	National Agricultural Statistics Service
NIH	National Institutes of Health
NMFS	National Marine Fisheries Service
NPR	National Performance Review
NSTC/OSTP	National Science and Technology Council/Office of Science and Technology Policy
OMB	Office of Management and Budget
USDA	U.S. Department of Agriculture

Part 1

Overview of Food Safety

Chapter 1

An Overview of Food Safety

Food safety is a matter that affects anyone who eats food. Whether or not a person consciously thinks about food safety before eating a meal, a host of other people have thought about the safety of that food, from farmers to scientists to company presidents to federal government officials and sanitarians. This chapter serves as a broad introduction to food safety and the concerns facing those who work with food.

After defining safe food and foodborne illness, this chapter examines the various chemical, microbiological, and physical hazards to the food supply, presenting the hazards in this order:

I. Chemical hazards
   1. Food additives
   2. Food allergens
   3. Antibiotics in animals
   4. Naturally occurring toxins
   5. Pesticides

II. Microbiological hazards
   1. Bacteria
   2. Viruses
   3. Protozoa and parasites
   4. Bovine spongiform encephalopathy (BSE)

III. Physical hazards
   1. Food Defect Action Levels

A table of the most important foodborne pathogens highlights their sources, along with foods involved and symptoms of foodborne illness. Next follows a discussion of the factors that influence foodborne illness, namely:

1. Demographics
2. Consumer lifestyles and demands
3. Food production and economics
4. New and evolving pathogens

A history of food safety concentrates on scientific discoveries from the 1600s to modern times. The chapter ends with a look at food preservation techniques that humankind has practiced over the millennia to make food safer. These techniques range from the earliest methods of drying to newer high-tech methods such as food irradiation, and newer lower-tech methods such as using natural antimicrobials.

SAFE FOOD DEFINED

The concept of safe and wholesome food encompasses many diverse elements. From a nutritional aspect, it is food that contains the nutrients humans need and that helps prevent long-term chronic disease, promoting health into old age. From a food safety aspect, it is food that is free not only from toxins, pesticides, and chemical and physical contaminants, but also from microbiological pathogens such as bacteria and viruses that can cause illness. This book is concerned with the food safety aspect of food, leaving the diet and nutritional properties of food for experts in nutrition.

While America's food supply is among the safest in the world, there are still numerous threats to the safety of the food supply. Some of these threats have been around since ancient times, while others are newer, the result of changing lifestyles, production practices, and even evolution of microorganisms themselves. Ensuring the safety of food is a shared responsibility among producers, industry, government, and consumers.

A major focus of this book is microbial foodborne illness, a widespread, but often unrecognized, sickness that affects most people at one time or another. It is caused by eating food that is contaminated with pathogens such as bacteria, viruses, or parasites. At least four factors are necessary for foodborne illness to occur: (1) a pathogen; (2) a food vehicle; (3) conditions that allow the pathogen to survive, reproduce, or produce a toxin; and (4) a susceptible person who ingests enough of the pathogen or its toxin to cause illness. The symptoms often are similar to those associated with the flu-nausea, vomiting, diarrhea, abdominal pain, fever, headache. Most people have experienced foodborne illness, even though they might not recognize it as such, instead blaming it on the "stomach flu" or "24-hour bug." Symptoms usually disappear within a few days, but in some cases there can be more long-lasting effects such as joint inflammation or kidney failure. In the most severe cases people die from foodborne illness. Every year more than 5,000 Americans die from eating contaminated food (Mead 1999).

It is difficult to trace a bout of foodborne illness back to a particular food because illness can occur anywhere from an hour to several days, or even weeks, after eating the contaminated food. Epidemiologists faced with tracing a foodborne illness outbreak may have to interview dozens of people, asking them to recall everything they ate for the past week. It is difficult for people to remember everything they ate yesterday, much less one week ago. Further complicating the picture is that one person may eat the contaminated food and not become ill, while someone else in a higher-risk group does. In 81 percent of foodborne illnesses the cause remains unknown (Mead 1999).

Food Hazards

Experts describe food safety problems in terms of hazards, with those hazards categorized as chemical, microbiological, or physical. They have long considered the most dangerous hazards to be those of microbiological origin, followed by those of naturally occurring toxins (Wodicka 1977; Cliver 1999). However, pesticides and additives have been prominent subjects for the media, which may lead some people to focus on those hazards more than others. But as more stories emerge of people becoming ill from bacterial contamination, the public is increasingly aware of the importance of microbiological hazards. People do die from microbial hazards, but deaths due to consuming pesticide residues or food additives are rare.

Water is a food, and also is subject to microbial contamination. Some pathogens, such as *Cryptosporidium parvum*, are more waterborne than foodborne. While this chapter does discuss microbial contamination of water, it is beyond the scope of this book to consider waterborne hazards primarily caused by pollution, such as heavy metals, or pathogens that follow pathways other than the digestive tract.

Chemical Hazards

Chemical hazards include agricultural chemicals such as pesticides, herbicides, rodenticides, insecticides, fertilizers, antibiotics and other animal drugs, cleaning residues, naturally occurring toxins, food additives, allergens, and toxic chemicals from industrial processes that can enter the food chain directly during processing or indirectly through plants and animals. The Environmental Protection Agency (EPA) controls chemicals applied at the farm; the United States Department of Agriculture (USDA) controls antibiotics and animal drugs; and the Food and Drug Administration (FDA) controls additives and residual chemicals on processed foods.

Food Additives

The use of food additives dates back to ancient times. Examples of these early additives are salt to preserve meats and fish, herbs and spices for seasoning foods, sugar to preserve fruits, and vinegar to preserve vegetables. Today manufacturers use more than 3,000 food additives. A commonly used definitition of a food additive is any substance added to a food either directly or indirectly through production, processing, storing, or packaging. Food additives serve a number of functions:

Preservatives to keep food fresh and to prevent spoilage. This is important, as in our modern lifestyle food is rarely eaten at the time or place it is produced. Calcium propionate inhibits molds and is often added to bread products for this purpose.

Nutrients to improve or maintain the nutritional quality of foods. Most salt contains iodine to prevent goiter, a condition resulting from iodine deficiency.

Processing aids to maintain product texture such as retaining moisture, preventing lumping, or adding stability. Powdered foods such as cocoa contain silicon dioxide to prevent clumping when water is added.

Flavors to enhance or change the taste or aroma of a food. These include spices, herbs, flavor enhancers, natural and synthetic flavors, and sweeteners.

Colors to give foods an appealing look. Many of the colors we associate with foods are from added colorings, such as caramel to make cola drinks brown and annatto to make margarine yellow.

Food additives are derived from naturally occurring and synthetic materials. Scientists can now synthesize in the laboratory many additives that used to be derived from natural substances, creating a larger and cheaper supply. Americans consume from 140 to 150 pounds of additives a year, mostly due to additives such as sugar, corn sweeteners, salt, pepper, vegetable colors, yeast, and baking soda. Food additives allow us to enjoy safe, wholesome, tasty foods year-round without the inconvenience of growing our own foods or shopping daily. Convenience foods are made possible by the use of food additives.

FDA approves all food additives before they can be added to foods. USDA authorizes additives used in meat and poultry products. Before manufacturers may use an additive, they must prove that the additive does what it was intended to do and that it will not be harmful to humans at the expected level of consumption. Two groups of additives are not subject to FDA's strict approval process—those that are prior sanctioned and those that are generally recognized as safe (GRAS). Prior sanctioned substances were already approved by FDA before the 1958 Food Additives Amendment to the Food, Drug and Cosmetic Act. GRAS substances, including salt, sugar, spices, and vitamins, have been used extensively in the past with no known harmful effects, and therefore experts believe them to be safe. FDA may also label an additive as GRAS based on scientific evidence that it is safe. FDA and USDA continue to monitor prior sanctioned and GRAS substances to ensure that they really are safe as new evidence emerges. In addition, FDA operates the Adverse Reaction Monitoring System (ARMS) to investigate all complaints related to specific foods, food and color additives, or vitamin and mineral supplements.

While the overwhelming majority of additives are safe for all people, small segments of the population are sensitive to some. Sulfites are an example of this; they cause hives, nausea, shortness of breath, or shock in some people. For this reason, in 1986 FDA banned the use of sulfites on fresh fruits and vegetables, such as in salad bars where they were used to keep lettuce and other produce looking fresh. Product labels must list sulfites if they are added. In the 1970s it was thought by some individuals that additives may contribute to childhood hyperactivity, but studies conducted since then have found no link.

Food Allergens

Up to 6 percent of children and 2 percent of adults suffer from food allergy-the body's immune system reacting to certain substances in food, usually a protein. The immune system misinterprets a chemical component of a food as harmful and releases histamines and other chemicals to combat it, which results in hives, swelling, itching, vomiting, diarrhea, cramps, or difficulty breathing. Severe reactions may cause anaphylaxis, which can result in death. Eight foods—egg, wheat, peanuts, milk, soy, tree nuts (such as walnuts and almonds), fish, and shellfish—cause 90 percent of all food allergies. The only way to prevent an allergic reaction is to avoid that food entirely.

Food intolerance often is confused with food allergy since the symptoms are often the same. Food intolerance is an adverse reaction to a food that does not involve the immune system. Lactose intolerance is an example of food intolerance. A person with lactose intolerance lacks an enzyme needed to digest a form of sugar present in milk. Consuming milk products causes symptoms such as gas, bloating, and abdominal pain, but does not involve any immune system response. If a person has a true allergy to milk, the only way to avoid milk allergy symptoms is to avoid all milk products entirely. Special drops or tablets that help digest the sugar in milk are available for those suffering from lactose intolerance, allowing them to consume milk products. (FAN 2000)

To avoid substances to which they are allergic, consumers must know exactly what is in foods. The Food, Drug and Cosmetic Act requires a complete listing of food ingredients on food labels. Many food products are recalled due to improper food labeling, such as ice cream with a label omitting peanuts, or processed foods that do not declare soy products as an ingredient. Common food allergens can also show up in restaurant foods in unexpected places, for example, peanut butter in Asian noodles or egg products in meatballs.

Recent cases of students who suffered allergy attacks from peanuts have prompted school officials to ban peanut products from some school cafeterias. This is a difficult task, as not only would this outlaw the popular peanut butter and jelly sandwich, but also any snacks or candies that contain peanuts. While it may be possible to control which foods are sold in schools, it is almost impossible to regulate foods students bring from home. Educating students who have food allergies to read carefully food ingredient labels and not to accept foods if they do not know what the ingredients are is key to reducing food allergy attacks.

Drugs, Hormones, and Antibiotics in Animals

The use of drugs to control and treat animal disease, and of hormones to promote faster, more efficient growth of livestock is a common practice. An estimated 80 percent of U.S. livestock and poultry receive some animal drugs during their lifetime. This includes topical antiseptics, bactericides, and fungicides to treat skin or hoof infections and cuts; hormones and hormone-like substances to improve growth; antiparasite drugs; and antibiotics. Improper use of animal drugs may cause residues in the edible tissues of slaughtered animals that could be hazardous to consumers. Before a new animal drug can be marketed in the United States, the FDA Center for Veterinary Medicine (CVM) must approve it on the basis of quality, safety, and efficacy. When the drug is for use in food-producing animals, not only must animal drug manufacturers prove that the drug is safe for the animal, but also that the food products derived from the treated animals are safe for human consumption. FDA establishes tolerances to include a safety factor to assure that the drug will have no harmful effects on consumers of the food product. FDA and USDA work together to monitor the use of animal drugs, identify improper use, and take enforcement action if necessary.

There are two issues of concern related to the use of drugs in food animals. The first is the presence of drug residues in meat or milk obtained from an animal that has been given an animal drug. Some of these residues may be allergenic, toxic, or carcinogenic to humans in large enough doses. According to the National Research Council's (NRC) 1999 report, *The Use of Drugs in Food Animals: Benefits and Risks*, FDA programs monitoring drug residues in animals are effective in protecting consumers from this danger. Because very few illegal drug residues are detected in meat, milk, or eggs, the health risk posed by drug residues is minimal.

Many food safety experts consider the second problem, antibiotic drug residues in farm animals, to be a problem of larger concern. Antibiotics for farm animals have two purposes. First, they are used to prevent and treat diseases, just as they are in humans. The second reason for administering antibiotics to farm animals is to improve growth and to promote feed efficiency—the production of more meat or milk with less input of feed. This is called a subtherapeutic dose, since it is given in doses lower than those required to treat an infection. Subtherapeutic use of antibiotics controls intestinal bacteria that interfere with an animal's ability to absorb nutrients. It also controls infections before they become noticeable, thus making animals healthier and allowing them to use nutrients for growth and production rather than to fight infections. Antibiotic use is one reason why the U.S. food supply is so abundant and affordable.

Bacteria will inevitably become resistant to the antibiotics used to kill them. This is because antibiotics do not generally kill 100 percent of their target bacteria. A few will always survive and pass that resistance on to successive generations of bacteria, and in some cases, to other unrelated bacteria. Eventually the genetic make-up of the bacterial strain changes enough so that the drug is no longer effective. This happens with human pathogens such as tuberculosis, as well as with pathogens that infect animals. The most common cause of antibiotic resistance is overuse of antibiotics. Most animal bacterial diseases cannot be passed on to humans, but there are notable exceptions—*Campylobacter* and *Salmonella*. Already these two bacteria have developed resistance to some drugs, particularly the fluoroquinolones, used to combat them. There is some evidence of a relationship between the use of fluoroquinolone drugs in poultry and other food-producing animals and the emergence of fluoroquinolone-resistant *Campylobacter* and *Salmonella* in humans (WHO 1998). The possibility exists that as pathogens in farm animals become resistant to antibiotics, if those same pathogens are passed on to humans, they will not respond to drug treatments. The NRC report states that there is a link between the use of antibiotics in food animals, the development of resistant microorganisms in those animals, and the spread of those resistant pathogens to humans. However, the report goes on to say that the incidence of this happening is very low, and that there are not enough data to determine whether the incidence is changing. The report concludes that alternatives to antibiotic use for maintaining animal health and productivity should be developed. The National Antimicrobial Resistance Monitoring System (NARMS), established in January 1996 as a collaborative effort among FDA, USDA, and the Centers for Disease Control and Prevention (CDC), seeks to gather more data on antimicrobial resistance to clarify the potential risks.

Naturally Occurring Toxins

In addition to synthetic chemicals such as pesticides, the food supply contains many naturally occurring toxins. In comparison to synthetic chemicals, scientists know very little about these natural toxins in terms of their toxicity and quantity in foods. They pose a greater risk than the synthetic chemicals because we eat at least 10,000 times more of them. Every food is a complex mixture of chemical compounds, some beneficial such as vitamins and minerals, but also some that are harmful. Even vitamins and minerals can be toxic if taken in great enough quantities. For example, vitamin A, a necessary vitamin, may be toxic in an amount only 15 times the recommended dietary allowance. Plants and animals developed toxic substances as protection against insects, microorganisms, grazing animals, and other potential dangers.

One of America's most loved foods, the potato, contains a very toxic substance called solanine. This naturally occurring toxin is present in larger amounts in the peel and in the eyes than in the potato. In the amounts normally eaten, solanine does not cause illness, but a diet of certain varieties of potato peels and eyes might contain enough solanine to cause illness and possibly even death. Solanine acts as a natural pesticide that protects the potato from the Colorado beetle, the leaf hopper, and other potato pests. In another instance, herbal teas are enjoying a renewed popularity in the United States. Consumers view these teas as a natural way of improving their health or treating diseases. However, chemicals in herbal teas can and have caused illness and death. Herbal teas are touted as the answer to many chronic ailments and as such are consumed at much higher levels than they were traditionally, which may lead to natural, but still harmful, side effects. In societies where herbal use is steeped in tradition, knowledge about the benefits and dangers of herbal remedies passes from generation to generation. Very few of the herbs used in natural herbal teas have been studied or tested for safety. One of these is ephedra, commonly known as Ma Huang, an ingredient in many herbal teas marketed as weight loss products. Ephedra is an amphetamine-like compound with potentially powerful stimulant effects on the nervous system and heart. More than 800 adverse events associated with the use of ephedrine-containing products have been reported to the Food and Drug Administration. These range from episodes of high blood pressure, heart rate irregularities, insomnia, nervousness, tremors and headaches to seizures, heart attacks, strokes, and death (FDA 1997). People who shun prescription drugs as unnatural or too strong with too many side effects may think nothing of drinking herbal teas, some of which can provoke very strong drug-like reactions and adverse effects in the body.

Seafood products contain some naturally occurring marine toxins that present unique food hazards. Molluscan shellfish, which includes oysters, clams, scallops, and mussels, can pick up toxins from algae that they feed on, and cause paralytic shellfish poisoning (PSP), neurotoxic shellfish poisoning (NSP), amnesic shellfish poisoning, and diarrhetic shellfish poisoning (DSP). The most serious is PSP, with symptoms ranging from tingling, burning, or numbness in the mouth or throat to paralysis, respiratory failure, and in severe cases, death. The algae that produce these toxins can be found during the warmer months anywhere. State authorities monitor harvest waters and close them to shellfish harvesting if algae is present. Since these toxins are not destroyed by heat, and can't be detected visually, the best control is for people to consume shellfish only from approved waters.

Tropical and subtropical reef fish such as grouper, barracuda, snappers, jacks, and king mackerel can accumulate ciguatera toxin by feeding on smaller fish that have ingested toxin-forming algae. Ciguatera can cause nausea, vomiting, diarrhea, and headaches in humans. Tuna, mahi mahi, bluefish, and mackerel have been the sources of scromboid poisoning, a type of foodborne illness caused by the consumption of scombroid and scombroid-like marine fish species that have begun to spoil. This occurs when the amino acid histidine breaks down into histamine, usually as a result of inadequate refrigeration. Scromboid symptoms include a rash, burning or peppery taste sensations about the mouth and throat, dizziness, nausea, headache, itching, and swelling of the tongue. Puffer fish, known as fugu in Japan, is a great and dangerous delicacy in that country. An extremely toxic poison called tetrodotoxin accumulates in the internal organs of the fish. Only specially trained and licensed chefs are allowed to prepare fugu fish, as improperly prepared fugu causes paralysis, respiratory failure, convulsions, and cardiac arrhythmia within 20 minutes. Death is not uncommon.

Fungi, which include mushrooms and molds, also produce toxins that are harmful to humans. Molds produce toxins called mycotoxins, with the major mycotoxin-producing molds being *Aspergillus*, *Fusarium*, and *Claviceps* species. Molds usually grow on damp cereal grains such as rye, wheat, corn, rice, barley, and oats, or oilseeds (peanuts), and then excrete their mycotoxins during their life cycle. Most of these mycotoxins are very resistant to heat, so cooking does not reduce their harmfulness. The only way to prevent intoxication is by preventing the mold from contaminating the product during harvesting, drying, storage, and processing.

One mold in particular, *Claviceps purpurea*, has been implicated in a number of historical events. Eating rye and other cereal grains contaminated with *Claviceps purpurea* results in the disease ergotism. This disease was first recorded in 857 in the Rhine Valley and has been recorded numerous times since, sometimes affecting up to 40,000 individuals at once. Rye is particularly susceptible to ergot contamination. Cold and damp growing or storage conditions also promote the formation of ergot. Ergot is the source of lysergic acid diethylamide (LSD); it and many other ergot derivatives are hallucinogens. The symptoms of ergotism are varied, but include central nervous system disorders such as muscle spasms, confusions, delusions, convulsive fits, hallucinations, visions, sensations of flying through the air, and psychosis. Other common symptoms are a prickly sensation in the limbs, feelings of intense alternating heat and cold, and increased appetite between episodes of fits. Linnda Caporael and Mary K. Matossian propose that the witch trials of 1692 in Salem, Massachusetts, could very well have been the result of ergot poisoning. They link the weather, crop, and economic conditions from the years 1691 and 1692 to an increased consumption of bread made from rye that could have been contaminated with ergot. The symptoms exhibited by those accused of being bewitched are suspiciously similar to the symptoms of ergotism. In another interesting footnote to history, Peter the Great had to cancel his plans to attack the Ottoman Empire in 1722 because his troops and their horses consumed rye contaminated with ergot, which caused hundreds either to die or go mad (Caporael 1976; Matossian 1989).

Fortunately the body has a very efficient mechanism to destroy many naturally and synthetic chemicals—the liver. The liver is capable of eliminating small quantities of many poisons, which allows humans to safely consume otherwise toxic chemicals. However, large quantities of toxins and chemicals can easily overwhelm the body's defenses. We often think of naturally occurring compounds as relatively safe, but in reality some are among the most toxic substances known.

Pesticides

Pesticides prevent, destroy, or control pests. Pests are any organism that causes damage to plants, animals, or foods, such as bacteria, viruses, rodents, worms, fungi, insects, or weeds. The term pesticide is very broad and includes herbicides (to control weeds), insecticides (to control insects), fungicides (to control mold, mildew, and fungi), rodenticides (to control rodents), and disinfectants (to control bacteria and viruses). Three-quarters of the pesticide use is for agriculture (mainly on crops in the field), but it is also used post-harvest during transportation and storage to prevent mold growth or insect infestation. While we may not think of household cleaners, pet flea collars, lawn and garden products, and insect repellants as pesticides, they are. About 350 pesticides are used on the foods we eat, and to protect our homes and pets (EPA 1999).

Since the beginnings of agriculture humankind has used pesticides in an attempt to control nature to ensure good crop yield. Egyptian records from 1500 B.C.E. contain instructions for preparing insecticides to control lice, fleas, and wasps. The

Greeks were using sulfur by 1000 B.C.E. to control insects, as did European farmers in the eighteenth century. The Chinese controlled insects with a mixture of arsenic and water. In 1865 farmers discovered Paris green, a mixture of copper and arsenic, as a way to control the Colorado potato beetle. A similar substance called Bordeaux mixture saved the grape industry in France from a fungal disease in the 1880s (Bohmont 1997). While we may think of pesticides as synthetic chemicals, the above examples show that many natural compounds also act as pesticides. The first synthetic insecticides and herbicides were produced in the early 1900s. Currently federal pesticide law registers 21,000 pesticide products and 860 active ingredients (Curtis 1995). See chapter 2 for a discussion of pesticide regulation.

Pesticide use has both advantages and disadvantages. In comparison with other nations, the United States has an abundant and affordable food supply. American consumers spend only about 11 percent of their income on food, less than consumers in any other country (see table 1-1, below). One reason for this abundance and low cost is improved crop yields, much of which is due to pesticide use. In 1850 each farmer in the United States produced enough food and fiber for four people; by 1990 that number grew to 79 (Bohmont 1997). The American diet consists of more fruits and vegetables in part because of this increased harvest, which leads to an improvement in public health. Experts agree that the benefits from eating a diet rich in fruits and vegetables far outweigh the potential risks from pesticides. Even with modern methods of pest control, U.S. farmers still lose from 25 to 30 percent of their crop to pests. Globally pests destroy up to 45 percent of the world's crops (Bohmont 1997). In addition to the benefit of increased yield, pesticide use in the United States satisfies the consumer's demand for uncontaminated and unblemished food.

Table 1-1
Percent of Income Spent on Food in Selected Countries

United States	10.9
United Kingdom	11.2
Sweden	14.6
France	14.8
Australia	14.9
New Zealand	15.4
Italy	17.2
Germany	17.3
Japan	17.6
Spain	18.2
Israel	20.5
Mexico	24.5
South Africa	27.5
India	51.3

Source: American Farm Bureau Federation. September 12, 2000. Farm Facts. http://www.fb.org/brochures/farmfacts/.

But pesticides can be dangerous to human health and to the environment. Most pesticides break down quickly in the environment, but some may still be present years later, sometimes at a great distance from their original application. Pesticides sprayed on plants can move through the air and end up in the soil or water. Pesticides applied to the soil may end up in rivers and lakes or move down through the soil to contaminate ground water. As an example, DDT, which the United States banned from use more than 20 years ago, is still showing up in the Great Lakes ecosystem, presumably through rainfall and dust from countries that still use it.

In addition to being potentially risky, pesticides are expensive. Farmers today are reducing pesticide use in several ways. Many farmers are turning to integrated pest management (IPM) techniques to reduce the need for pesticides. Examples of IPM include using ladybugs or other "good bugs" to destroy unwanted insects, adjusting planting times to avoid pest infestations, disrupting insect reproduction cycles, and destroying areas where pests breed and live. Although pesticides are still used in conjunction with many IPM techniques, the amount used is less. In 1993 the federal government set a national goal that 75 percent of all farms in the United States use IPM techniques by the year 2000. Researchers are also using biotechnology to develop crops that are more resistant to insects and viruses, which reduces the need to apply insecticides.

Microbiological Hazards

Microbiological hazards include disease-causing bacteria, viruses, and parasites. Table 1-2 lists these organisms, along with their sources and their symptoms. Many of these microorganisms occur naturally in the environment and can be foodborne, waterborne, or transmitted from a person or an animal. Cooking kills or inactivates most pathogens, while proper cooling and storage can control them before or after cooking.

Bacteria

Bacteria are single-celled organisms so small they can only be seen with a microscope. Bacteria are everywhere and most are not pathogenic (disease-causing). The human gastrointestinal tract is home to more than 300 species of bacteria (Doyle 2000). Fortunately, only a few of these cause illness. Some bacteria are beneficial and are used in making foods such as yogurt, cheese, and beer. Others cause food to spoil, but do not cause human sickness. This difference between spoilage bacteria and pathogenic bacteria is important in the prevention of foodborne illness. Since pathogenic bacteria generally cannot be detected by looks, smell, or taste, we rely on spoilage bacteria to indicate that a food should not be eaten. Not many people will eat food that has become slimy or that smells bad. Pathogenic bacteria cause foodborne illness in three different ways (Acheson 1998):

Infection. Some bacteria damage the intestines directly. This type of illness occurs from eating food contaminated with live pathogenic bacteria. Cells that are alive and reproducing are vegetative cells. Many bacteria are killed in the acidic environment of the stomach, but some survive, pass through to the small intestine, and begin to grow in number. When the bacteria have multiplied to a high enough number (this depends on the strain of bacteria, its virulence or strength, and the health and susceptibility of the individual), the person becomes ill. *Salmonella* is a classic example of this kind of bacteria. *Salmonella* exists in the intestinal tracts of animals, including food-producing animals as well as turtles, cats, dogs, birds, rodents, and wild animals. Raw milk and eggs are also sources of *Salmonella*. While heat easily destroys *Salmonella*, inadequate cooking allows some of the organisms to survive. Often *Salmonella* is spread through cross-contamination. This could happen when a cook prepares a piece of raw poultry on a cutting board and then uses the same cutting board without cleaning it to prepare another food that will not be cooked, such as a salad. The second food will not receive any heat treatment to kill the bacteria. *Salmonella* can reproduce very quickly; they double their number almost every 20 minutes. When the number of *Salmonella* are very high, there is a better chance that some of them will survive the harsh environment of the stomach and make it to the small intestine. Once there, they will continue to multiply, eventually causing damage to the intestine and symptoms of foodborne illness. With some bacteria the infectious dose, the number of bacteria necessary to cause illness, is very high, in the millions; while in others it can be as low as 10 organisms.

Intoxication. Some bacteria produce harmful toxins or other chemicals that are then present in the food. It is not the bug itself that causes illness, but rather the toxin the bacteria produce. This can happen even if the pathogen itself has been killed, as long as it had sufficient time to produce enough toxin before dying. *Staphylococcus aureus* is an example of this type of bacteria. *Staphylococci* exist in air, dust, sewage, water, milk, animals, humans, and in food or on food equipment. They are present in the nasal passages and throats and on the hair and skin of 50 percent or more of healthy individuals. Illness is caused by ingesting toxins produced in food by some strains of *S. aureus*, usually because the food has not been kept hot enough or cold enough. Although cooking easily destroys the bacteria, the toxin produced by the bacteria is very resistant to heating, refrigeration, and freezing. It is not possible to detect the presence of the toxin in food by smell, appearance, or taste. The likelihood of illness increases with the amount of time the bacteria are left at an improper temperature.

Toxico-infection. Some bacteria enter the intestines live, survive the acidic environment of the stomach, and then produce a harmful toxin inside the human digestive system. Toxico-infection is a combination of the previous two examples in that live cells must be consumed, but the toxin is produced in the intestine and it is the toxin that really causes the illness. An example of an organism that causes foodborne illness in this manner is *Clostridium perfringens.* Like many bacteria, this organism is widely distributed in the environment in soil, water, dust, and in the intestines of domestic and wild animals. Large numbers of the bacteria, usually in the millions, need to be ingested to cause illness. These bacteria produce a spore, which is a dormant form of the organism. Vegetative cells may form a spore when the conditions for survival are not optimal for the cell, such as high heat or lack of water and food. Heat often does not destroy spores. Once the conditions are conducive to growth again, the spore will again become a vegetative cell. A typical case of foodborne illness occurs when a piece of meat is cooked, but the spores survive. Then, if the meat is not cooled properly the spores revert back to their non-dormant vegetative form and reproduce to high numbers. When food contaminated with *C. perfringens* is eaten, the organism grows in the small intestine and produces a toxin that causes illness.

Some bacteria use a combination of the above methods to cause illness. Just how many bacteria or how much toxin needs to be consumed before a person becomes ill depends on a number of factors that will be covered later in the section on factors that contribute to foodborne illness. Onset time, the time between when a person eats the food and when the symptoms start, is also highly variable. Most animals, including humans, are carriers of all kinds of bacteria, some of which do cause foodborne illness. Additionally, since many bacteria occur everywhere in nature—in the soil, air, water, etc.—it is not possible to totally eliminate harmful bacteria from the food supply. Bacteria need certain elements to survive and grow:

Water. Bacteria need water in order to carry out the biologic processes of life, much as humans do. Drying foods and adding salt or sugar to a food, which bind the available water, inhibit microbial growth. This is why foods such as dry pasta do not spoil as easily as a piece of meat. The amount of available water in a food is called water activity (A_W).

Table 1-2
Major Foodborne Illness Pathogens

Organism name	Source and Food Involved	Symptoms
Bacteria		
Bacillus cereus	**Source:** Soil, dust. **Foods involved:** Rice dishes, pasta, sauces, puddings, soups, casseroles, pastries, meats, milk.	**Onset:** 6-15 hours after eating. **Duration:** 24 hours. **Symptoms:** Watery diarrhea, abdominal cramps, nausea, vomiting.
Campylobacter jejuni	**Source:** Soil, water, intestinal tracts of animals . **Foods involved:** Raw or undercooked poultry and meat, unpasteurized milk and dairy products.	**Onset:** 2-5 days after eating. **Duration:** 2-10 days. **Symptoms:** Diarrhea (sometimes bloody), abdominal pain, fever, headache. Possible complications of meningitis and arthritis.
Clostridium botulinum	**Source:** Spores of these bacteria are wide-spread in the soil and intestinal tracts of animals. Produces a very potent toxin in an anaerobic (oxygen less) environment. **Foods involved:** Improperly processed canned goods, especially low acid foods and meats; garlic in oil products; smoked fish.	**Onset:** Generally 12-36 hours after eating, but range is 4 hours to 8 days. **Duration:** Several days to a year. **Symptoms:** Muscle weakness, dizziness, double vision, difficulty speaking and swallowing, progressive paralysis of the respiratory system that could lead to death.
Clostridium perfringens	**Source:** Sewage, soil, dust, water, intestinal tracts of animals and humans, . **Foods involved:** Improperly held, cooled or reheated foods. Meat, poultry, stews, casseroles, gravies.	**Onset:** 8-24 hours after eating. **Duration:** 24 hours. **Symptoms:** Intense abdominal pain, diarrhea.
Escherichia coli O157:H7	**Source:** *E. coli* is a normal inhabitant of the intestines of all animals, including humans. *E. coli* O157:H7 is a rare variety of *E. coli* that produces large quantities of toxins that cause severe damage to the lining of the intestine. **Foods involved:** Undercooked or raw ground beef, raw milk and cheeses made from raw milk, unpasteurized juices.	**Onset:**3-8 days after eating. **Duration:** The illness usually lasts for an average of 8 days. **Symptoms:** Severe cramping, abdominal pain, and diarrhea which is initially watery but becomes bloody. Occasionally vomiting occurs. Low fever may be present Some victims, particularly the very young and very old, develop hemolytic uremic syndrome (HUS), characterized by renal failure and hemolytic anemia. Can cause death.
Listeria monocytogenes	**Source:** Soil, water, intestinal tracts of animals. Can grow at low temperatures and can withstand heat, cold, and drying better than most pathogens. **Foods involved:** Unpasteurized milk, soft cheeses, undercooked meat and poultry, hot dogs, luncheon meats, chilled ready-to-eat foods, raw vegetables if fertilized with manure containing the organism.	**Onset:** 1 day to 3 weeks after eating. **Duration:** Unknown. **Symptoms:** Fever, headache, nausea, vomiting. Primarily affects immuno-compromised persons and pregnant women. Can cause fetal death, as well as meningitis, encephalitis, and septicemia.

Salmonella	**Source:** Intestinal tract of animals and humans. **Foods involved:** Undercooked eggs, raw meats and poultry, unpasteurized milk and dairy products, shrimp, custards, sauces, cream desserts.	**Onset:** Generally 6-48 hours after eating. **Duration:** 1-2 days or may be prolonged, again depending on host factors and ingested dose. **Symptoms:** Nausea, vomiting, abdominal cramps, diarrhea, fever, headache. Arthritis symptoms may follow 3-4 weeks after onset of above symptoms.
Shigella	**Sources:** Principally a disease of humans and other primates. The organism is frequently found in water polluted with human feces. **Foods involved:** Salads (potato, tuna, shrimp, macaroni, and chicken), raw vegetables, milk and dairy products, poultry. Contamination of these foods is usually through fecally contaminated water and unsanitary handling by food handlers.	**Onset:** 12-48 hours after eating. **Duration:** 1-2 days, may have symptoms for months. **Symptoms:** Abdominal cramps, diarrhea, fever, sometimes vomiting, stools may contain blood, pus, or mucus. Arthritis is a possible complication following illness.
Staphylococcus aureus	**Source:** Humans and animals are the primary carriers. Staphylococci are present in the nasal passages and throats and on the hair and skin of 50 percent or more of healthy individuals. **Foods involved:** Meat and poultry products, eggs, salads (potato, tuna, shrimp, macaroni, and chicken), cream-filled desserts, sandwich fillings, milk and dairy products. Foods that require considerable handling during preparation and that are kept at slightly elevated temperatures after preparation are frequently involved in staphylococcal food poisoning.	**Onset:** Generally ½-8 hours after eating. **Duration:** 1-2 days. **Symptoms:** Diarrhea, vomiting, nausea, abdominal pain, cramps, and prostration. Rarely fatal.
Vibrio vulnificus	**Source:** Seawater contaminated with human feces. **Foods involved:** Raw or undercooked oysters, clams, shrimp, crabs.	**Onset:** 2-76 hours after eating. **Duration:** 1-8 days. **Symptoms:** Chills, fever, and/or prostration. People with liver conditions, low stomach acid, and weakened immune systems are especially susceptible. Death in those individuals is about 50 percent.
Vibrio parahaemolyticus	**Source:** Marine coastal environment. **Foods involved:** Raw or improperly cooked fish and shellfish. Infection is more likely in the warmer months of the year.	**Onset:** 4-96 hours after eating. **Duration:** Average is 2.5 days. **Symptoms:** Diarrhea, abdominal cramps, nausea, vomiting, headache, fever, and chills.
Vibrio cholerae	**Source:** Shellfish harvested from U.S. coastal waters frequently contain *V. cholerae*. **Foods involved:** Raw or improperly cooked shellfish.	**Onset:** 48 hours after eating. **Duration:** 6-7 days. **Symptoms:** Diarrhea, abdominal cramps, and fever.
Yersinia enterocolitica	**Source:** Soil, water, intestinal tract of animals, especially pigs. **Foods involved**: Meats, oysters, fish, and raw milk.	**Onset:** 24-48 hours after eating. **Duration:** 2-3 weeks. **Symptoms:** Fever, abdominal pain, diarrhea and/or vomiting, may mimic appendicitis. Sometimes misdiagnosed as Crohn's disease. The major complication is the performance of unnecessary appendectomies, since one of the main symptoms of infections is abdominal pain of the lower right quadrant.

Protozoa and Parasites		
Anisakis sp. and related worms	**Source:** Parasites are in the flesh of fish. **Foods involved:** Fish - especially cod, haddock, fluke, pacific salmon, herring, flounder, and monkfish.	**Onset:** 1 hour to 2 weeks after eating. **Duration:** Varies, worm must be coughed up or removed surgically. **Symptoms:** Acute abdominal pain, much like acute appendicitis accompanied by a nauseous feeling.
Cryptosporidium parvum	**Source:** This single-celled protozoa infects humans and other animals. **Foods involved:** Contaminated water or any food contaminated by fecal matter.	**Onset:** 1-12 days. **Duration:** 2-4 days, up to 4 weeks. **Symptoms:** Severe watery diarrhea.
Cyclospora cayetanensis	**Source:** Very little is known about this organism. **Foods involved:** Contaminated water, as well as various types of fresh produce treated with contaminated water.	**Onset:** 1 week. **Duration:** Days to weeks, may reoccur. **Symptoms:** Watery diarrhea, loss of appetite, weight loss, bloating, increased flatus, stomach cramps, nausea, vomiting, muscle aches, low-grade fever, and fatigue.
Giardia lamblia	**Source:** Single-celled protozoa that lives in the intestines of people and animals. **Foods involved:** Most frequently associated with consumption of contaminated water.	**Onset:** 1-2 weeks after infection. **Duration:** 4-6 weeks, but sometimes months to years. **Symptoms:** Diarrhea, abdominal cramps, nausea. Especially infects hikers, children, travelers, and institutionalized patients.
Trichinella spiralis	**Source:** Worm larvae in animal meat. **Foods involved:** Undercooked pork and wild game meats.	**Onset:** 8-15 days **Duration:** Days to weeks. **Symptoms:** Muscle pain, vomiting, nausea.
Virus		
Hepatitis A virus	**Source:** Hepatitis A virus is excreted in feces of infected people. **Foods involved:** Water, shellfish, and salads are the most frequent sources. Contamination of foods by infected workers in food processing plants and restaurants is common.	**Onset:** 10-50 days after exposure. **Duration:** 1-2 weeks, or several months if symptoms are severe. **Symptoms:** Fever, malaise, nausea, anorexia, and abdominal discomfort. After 3-10 days patient develops jaundice with darkened urine. Severe cases can cause liver damage and death.
Norwalk virus	**Source:** Human fecal contamination. **Foods involved:** Water is the most common source of outbreaks and may include water from municipal supplies, wells, recreational lakes, swimming pools, and water stored aboard cruise ships. Salads and raw or undercooked shellfish are the foods most often implicated in Norwalk outbreaks.	**Onset:** 24- 48 hours after eating or drinking. **Duration:** 24-60 hours. **Symptoms:** Nausea, vomiting, diarrhea, and abdominal pain. Headache and low-grade fever may occur. Only the common cold is reported more frequently than viral gastroenteritis as a cause of illness in the U.S.

Natural Toxins		
Ciguatera	**Source:** Fish accumulate this toxin from eating algae in tropical waters. **Foods involved:** Marine finfish most commonly implicated in ciguatera fish poisoning include the groupers, barracudas, snappers, jacks, mackerel, and triggerfish.	**Onset:** Within 6 hours after eating. **Duration:** Several days to months. **Symptoms:** Numbness and tingling, nausea, vomiting, diarrhea, headache, acute sensitivity to temperature extremes, vertigo, muscular weakness, arrhythmia, bradycardia or tachycardia, and reduced blood pressure.
Scombrotoxin	**Source:** From consumption of foods that contain high levels of histamine. **Foods involved:** Fishery products that have been implicated in scombroid poisoning include the tunas (e.g., skipjack and yellowfin), mahi mahi, bluefish, sardines, mackerel, amberjack, and abalone.	**Onset:** 30 minutes after eating. **Duration:** 3 hours to several days. **Symptoms:** Tingling or burning sensation in the mouth, rash on the upper body, drop in blood pressure. Frequently headaches and itching of the skin are encountered. The symptoms may progress to nausea, vomiting, and diarrhea and may require hospitalization.
Shellfish toxins	**Source:** Many different toxins cause shellfish poisoning. Shellfish accumulate the toxins from feeding on "red tide" algae. **Foods involved:** mussels, clams, oysters, and scallops.	**Onset:** Few minutes to a few hours, depending on the toxin. **Duration:** Varies with toxin. **Symptoms:** Tingling, burning, numbness, drowsiness, incoherent speech, difficulty breathing, lack of muscle coordination.
Tetrodotoxin	**Source:** This toxin is one of the most potent toxins in nature. **Foods involved:** Pufferfish, also known as fugu.	**Onset:** 20 minutes to 3 hours after eating. **Duration:** Varies. **Symptoms:** Headache, epigastric pain, nausea, diarrhea, and/or vomiting may occur. The second stage of intoxication is characterized by increasing paralysis. Many victims are unable to move, even sitting may be difficult. There is increasing respiratory distress. Paralysis increases and convulsions, mental impairment, and cardiac arrhythmia may occur. Death usually occurs within 4-6 hours, with a known range of about 20 minutes to 8 hours.
Mycotoxins		
Aflatoxin	**Source:** Produced by certain strains of the fungi *Aspergillus flavus* and *A. parasiticus* that grow in fields or during storage. **Foods involved:** In the United States, aflatoxins have been identified in corn and corn products, peanuts and peanut products, cottonseed, milk (from cows eating moldy feed), and tree nuts such as Brazil nuts, pecans, pistachio nuts, and walnuts.	**Onset:** Varies with dose. **Duration:** Varies. **Symptoms:** Acute short term - fever, jaundice, swelling, vomiting, pain, enlarged liver. Chronic long term - cirrhosis and cancer of the liver.
Ergot	**Source:** Toxin produced by the fungus *Claviceps purpurea*. **Foods involved:** Rye, wheat, barley, oats.	**Onset:** Varies with dose. **Duration:** Varies with dose. **Symptoms:** Gangrene, convulsions, dementia.

Food. Bacteria prefer foods that are high in protein such as meats, dairy products, and seafood. High-fat foods can protect bacteria from acidic juices in the stomach, and can help the bacteria to survive and pass into the small intestine. Foods with a high water and protein content, which are more likely to foster the growth of pathogens are called potentially hazardous foods.

Proper temperature. While many pathogenic bacteria grow best at temperatures near human body temperature, they can survive and grow over a temperature range from 40 degrees F to 140 degrees F (or from 4 degrees C to 60 degrees C). This range is called the danger zone, and keeping foods out of the danger zone is one of the main ways of controlling bacterial growth. Bacteria do not grow as well at the extremes of this range, but they can still survive and grow at those extremes. Some bacteria can even grow at temperatures below or above the danger zone, but their growth is very slow at those temperatures. Refrigerator temperature is 40 degrees F (5 degrees C) to inhibit bacterial growth.

Time. Some bacteria grow very quickly; it only takes 20 to 30 minutes for their numbers to double. Table 1-3 shows the number of bacteria that would be present after 10 hours for an organism that reproduces every 20 minutes. Given the right conditions, a single cell can multiply to more than one billion cells in that amount of time, about the same amount of time it would take for the center of a big deep pot of chili to cool below 40 degrees F. For most bacteria, large numbers of them must be consumed before illness occurs. There are exceptions to this, such as *E. coli* 0157:H7 in which consuming as few as 10 cells can cause foodborne illness.

Oxygen. Some microorganisms need oxygen to live, while others do not. Bacteria that need oxygen are called aerobic, those that do not are anaerobic. For example, *Clostridium botulinum*, the pathogen that causes botulism, only grows in the absence of oxygen. Many pathogenic bacteria, called facultative anaerobes, can grow with or without oxygen but have a preference.

Proper pH or acidity. Microorganisms prefer foods that are neutral (pH 7) or slightly acidic. Many foods fall into this category—eggs, meat, poultry, fish, sauces, soups, gravies.

Viruses

Several viruses also cause foodborne illness. Viruses differ from bacteria in that they are smaller, require a living animal or human host to grow and reproduce, do not multiply in foods, and are not complete cells. Ingestion of only a few viral particles is enough to produce an infection. Humans are host to a number of viruses that

Table 1-3
Multiplication Rate for a Bacterium that Reproduces Every 20 Minutes

Time	Number of Bacteria
20 minutes	2
40 minutes	4
1 hour	8
2 hours	64
3 hours	512
4 hours	4,096
5 hours	32,768
6 hours	262,144
7 hours	2,097,152
8 hours	16,777,216
9 hours	134,220,000
10 hours	1,073,700,000

reproduce in the intestines and then are excreted in the feces. Thus, transmission of viruses comes from contact with sewage or water contaminated by fecal matter or direct contact with human fecal material. Raw or undercooked molluscan shellfish (oysters, clams, mussels, and scallops) are the food most often associated with foodborne viral diseases. Human pathogenic viruses are often discharged into marine waters through treated and untreated sewage. As shellfish filter contaminants from these polluted waters, they store them within their edible tissues. Shellfish grown and harvested from polluted waters have been implicated in outbreaks of viral diseases. In spite of this, surveys done in Virginia and Florida estimated that 850,000 and three million people respectively, consume raw oysters (Wittman 1995). The other main source of transmission is from infected food workers who have poor personal hygiene. An infected worker can transfer viral particles to any food. Therefore, proper handwashing and using a clean water supply are vital to controlling the spread of foodborne viruses.

Scientists do not know as much about viruses as they do about bacterial pathogens. One problem has been a lack of good laboratory methods to detect viruses. Without rapid, easy, inexpensive testing methods it has not been possible to study how viruses are transmitted, the number of people who become ill from foodborne viral infections, or the best methods to control viruses. Because of these problems, health care providers often do not order tests to detect viral infections, which causes foodborne illness from viruses to be even more underreported than for bacteria. Epidemiologists estimate that 67 percent of foodborne illnesses can be attributed to viruses, although only a small percentage of total foodborne illness deaths are due to viruses (Mead 1999).

Hepatitis A is a virus commonly associated with foodborne infections. The incubation period for hepatitis A, before a person develops any symptoms, is anywhere from 10 to 50 days. It is during this period before symptoms appear that a carrier is most infectious and most likely to spread the disease. Hepatitis A, and many other viral and bacterial pathogens, is most often transmitted via a fecal-oral route. The fact that a person is infectious even before they know they have the disease makes it difficult to control. An outbreak of hepatitis A associated with eating clams in China in 1988 sickened 292,000 people. Since 1996 a vaccine offering lifetime immunity to hepatitis A has been available, but rarely used in the United States.

Protozoa and Parasites

Some parasites also cause foodborne illness. Parasites must live on or inside a living host to survive. The most common foodborne parasites are *Anisakis simplex, Cryptosporidium parvum, Toxoplasma gondii, Giardia lamblia*, and *Cyclospora cayetanensis. Giardia, Cryptosporidium*, and *Toxoplasma* are all protozoa, or single-celled organisms. *Cyclospora* was not known to cause human sickness until 1979, when the first cases were reported. Since then fresh produce has been associated with several outbreaks of foodborne illness from *Cyclospora. Giardia* has been identified more than any other pathogen in waterborne disease outbreaks, but there also have been foodborne *Giardia* outbreaks. *Cryptosporidium* is also primarily a waterborne pathogen. An estimated 21 percent of waterborne outbreaks from drinking water are due to parasitic agents, mainly *Giardia* and *Cryptosporidium.* These two parasites are the most common cause of human parasitic infections in the United States. *Toxoplasma gondii* is common in warm-blooded animals, including cats, rats, pigs, cows, sheep, deer, chickens, and birds. It can be found in feces and raw meat from these animals. While not a problem for healthy adults, it can cause a very severe infection in unborn babies and in people with immune system disorders. *Anisakis simplex* and related worms are found in raw or undercooked seafood. Although currently rarely diagnosed in the United States, it is expected that with the increase in consumption of raw fish in the country, anisakiasis will increase. As with viruses, parasitic infections are underreported due to poor testing and diagnostic methods.

Trichinosis, caused by the parasitic worm *Trichinella spiralis* and associated with eating undercooked pork, is now relatively rare in the United States. The reported incidence of trichinosis has declined from an average of 400 cases per year in the late 1940s to 13 cases in 1997. This decline is due to laws that prohibit feeding garbage to hogs, the increased freezing of pork (freezing kills the parasite), and the practice of thoroughly cooking pork. The largest outbreak recently, in which 90 persons were infected, occurred in 1990 and was caused by the ingestion of a Southeast Asian dish that is made from raw pork sausage. Other recent cases have been associated with eating undercooked horse meat and undercooked wild game such as cougar, boar, bear, and walrus.

Bovine Spongiform Encephalopathy (BSE)

Bovine spongiform encephalopathy, or mad cow disease, is a fatal brain disease of cattle. The brain of affected animals appears sponge-like under a microscope. BSE first appeared in the United Kingdom in 1986. Since then more than 173,000 cattle in the United Kingdom have become infected. All these cattle and the herds to which they belonged were destroyed. New cases have dropped significantly since the U.K. government enacted measures to stop its spread. Scientists believe the disease may have first been transmitted through feeding cattle protein made from sheep carcasses infected with scrapie, the sheep form of the disease. Meat-and-bone meal made from infected animals and used as a protein source for cattle feed may also have been a causative factor and was a common practice for several decades. In the early 1980s a change in the manufacturing process that eliminated steam heat treatment may have played a role in the appearance of the disease. Although BSE has not been found in cattle in the U.S., spongiform encephalopathies affect other animals too, and have been found in the United States in sheep (called scrapie), mink, elk, deer, cats, and humans.

The human form is Creutzfeldt-Jakob disease (CJD). It is a rare disease that occurs in approximately one person per million. A new type of CJD, new variant or nvCJD, has been linked to BSE exposure. This new variant of CJD differs from the traditional type mainly in that it affects younger people. To date, approximately 100 cases of nvCJD have been diagnosed, all in Europe. Although scientists know little about the origin, transmission, and nature of spongiform encephalopathies, the most accepted theory is that the causative agent is a prion, a type of pathogenic protein. In 1997 Stanley B. Prusiner from the University of California, San Francisco, won the Nobel Prize for his work on prions. Infective prions are thought to be found only in the brain tissue, spinal cord, and retina of infected animals, not in meat or milk products. Gelatin and beef tallow both undergo a manufacturing process thought to produce a product free of the BSE causative agent. In Papua New Guinea CJD is known as kuru and is believed to have been transmitted through cannibalism. Scientists were puzzled as to why kuru affected mostly women, until they discovered that during funeral ceremonies women traditionally ate the dead person's brain, while men ate the muscle. This tradition has recently been curtailed.

So far there have been no cases of BSE or nvCJD in the United States. The USDA Animal and Plant Health Inspection Service has monitored American cattle for BSE for the past 10 years, with all tests for the disease negative. No beef has been imported from Britain since 1985, and since 1989 there has been a ban on imported cattle from any country where BSE exists. FDA prohibits the use of most mammalian protein in the manufacture of animal feed given to cattle and other ruminants. Much research still needs to be done to better understand this relatively new disease.

Physical Hazards

Physical hazards are foreign objects such as insects, dirt, jewelry, and pieces of metal, wood, plastic, glass, etc. that inadvertently get into a food and could cause harm to someone eating that food. FDA has established maximum levels of natural or unavoidable defects in foods for substances that present no major human health hazard. These are called Food Defect Action Levels. This is the maximum amount of unavoidable defects that might be expected to be in food when handled under good manufacturing and sanitation practices. They are allowed because it is economically impractical, and sometimes impossible, to grow, harvest, or process raw products that are totally free of natural defects. Unavoidable defects include insect fragments, larvae, and eggs; animal hair and excreta; mold, mildew, and rot; shells, stems, and pits; sand and grit. The allowable levels of these substances are set at very specific levels deemed not to be a threat to human health. If a food contains more than these allowable levels, it is considered adulterated. While it may be unpleasant to find such substances in food, eating them at such low levels is not a health hazard and will not lead to illness.

FACTORS THAT CONTRIBUTE TO FOODBORNE ILLNESS

More than a million pounds of beef recalled and destroyed. One child dead and others sick from drinking fresh juice. In Milwaukee 400,000 people sick with diarrhea and vomiting. Thirty-five percent of residents in a nursing home sick with salmonellosis and four die. Raspberries causing sporadic foodborne illness for three years in a row. Such news stories of people getting sick from food are no longer new to us. Why are we hearing more about foodborne illness today than we did in the past? If foodborne disease is on the rise, what factors account for this increase?

News travels fast these days, both electronically and through the news media. What were once isolated events and stories, now reach millions within hours. Diagnostic techniques are constantly improving, which allows for identification of diseases, foodborne and otherwise, that would have been of unknown origin in the past. But even considering these facts, public health officials believe that the risk of foodborne illness has increased over the past 20 years (GAO 1996). Changes in demographics, consumer lifestyles and demands, and food production and economics are changing how food is produced and eaten. In addition, the microbial world is evolving. The next few pages examine factors influencing foodborne illness and food safety problems in the United States.

Demographics

The proportion of the population at serious risk of foodborne illness is increasing with the aging of the U.S. population and the growing number of people with weakened immune systems. Susceptibility to foodborne pathogens varies within the population. Thus, two people could eat the exact same food and amount; one may become ill while the other does not. People who are at higher risk of becoming seriously ill include infants, young children, the elderly, pregnant women, those taking certain medications and those with diseases such as AIDS, cancer, and diabetes that weaken their immune systems. Twenty-five percent of Americans fall into this category, and the size of this vulnerable population is growing. Demographers predict that the proportion of people over 60 years old in industrialized countries such as the United States will rise from the current 17 percent of the population to 25 percent by 2025 (Kaferstein 1999). Nursing home residents are particularly susceptible to foodborne illness as the weakening of the immune system that comes with age, and the use of antibiotics and other drugs give pathogens a chance to take hold. Foodborne illnesses are more likely to be fatal in a nursing home than in the general population. In a recent survey 89 percent of deaths with diarrhea as an underlying cause were adults 55 and over or children under the age of five (Morris 1997).

While anybody can get sick from eating contaminated food, the length of time it takes before they become ill and how ill they become depends on a number of factors. Most important among these are age, amount of contamination consumed, and health status of the individual. The body has a number of defenses to protect itself against harmful bacteria. The acidic gastric juices of the stomach are one of the first defenses against foodborne pathogens, as many bacteria cannot survive in an acidic environment. Very young infants and aging adults produce less, or less acidic, gastric juices than younger, healthy adults. The normal bacteria present in the gastrointestinal system form another protective barrier against foodborne illness by preventing harmful bacteria from colonizing the gut. Thus antibiotics, which do not discriminate between good and bad bacteria, but rather destroy them all, can also increase a person's susceptibility to foodborne illness. Without the protective bacteria that are normally present in the gastrointestinal tract, pathogenic bacteria can more easily invade and cause illness. Finally, the human immune system, not fully developed at birth, gradually reaches maturity in puberty and then slowly begins to decline after about 50 years of age.

Consumer Lifestyles and Demand

The pace of life in the United States has quickened. We often eat meals on the run, since we do not have time to prepare food at home. This means that by the time you eat your food, whether it is a restaurant meal or convenience food, it may have been transported, cooked, cooled, stored, transported again, reheated, and touched by numerous individuals. Each processing step introduces new hazards that could allow for the survival and growth of pathogenic bacteria that ultimately lead to foodborne illness. Two out of three people ate their main meal away from home at least once a week in 1998. The typical consumer over eight years of age ate food away from home at least four times per week (Collins 1997). Each time you eat food out you are placing your trust in that food establishment and its workers to handle your food properly. Americans spend 50 cents of every food dollar on food prepared outside the home—from supermarkets, restaurants, or institutions.

Add to this the abuse that occurs after a consumer purchases food and takes it home, and the likelihood of illness increases. Approximately 20 percent of reported foodborne illness cases occur from food cooked at home. Experts believe that this number is actually much higher (estimates range from 32 to 80 percent), but that most people do not report cases of illness caused by foods cooked at home (Knabel 1995; Doyle 2000). Americans are cooking less, and that also means they pass on less knowledge of cooking to their children, who are nevertheless increasingly responsible for preparing meals. Young cooks are receiving less training in food preparation than previous generations. This has grave implications for the future of food safety. In a survey of consumer food safety knowledge and practices, 86 percent of respondents knew that they should wash their hands before preparing food, but only 66 percent reported actually doing so. Only 67 percent of respondents reported washing or changing cutting boards after cutting raw meat or poultry. Older adults practiced safe behaviors more often than did younger adults (Altekruse 1995). In an Australian study in which researchers asked people about their food safety and kitchen habits, and then filmed them preparing food, there were large differences in what people said they did and what they actually did. Almost half the people who said they washed their hands after handling raw meat did not, and when they did it was often without soap. Nineteen percent of the households that claimed to have soap in the kitchen did not (Jay 1999).

Consumers are increasingly demanding fresh and natural products, and products with fewer preservatives. Without the traditional preservatives and processing methods that prevent microbial growth, modern all-natural and fresh products are more perishable. Food processing, mainly canning, freezing, and pasteurizing, not only extend the shelf life of foods, but also inhibit bacterial growth, making food safer. As an example, fresh apple cider has been associated with several foodborne disease outbreaks. An outbreak of *E. coli* O157:H7 in which a child died was associated with raw unpasteurized apple juice from a company that built its reputation on the naturalness of its products. This company now uses only pasteurized apple juice in its products (Odwalla Web site 2000). While pasteurization will kill harmful bacteria, advocates of fresh juice argue that pasteurization diminishes taste. To inform consumers of the risk posed by fresh, unprocessed juices, FDA revised its food labeling regulations. Fruit and vegetable juice products that have not been processed to prevent, reduce, or eliminate pathogenic microorganisms that may be present must have a warning statement to that effect on the label.

As the role of fresh fruits and vegetables in a nutritious diet has become evident, people are including them in their diet more. In 1993 Americans ate 27 percent more fresh produce than they did in 1973. An increase in the number of foodborne illness outbreaks associated with fresh produce has accompanied this increase in consumption. In the last 20 years the number of identifiable outbreaks in which produce was the food vehicle doubled (Tauxe et al. 1997). We also want produce year-round, which makes us dependent on foreign imports to meet that demand. Most produce only grows in the United States in certain seasons; yet this seasonal availability has almost disappeared from our supermarkets. Corn, berries, lettuce, peaches, and tomatoes, to name a few, are available year-round, or at least much longer than their growing season. From 1996 to 1998 *Cyclospora cayetanensis* sickened more than 2,400 people throughout 20 states and Canada. The only common food vehicle among these individuals was raspberries imported from Guatemala. Smaller outbreaks of *Cyclospora* have been traced to basil and mesclun lettuce grown in the United States. Very little is known about *Cyclospora*, and although there are tests to identify it in stool samples, so far there are no good tests to identify it in foods. This lack of ability to test for the organism in food samples complicates the recommendations public health officials should make to the public.

Food Production and Economics

In the past, outbreaks of foodborne illness were relatively small and local. Illness could be traced back to local events such as weddings, church dinners, and other gatherings where a large number of people ate the same food. Most of the victims lived in the same area and knew each other. That picture has changed today for several reasons.

Today's food is produced in vastly different ways from even several decades ago. Food used to be grown, produced, and distributed on a local basis. Food production is now centralized and on a larger scale than in the past. Products made in a single processing plant in mass quantities are shipped all over the country, sometimes the world. A mistake made in the processing will be felt nationwide instead of just locally. This is precisely what happened with Schwan's ice cream in 1994. A study in the *New England Journal of Medicine* reported that an estimated 224,000 people throughout the nation became ill from *Salmonella enteritidis* after eating ice cream produced on certain dates at an ice cream processing facility in Minnesota. Several suppliers shipped ingredients for the ice cream in bulk to the plant by tanker truck. The most likely cause of the outbreak was determined to be contamination of the ice cream premix during transport in tanker trailers that had previously carried unpasteurized liquid eggs, a known source of *Salmonella enteritidis* (Hennessy 1996). Recalls from processing plants are on a larger and larger scale. In 1997 Hudson Foods recalled 25 million pounds of ground beef produced at its large Nebraska facility due to the presence of *E. coli* 0157:H7. This is a scale unprecedented a generation ago.

Even the manner in which farmers raise animals can contribute to an increase in food safety problems. A large number of animals are often crowded together, which increases their stress levels and weakens their immune systems. This crowding also facilitates the spread of disease from one animal to another. In the past a sick animal was fairly isolated and would not pass on illness to the rest of the flock or herd. But with animal-to-animal contact, disease can quickly spread.

Many pathogens that cause foodborne illness in humans are present in the animals we consume. However, the pathogens do not cause illness in the animals themselves, making it difficult to distinguish which animals are carrying pathogens and which are not. Cattle infected with *E. coli* O157:H7 appear just as healthy as those that are not. Little is known on how these animals become infected and how they transmit these pathogens. Research into food safety is expanding to investigate what animals eat and drink and how that ultimately affects humans (Tauxe 1997).

New and Evolving Pathogens

As recently as 50 years ago scientists had identified four foodborne pathogens. Today five times that number are on the list. Twenty years ago scientists did not even recognize three of the four pathogens that the Centers for Disease Control and Prevention considers the most important in causing foodborne illness—*Campylobacter jejuni*, *Listeria monocytogenes*, and *E. coli* O157:H7. *Cyclospora cayetanensis* first appeared in 1979 and is still not well understood. It is likely that scientists will discover new foodborne pathogens as laboratory techniques improve.

As living organisms, pathogens are constantly evolving. With better ability to trace outbreaks, scientists are discovering that some bacteria survive in environments previously thought safe. For example, *E. coli* O157:H7, originally called hamburger disease because of its presence in undercooked ground beef, has shown up in food as diverse as salami, apple cider, raw milk, and lettuce. It also survives in lower pH conditions than originally thought, which leads to outbreaks in acidic foods such as salami and apple cider. It is now known that *Yersinia enterocolitica* and *Listeria monocytogenes* can survive and multiply at refrigeration temperatures.

Some foods long considered safe recently have been implicated in foodborne outbreaks. For years scientists believed the inside of an egg was sterile and that *Salmonella enteritidis* was not of concern. In 1989, however, they discovered that chickens infected with *Salmonella* pass this infection along in their eggs, so that the bacteria can be inside the raw egg, making it unsafe to eat raw or undercooked eggs. Knowledge of this fact caused food safety experts to advise people to cook eggs thoroughly or to use liquid pasteurized eggs. This means icings, egg drinks, ice cream, cookie dough, sauces, or salad dressings that contain raw eggs could be infected with the bacteria. Recently a private company developed a process to pasteurize whole eggs still in the shell, which could make these uncooked foods safe to eat again.

One of the largest outbreaks in the United States came not from food, but from the water supply. In Milwaukee, Wisconsin, an estimated 403,000 people became ill with watery diarrhea in April 1993. Ultimately it was found that *Cryptosporidium parvum*, a one-celled parasite first documented to infect humans in 1976, was the culprit. While in healthy people cryptosporidiosis is only moderately serious with watery diarrhea lasting seven to 14 days, in the immunocompromised it can lead to severe prolonged diarrhea and even death. In this outbreak 4,400 people were hospitalized. Although *Cryptosporidium* had previously been found in surface water, it was not expected to be found in treated water from a municipal water supply that met state and federal standards for acceptable water quality (MacKenzie 1994). Increased awareness of the parasite has led to increased testing for it and, not surprising, increased prevalence has been discovered. In addition to drinking water outbreaks, *Cryptosporidium* is associated with swimming pools and amusement park wave pools. This is particularly important because *Cryptosporidium* is highly resistant to chlorine and other chemical disinfectants. This is a new parasite showing up in new environments with new resistance capabilities.

Bacteria have evolved to thwart attempts to eliminate them. Some pathogens are now becoming resistant to common antimicrobial agents. It is thought that the resistance may be due to the use of these antibiotics in animals. We are seeing this same adaptability in foodborne bacteria. *Salmonella typhimurium* DT104 is widely distributed in wild and farm animals, especially in Europe and is resistant to several common antibiotics. There has been a parallel increase of people getting sick from this type of drug-resistant *Salmonella*.

HISTORY OF FOOD SAFETY

Very little about foodborne illness or food safety is found in historical records. Scientists did not begin to understand bacteria, and their relationship to disease, until the late nineteenth century. People did recognize that food spoils, but the reasons for that and the potential for becoming ill from food were not known. Perhaps the absence of food safety from historical chronicles is an indication that it was less of a concern than were other problems in the past. Even early food regulations were not aimed at making food safer, but rather at preventing economic fraud. So, a history of food safety really does not exist, but numerous discoveries, inventions, and regulations have led to the present knowledge and state of affairs in food safety. Chapter 1, in the section on food preservation, covers many of the inventions contributing to food safety; chapter 4 provides extensive coverage of the history of food regulations; and the chronology in chapter 3 presents other details of food safety history.

Food preservation methods such as drying, smoking, freezing, marinating, salting, and pickling had their beginnings thousands of years ago. Whether these methods were employed solely to keep food for later use, to improve flavor, or for other reasons is not known. But they also had the effect of keeping food safer. Even cooking can be viewed as an ancient method of making food safer. The Chinese Confucian Analects of 500 B.C.E. warned against consumption of sour rice, spoiled fish or flesh, food kept too long or insufficiently cooked food. The Chinese disliked eating uncooked food believing, "Anything boiled or cooked cannot be poisonous." Among the earliest of food safety manuals was one published in China in the year 2 (Needham 1962). It is possible that the practice of drinking tea originated because tea required using hot water, which would make it safer than using unheated contaminated water (Trager 1995). Doubtless other cultures in antiquity, while oblivious to the causes or prevention of foodborne disease, experienced it and prescribed methods to avoid it.

Early scientists grappled with the nature of disease and bacteria, which would set the stage for later discoveries. Much of the present knowledge about pathogens that cause foodborne illness is built on a foundation of scientific discoveries spanning back over three centuries. Aristotle (384–322 B.C.E.) and his Greek philosopher/scientist predecessors believed in the spontaneous generation of organisms—that insects and animals arose spontaneously from soil, plants, or other species of animals. Francisco Redi, an Italian physician and poet, set out to disprove this theory in 1668. He believed that maggots did not arise spontaneously in meat, which challenged the common wisdom of the day. He prepared eight flasks with meat in them; four sealed and four left open to the air. No flies could land on the meat in the sealed flasks, thus no maggots grew. The clear conclusion was that maggots did not form by spontaneous generation, but that flies laid eggs that were too small to be seen. This, however, was not enough to convince skeptics. Italian biologist Lazzaro Spallanzani in 1768 disproved the spontaneous generation theory. Even though Redi proved that insects did not arise from spontaneous generation, scientists still believed that microorganisms did. In his experiments, Spallanzani boiled solutions that would normally breed microorganisms for prolonged periods of time, which killed any microorganisms that might be in the solution, on the walls of the flask, or in the air inside the flask. Then he sealed the flasks to prevent any new spores or microorganisms from entering. No microorganisms grew no matter how long he left them standing. The fact that no new microorganisms appeared meant that there was no spontaneous generation (Satin 1999).

The discovery of bacteria in the late nineteenth century, the increased understanding of bacteria's role in disease, and the realization that there is a connection between human diseases and animal diseases led to the ideas that cleanliness is important and that unsanitary conditions can contribute to disease. In 1847 Hungarian physician Ignaz Semmelweiss wondered why women who bore their children in hospitals died of fever during childbirth, while those who gave birth at home usually did not. Noting that doctors went straight from the operating room to laboring mothers, he concluded that the doctors themselves were carrying disease to the women from the dissecting room. In those days the doctors didn't wash their hands, but wiped them on their aprons, which were already coated with body fluids. Semmelweiss ran experiments in which he had the doctors wash their hands with soap and water, and then rinse them in a chlorinated lime solution before entering the maternity wards. Death rates plummeted from 10 percent to 1.5 percent, only to climb again when the experiments were discontinued. Thereafter, he forced doctors to wash their hands before treating patients. Unfortunately, the validity of his work was not recognized at the time. His colleagues greeted his theory with ridicule, refusing to believe that their own hands were a vehicle for disease. Instead they attributed the deaths to a phenomenon arising from the "combustible" nature of the pregnant women. Historians attribute Semmelweiss's eventual despondency to the ridicule of his theories and attacks on his character. He was committed to an insane asylum, where he died of blood poisoning (Britannica.com Inc.). Lack of personal hygiene remains one of the main causes of foodborne illness 150 years later.

In a classic case of epidemiologic sleuthing, Dr. John Snow demonstrated in 1848 how cholera spread throughout London. He noticed that people who obtained their water from a particular well were more likely to become ill than those drawing their water from another well. He persuaded city officials to remove the pump handle from that particular well, which forced inhabitants to draw water from another well. The number of cholera cases dropped immediately (Frerichs 1999). Louis Pasteur further elucidated the linkage among spoilage, disease, and microorganisms with his work on fermentation and pasteurization in the 1860s and 1870s. In 1872 German scientist Ferdinand Julius Cohn published a three-volume treatise on bacteria, and essentially founded the science of bacteriology. He was the first to attempt to classify bacteria into genera and species, and the first to describe bacterial spores. But this new field of bacteriology needed bacteria on which to conduct experiments and to study. It took Robert Koch in the 1880s to perfect the process of growing pure strains of bacteria in the laboratory. At first he used flat glass slides to grow the bacteria. His assistant, Julius Richard Petri, suggested using shallow glass dishes with covers, now commonly called Petri dishes. Koch also established strict criteria for showing that a specific microbe causes a specific disease. These are now known as Koch's Postulates. Using these criteria scientists can identify bacteria that cause a number of diseases, including foodborne diseases. In 1947 Joshua Lederberg and Edward Lawrie Tatum discovered that bacteria reproduce sexually, and opened up a whole new field of bacterial genetics (Asimov 1972).

Even though Anthony van Leeuwenhook, a Dutch biologist and microscopist, had improved the microscope to the degree that small microscopic organisms could be seen for the first time as far back as 1673, the discovery of foodborne disease–causing microorganisms developed slowly. In 1835 James Paget and Richard Owen described the parasite *Trichinella spiralis* for the first time. German pathologists Friedrich Albert von Zenker and Rudolph Virchow were the first to note the clinical symptoms of trichinosis in 1860. However, the association between trichinosis and the parasite *Trichinella spiralis* was not realized until much later. In 1855 the non-pathogenic form of *Escherichia coli* was discovered. It later became a major research tool for biotechnology. Englishman William Taylor showed in 1857 that milk can transmit typhoid fever. In1885 USDA veterinarian Daniel Salmon described a microorganism that caused gastroenteritis with fever when ingested in contaminated food. The bacteria were eventually named *Salmonellae* (Asimov 1972). August Gärtner, a German scientist, was the first to isolate *Bacillus enteritidis* from a case of food poisoning in 1888. The case was the result of a cow with diarrhea slaughtered for meat; 57 people who ate the meat become ill (Satin 1999). Emilie Pierre-Mare van Ermengem, a Belgian bacteriologist, was the first to isolate the bacterium that causes botulism, *Clostridium botulinum*, in 1895. The case concerned an uncooked, salted ham served at a wake in Belgium. Twenty-three people became ill; three died. Van Ermengem isolated *C. botulinum* from both the ham and one of the victim's intestines. He demonstrated that the organism grows in an oxygen-free environment, and that it produces a toxin that causes the illness. In a perhaps overzealous use of the scientific method, M.A. Barber demonstrated that *Staphylococcus aureus* causes food poisoning. He became ill after each of three visits to a farm in the Philippines in 1914. Suspecting cream from a cow with an udder infection, Barber took home two bottles of cream, let them sit out for five hours, drank some of the cream, and became ill two hours later with the same symptoms he experienced on the farm. He isolated a bacterium from the milk, placed it in a germ-free container of milk, waited a while, and then convinced two hapless volunteers to drink the milk with him. They all became ill with the same symptoms (Asimov 1972). In 1945 *Clostridium perfringens* was first recognized as a cause of foodborne illness. It wasn't until the years between 1975 and 1985 that some of today's major foodborne pathogens—*Campylobacter jejuni*, *Yersinia enterocolitica*, *Escherichia coli* O157:H7, and *Vibrio cholerae*—were first recognized.

THE ROLE OF FOOD PRESERVATION IN FOOD SAFETY

Since the earliest times humankind has searched for ways to make the food supply safer and to make food last longer. Without the use of some preservation technique, the natural microorganisms that are present everywhere in the environment will grow and multiply in foods. Preservation aims either to destroy or inhibit the growth of harmful microorganisms in food by making an environment unsuitable for them.

The earliest recorded instances of food preservation date back to ancient Egypt and the drying of grains and subsequent storage in sealed silos. The stored grain could be kept for several years to insure against famine in case the Nile River flooded. People in many parts of the world developed techniques for drying and smoking foods as far back as 6000 B.C.E. Microorganisms need water to carry out their metabolic processes. Many preservation techniques that are familiar to us, such as drying, smoking, and salting, seek to reduce available water in a product. Freezing foods and making foods more acidic through fermentation and pickling also inhibit microorganism growth. Salting was so important in Roman life that Roman soldiers received "salarium," or salt, as payment. This is the origin of today's term "salary."

Large-scale deployment of armed forces led to the need for more advanced methods of food preservation to keep food safe for troops in the field. Napoleon's realization that armies do indeed travel on their stomach caused him to offer a prize for an improved food preservation method. In response to this need, Nicolas Appert, a French candy maker, developed a process by which he placed food in bottles, sealed the bottles, and then heated them for hours in boiling water. When Appert published his method in 1810 he had no knowledge of bacteria. It took another 50 years and Louis Pasteur to elucidate the relationship between microorganisms and the spoilage of food. What Appert developed is essentially the process for canning food. Over the years, food scientists have made many improvements in the canning process, but the basic idea of using high heat remains the same. As testimony to the durability of canned foods, a can of meat from Captain Parry's 1824 expedition to the Northwest Passage opened 114 years later in 1938 was still perfectly safe and edible (Thorne 1986, 23).

Most American homes have a device that is extremely useful for keeping foods safe—the refrigerator. Although refrigeration was developed in the early 1800s, refrigerators were not readily available for home use until the 1930s. Most pathogenic bacteria do not grow at all, or grow very slowly, at refrigerated temperatures. However, spoilage bacteria, those that cause food to smell or taste bad, can grow in the refrigerator. While spoilage bacteria cause foods to become of unacceptable quality, they do not cause illness. Spoilage bacteria serve a good purpose in that they prevent people from eating food that may contain harmful bacteria.

Freezing, except in cold climates, did not fully develop until the 1950s. Freezing keeps food safe by slowing the movement of molecules, causing microbes to enter a dormant stage. Freezing preserves food for extended periods of time because it prevents the growth of microorganisms that cause both food spoilage and foodborne illness; so frozen food is theoretically safe forever. The quality of frozen food, however, diminishes quickly with time. For example, when air reaches the surface of food, it causes dry grayish-brown leathery spots to appear. A turkey kept in the freezer for 10 years would be perfectly safe, but may be dried to little more than skin and bones. One can only wonder about the quality of the meal served in 1799 by William Buckland, dean of Westminster, England, who reportedly served his unsuspecting dinner guests meat from a recently discovered frozen mammoth that was 100,000 years old (Wilson 1991, 113).

A method of making food safer that is well-known and accepted today is pasteurization. Pasteurization is the process of heating foods to a temperature for a designated period of time to destroy disease-causing and/or food spoilage bacteria. The amount of time the product is heated depends on the temperature; higher temperatures require less time. It is different from sterilization in that some spoilage bacteria survive. Pasteurization takes its name from its inventor, Louis Pasteur. The most familiar pasteurized product in the United States is milk. Before milk was routinely pasteurized it spread tuberculosis, brucellosis, typhoid fever, diphtheria, and scarlet fever. Pasteurized milk made its debut in the United States in the 1880s, but took 30 years to gain full acceptance. Milk is not the only pasteurized food product available in grocery stores. In the mid-1990s there were several high-publicity foodborne illness outbreaks traced back to unpasteurized juice. Now, 98 percent of all juices in the United States are pasteurized. Eggs are another product that has benefited from pasteurization. While estimates are that *Salmonella enteritidis* infects only one in 20,000 eggs, with a production rate of almost 60 billion eggs per year, that still leaves close to three million infected eggs. Egg products, which are eggs removed from their shells for use in processed foods and available in liquid, frozen, and dried forms, must be pasteurized by law. The latest product to undergo pasteurization is intact shell eggs. Shell eggs are pasteurized with a combination water bath and hot air treatment under relatively low temperatures but longer times so that the nature of the egg does not change.

A newer form of pasteurization is called ultrahigh temperature (UHT) pasteurization. The amount of bacteria killed with a heat method such as pasteurization depends on how high the temperature is, and how long the food is held at that temperature. For instance, heating to a lower temperature requires that the food be held at the low temperature for a longer time. But using very high heat means that the food can be kept at that heat for a shorter time. UHT pasteurization takes advantage of this principle by using a very high temperature for a very short time. This provides an almost sterile product with an increased shelf life, but without significant changes in color, flavor, or texture of the food. Many countries use UHT for processing milk, which allows consumers to purchase cartons of milk that do not need refrigeration.

Preservation techniques that limit the availability of water, such as drying, salting, and smoking, and those that use heat, such as canning and pasteurization, dramatically alter the nature of the food itself. These processes degrade the color, flavor, texture, and nutrients in food. Today's consumers want their food to appear fresh and natural, as close to just-picked or just-slaughtered as possible. They don't want preservatives and other chemicals added to their foods, and at the same time they want convenience. But not many American consumers are willing to shop for fresh produce or meats every day. A number of new techniques are in use or in development that try to meet this demand for food with fresher, more natural qualities. There are several methods of applying electricity instead of heat to pasteurize food; these techniques are referred to as cold pasteurization. Irradiation, ohmic heating, and high-intensity pulsed electric fields are some of these technologies.

One of the earliest examples of applying electricity to foods is ohmic heating. In this process, a continuous electric current, which generates heat, is passed through the food. Experiments with ohmic heating began in the early 1900s. This method of processing is useful for viscous liquids and foods containing particles. High-intensity pulsed electric fields (PEF) is another emerging nonthermal technique. Unlike ohmic heating, PEF does not cause an increase in the temperature of food. PEF involves applying a short burst of high voltage to a food placed between two electrodes, which destroys bacterial cell membranes. This process has the potential to be used on juices, cream soups, milk, and egg products—all products in which heat produces undesirable changes.

Food irradiation is another technology to make food safe that, like canning, got its start in feeding the military. After World War II, the U.S. Army began experiments irradiating fresh foods for troops in the field. All irradiation is energy moving through space in invisible waves. The length of the wave determines the nature of the energy. As the wavelength gets shorter, the energy of the wave increases. Microwaves have a relatively long wavelength, so they have lower energy that is strong enough to move molecules and cause heat through friction, but not strong enough to structurally change atoms in the molecules. Ionizing radiation has a shorter wavelength and therefore higher energy—enough energy to change atoms by knocking electrons from them to form ions, but not enough energy to split atoms and cause exposed objects to become radioactive. Food irradiation exposes foods to very high-energy, short-length invisible waves. Depending on the dose, irradiation performs different functions. Low doses delay ripening and sprouting in fresh fruits and vegetables, and control insects and parasites in foods. Medium doses extend the shelf life of foods and reduce both spoilage and pathogenic microorganisms by damaging the genetic material of bacteria so they can no longer survive or multiply. High doses disinfect certain food ingredients, such as spices, and sterilize meat, poultry, seafood, and prepared foods. NASA began irradiating foods for astronauts in 1972; a case of foodborne illness while in space could be deadly, since no medical care would be available. Similarly, some hospitals use irradiated foods to feed their more susceptible patients.

Irradiation is regulated in the United States as a food additive, therefore FDA approves the process. Each new food is approved separately with a specific dosage level. After FDA grants approval, guidelines are established. USDA writes the guidelines for irradiation of meat and poultry products. The latest approval for irradiation in the United States was granted in 2000 for eggs. A petition is pending for permission to irradiate ready-to-eat meat and poultry products. Foods that are irradiated must display the radura (see figure 1-1) and the words "treated with radiation" or "treated by irradiation." Although 40 countries currently permit irradiation of food, its usage has been slow to catch on in the United States. This is mainly due to high start-up costs and to fears about consumer acceptance of the process. When the technology was new, many thought irradiation meant the food would be radioactive. As consumers have become more educated, they have realized that is not the case. Opponents of irradiation argue that irradiating foods produces chemical changes in the food. Proponents of the technology answer that these same chemical changes occur when food is cooked. Recent outbreaks of *E. coli* O157:H7, *Listeria*, and other bacteria are creating a demand for irradiated products. Irradiated foods also retain their texture, color, and taste better than do foods that are preserved by heat treatments. Food irradiation is explored in more detail in chapter 2.

Applying high pressure uniformly throughout a food product is another method of nonthermal food preservation. This inactivates microorganisms, spores, and undesirable enzymes, and increases the shelf life of foods. Japan is a leader in this technology. Although this method was initially studied at the end of the nineteenth century, consumer demand has caused renewed interest in commercializing the process. Jams made by high-pressure processing retain the taste and color of fresh fruit, unlike conventionally cooked jams. High-pressure processing is currently used in yogurts, salad dressings, and citrus juices. It has the potential to be used for minimally processed meat and fish products, convenience foods with long shelf lives and fresh and natural colors, and frozen foods with improved quality. The major drawback to this method is that it is costly to implement. Future usage will depend on how much the consumer is willing to pay for more natural food.

Modified atmosphere packaging (MAP) is a process in which oxygen is removed from a food package and other gases, usually carbon dioxide and/or nitrogen, are added. Vacuum-packaging, in which oxygen is removed but no other gases are added is also a type of MAP. The role of oxygen in food is that of a spoiler, one that causes degradation and spoilage of foods. Thus eliminating or reducing the amount of oxygen in a package prolongs the shelf life of the product. Examples of MAP prod-

Figure 1-1
Radura Denoting Irradiated Food

Treated with irradiation

ucts are fresh-cut produce, ready-to-eat salads, fresh pasta, lunch meats, and other meat products. These are the convenience food products that consumers want. However, from a food safety standpoint, there are some dangers with MAP products. Because lack of oxygen suppresses most spoilage bacteria in MAP products, the odors that would normally warn consumers that a food is spoiled are not present. There are some pathogenic bacteria, notably *C. botulinum*, that do not need oxygen to survive. Without the competition for food and water from spoilage bacteria, these bacteria can thrive. Manufacturers combat this by adding other gases such as carbon dioxide, which lowers the pH; decreasing the available water in a food; adding salt; and keeping the temperature low. It is important for consumers to understand that these types of products must be kept at the proper temperatures to keep them safe.

Ultraviolet (UV) radiation is the major bacteria-destroying factor in sunlight. Scientists are using UV light to kill pathogenic microorganisms. The most prevalent use of this technology is to kill pathogens in water systems. It is environmentally friendly, safe, more cost-effective than chlorination, and doesn't affect the taste of water as chlorination does. One problem with this technique is that it doesn't penetrate substances very deeply, so action is limited to the surface. At high doses products develop off flavors and odors, but at low doses it can extend the shelf life of foods without damaging quality. It is used in dairy plants, in meat and vegetable processing plants, in the ice cream industry, and to sterilize packaging materials.

As consumers have become chemical- and preservative-phobic, food preservation using natural antimicrobials has evolved. This concept involves a more natural and milder alternative to making food safer. By their very nature of being milder, natural antimicrobials by themselves are not sufficient to control pathogens. However, when used in combination with other food preservation methods they can improve the safety of foods without the use of traditional chemical preservatives such as sorbate or benzoate, which consumers no longer consider natural and healthy. Nature contains many antimicrobial compounds. Those used in food processing are derived from either plants or microorganisms. Spices and herbs have long been used to inhibit yeasts, bacteria, and molds. However, the spices and herbs themselves are less effective than the active ingredients such as essential oils, organic acids, and phenols found in them. Scientists are working to more actively exploit these active ingredients rather than using the whole spice or herb. As part of their life cycle, microorganisms produce compounds that affect the growth of other microorganisms around them. Many of these compounds inhibit microbial growth to increase the competitive edge of the producing organism. Lactic acid bacteria are the most important of these natural antimicrobials. Lactic acid bacteria have been used for centuries in fermentation, cheeses, and sausages. Many natural antimicrobials also have the advantage of being regulated as generally recognized as safe (GRAS) substances.

SOURCES

Acheson, David, W. K., MD, and Robin K. Levinson. 1998. *Safe Eating*. New York: Dell.

Altekruse, Sean F., D. A. Street, Sara B. Fein, and Alan S. Levy. 1995. Consumer Knowledge of Foodborne Microbial Hazards and Food-handling Practices. *Journal of Food Protection* 59(3): 287–294.

American Dietetic Association (ADA). January 1996. Position of the American Dietetic Association: Food Irradiation. *Journal of the American Dietetic Association* 96(1): 69–72. http://www.eatright.org/airradi.html.

American Egg Board. Date unknown. *Egg Production Information.* http://www.aeb.org/eii/production.html.

American Farm Bureau Federation. September 12, 2000. Farm Facts. http://www.fb.org/brochures/farmfacts/.

Animal Health Institute. December 1998. *Antibiotics Info Kit.* Washington: Animal Health Institute. http://www.ahi.org/info/general/General_Template.htm.

Asimov, Isaac. 1972. *Asimov's Biographical Encyclopedia of Science and Technology*, rev. ed. Garden City, NY: Doubleday.

Barbosa-Canovas, Gustavo V., M. Marcela Gongora-Nieto, Usha R. Pothakamury, and Barry G. Swanson. 1999. *Preservation of Foods with Pulsed Electric Fields.* San Diego: Academic Press.

Bohmont, Bert L. 1997. *The Standard Pesticide User's Guide.* 4th ed. Upper Saddle River, NJ: Prentice-Hall, Inc.

Britannica.com Inc., 1999–2000. *Semmelweiss, Ignaz Philippe.* http://www.britannica.com/bcom/eb/article/5/0,5716,68445+1,00.html.

Brody, Aaron L., ed. 1994. *Modified Atmosphere Food Packaging.* Herndon, VA: Institute of Packaging Professionals.

Caporael, Linnda R. 1976. Ergotism: The Satan Loosed in Salem? *Science* 192: 21–26.

Centers for Disease Control and Prevention (CDC). June 13, 1997. Update: Outbreaks of Cyclosporiasis—United States and Canada 1997. *Morbidity and Mortality Weekly Report* 46 (23): 521–523. http://www.cdc.gov/epo/mmwr/preview/index97.html.

Cliver, Dean O. 1999. *Eating Safely: Avoiding Foodborne Illness.* 2nd ed. New York: American Council on Science and Health. http://www.acsh.org/publications/booklets/eatsaf.html.

Collins, Janet E. 1997. Impact of Changing Consumer Lifestyles on the Emergence/Reemergence of Foodborne Pathogens. *Emerging Infectious Diseases* 3(4): 471–479.

Curtis, C. R. 1995. *The Public and Pesticides: Exploring the Interface.* Columbus, OH: National Agricultural Pesticide Assessment Program, Ohio State University and USDA.

Doyle, Michael P., Kathryn L. Ruoff, Merle Pierson, Winkler Weinberg, Barbara Soule, and Barry S. Michaels. June 2000. Reducing Transmission of Infectious Agents in the Home. *Dairy, Food and Environmental Sanitation* 96(1): 330–337.

Environmental Protection Agency, Office of Pesticide Programs, The Food Quality Protection Act (FQPA) of 1996 Web site: http://www.epa.gov/oppfead1/fqpa/.

Environmental Protection Agency (EPA). January 1999. *Assessing Health Risks from Pesticides.* Washington: Environmental Protection Agency. http://www.epa.gov/pesticides/citizens/riskassess.htm.

Food Allergy Network (FAN). Last modified June 29, 2000. Answers to Frequently Asked Questions. Fairfax, VA: Food Allergy Network. http://www.foodallergy.org/questions.html.

Frerichs, Ralph R. 1999. *Snow on Cholera. Part 2: Broad Street Pump Outbreak.* Los Angeles: UCLA School of Public Health. Internet slide show. http://www.ph.ucla.edu/epi/snow/Snowpart2_files/frame.htm.

Giblin, James C. 1986. *Milk: The Fight for Purity.* New York: Thomas Y. Crowell.

Henkel, John. 1998. Irradiation: A Safe Measure for Safer Food. *FDA Consumer* 32(3): 12–17 May/June. http://vm.cfsan.fda.gov/~dms/fdirrad.html.

Hennessy, T. W., C. W. Hedberg, L. Slutsker, K. E. White, J. M. Besser-Wiek, M. E. Moen, J. Feldman, W. W. Coleman, L. M. Edmonson, K. L. MacDonald, and M. T. Osterholm. 1996. A National Outbreak of *Salmonella enteritidis* Infections from Ice Cream. *New England Journal of Medicine* 334(20): 1281–1286.

Hou, H., R. K. Singh, P. M. Muriana, and W. J. Stadelman. 1996. Pasteurization of Intact Shell Eggs. *Food Microbiology* 13(2): 93–101.

International Food Information Council (IFIC). January 1995. *IFIC review: On Pesticides and Food Safety.* Washington: International Food Information Council. http://ificinfo.health.org/review/ir-pest.htm.

Jay, L. S., D. Comar, and L. D. Govenlock. 1999. A Video Study of Australian Domestic Food-handling Practices. *Journal of Food Protection* 62(11): 1285–1296.

Kaferstein, F. K., and M. Abdussalam. 1999. Food Safety in the 21st Century. *Dairy, Food and Environmental Sanitation.* 19(11): 760–763.

Knabel, S. J. 1995. Foodborne Illness: Role of Home Food Handling Practices. *Food Technology* 49: 119–131.

Labuza, T. P., and A. E. Sloan. 1981. Forces of Change: From Osiris to Open Dating. *Food Technology* 35(7): 34–36, 38–40, 42–43.

Lewis, Carol. 1998. Critical Controls for Juice Safety. *FDA Consumer* 32(5): 16–19 September/October. http://vm.cfsan.fda.gov/~dms/fdjuice.html.

MacKenzie, W. R., N. J. Hoxie, M. E. Proctor, M. S. Gradus, K. A. Blair, D. E. Peterson, J. J. Kazmierczak, D. G. Addiss, K. R. Fox, and J. B. Rose. 1994. A Massive Outbreak in Milwaukee of *Cryptosporidium* Infection Transmitted through the Public Water Supply. *New England Journal of Medicine* 331(3): 161–167.

Matossian, Mary K. 1989. *Poisons of the Past.* New Haven: Yale University Press.

Matossian, Mary K. 1982. Ergot and the Salem Witchcraft Affair. *American Scientist* 70: 355–357.

Mead, Paul S., Laurence Slutsker, Vance Dietz, Linda F. McCaig, Joseph S. Bresee, Craig Shapiro, Patricia M. Griffin, and Robert V. Tauxe. 1999. Food-related Illness and Death in the United States. *Emerging Infectious Diseases.* Vol. 5(5). http://www.cdc.gov/ncidod/eid/vol5no5/mead.htm.

Mellon, Margaret. 1998–99. Prescription for Trouble. *Nucleus* Winter: 1–3.

Morris, J. Glenn Jr., and Morris Potter. October-December 1997. Emergence of New Pathogens as a Function of Changes in Host Susceptibility. *Emerging Infectious Diseases.* 3(4): 435–441.

National Research Council Committee on Pesticides in the Diets of Infants and Children. 1993. *Pesticides in the Diets of Infants and Children.* Washington: National Academy Press.

National Research Council (NRC). 1998. *Ensuring Safe Food: From Production to Consumption.* Washington: National Academy Press.

National Research Council Panel on Animal Health, Food Safety, and Public Health, Committee on Drug Use in Food Animals. 1999. *The Use of Drugs in Food Animals: Benefits and Risks.* Washington: National Academy Press. Executive summary: http://www.nap.edu/readingroom/books/foodanim/.

Needham, Joseph, and Lu Gwei-Djen. 1962. Hygiene and Preventive Medicine in Ancient China. *Journal of the History of Medicine and Allied Sciences* 17(4): 429–478.

Odwalla Web site. Accessed May 28, 2000. *Food Safety.* Half Moon Bay, CA: Odwalla. http://www.odwalla.com/news/safety.html.

Potter, Morris E. 1996. Factors for the Emergence of Foodborne Disease. In *Proceedings of the Fourth ASEPT International Conference, Food Safety 1996.* 185–195.

Rahman, Shafiur, ed. 1999. *Handbook of Food Preservation.* New York: Marcel Dekker.

Satin, Morton. 1999. *Food Alert! The Ultimate Sourcebook for Food Safety.* New York: Facts on File.

Tauxe, R., H. Kruse, C. Hedberg, M. Potter, J. Madden, and K. Waschsmuth. 1997. Microbial Hazards and Emerging Issues Associated with Produce. A preliminary report to the National Advisory Committee on Microbiologic Criteria for Foods. *Journal of Food Protection* 60(11): 1400–1408.

Tauxe, Robert V. 1997. Emerging Foodborne Diseases: An Evolving Public Health Challenge. *Emerging Infectious Diseases* 3(4): 425–433.

Thorne, Stuart. 1986. *The History of Food Preservation.* Totowa, NJ: Barnes and Noble Books.

Trager, James. 1995. *The Food Chronology.* New York: Henry Holt and Company.

U.S. Department of Agriculture Food Safety and Inspection Service. December 1995. *Focus on: Egg Products.* http://www.fsis.usda.gov/OA/pubs/eggprod.htm.

U.S. Food and Drug Administration (FDA). May-June 1998. Irradiation: A Safe Measure for Safer Food. *FDA Consumer.* http://vm.cfsan.fda.gov/~dms/fdirrad.html.

U.S. Food and Drug Administration (FDA). rev. May 1998. *The Food Defect Action Levels. Levels of Natural or Unavoidable Defects in Foods that Present No Health Hazards for Humans.* Washington: Department of Health and Human Services. http://vm.cfsan.fda.gov/~dms/dalbook.html.

U.S. Food and Drug Administration (FDA). November 6, 1997. *FDA Warns against Drug Promotion of "Herbal Fen-Phen."* FDA talk paper. Washington: U.S. Food and Drug Administration. http://vm.cfsan.fda.gov/~lrd/tpfenphn.html.

U.S. General Accounting Office. May 1996. *Food Safety: Information on Foodborne Illnesses.* Washington: U.S. General Accounting Office.

University of Georgia Cooperative Extension Service. August 1998. *Food Irradiation: Questions and Answers.* Athens: University of Georgia. http://www.foodsafety.org/ga/ga009.htm.

Wilson, C. Anne. 1991. *Waste Not, Want Not. Food Preservation from Early Times to the Present Day.* Edinburgh: Edinburgh University Press.

Wittman, R. J., and G. J. Glick. 1995. Microbial Contamination of Shellfish: Prevalence, Risk to Human Health and Control Strategies. *Annual Review of Public Health* 16: 123–140.

Wodicka, Virgil O. 1977. Food Safety: Rationalizing the Ground Rules for Safety Evaluation. *Food Technology* 31(9): 75–79.

World Health Organization (WHO). June 1998. Emerging and Other Communicable Diseases, Surveillance and Control. *Use of Quinolones in Food Animals and Potential Impact on Human Health. Report of a WHO meeting.* Geneva: World Health Organization. http://www.who.int/emc-documents/zoonoses/docs/whoemczdi9810.html.

CHAPTER 2

ISSUES IN FOOD SAFETY

This chapter examines genetic engineering as it pertains to agriculture and the controversies involved in the genetic engineering of food products, and including a discussion of the debate behind one product in particular, bovine somatotropin. Because it still engenders debate, although less now than in the past, food irradiation is also explored. Pesticides and water quality are covered with a focus on food safety rather than environmental issues. Finally, because eating out at restaurants has become such a central component of our lives, the chapter includes food safety issues in restaurants. Sources used are listed after each section for ease in locating materials on the following specific topics:

Genetically engineered foods
Bovine somatotropin
Food irradiation
Pesticide residues in foods
Drinking water quality
Restaurant food safety

GENETICALLY ENGINEERED FOODS

Genetic engineering techniques applied to agricultural products, both plant and animal, have been referred to by terms as varied as food biotechnology, frankenfoods, agricultural genetic engineering, genetically modified organisms (GMOs), transgenic, and genetically engineered (GE). By whatever name, it is the topic for the new millennium. Genetic engineering is simply altering the genetic material of an organism. The debate on the topic is anything but simple. It generates emotional and far-reaching opinions among consumers, researchers, and governments around the world. A simplistic view would be that grassroots consumer groups, organic farmers, religious groups, and Europeans oppose genetic engineering; while industry, academic groups allied and funded by industry, and the U.S. government support it. Caught in the middle is the U.S. consumer—lulled by the promise of low food prices and improved foods, frightened by new technology, consumed by the media, and confused by conflicting reports from scientists. Groups on either side of the issue can produce many well-known experts who cite studies supporting their view (IFIC 2000; BioDemocracy and Organic Consumers Association 1998).

The controversial methods of modern food biotechnology center around taking genes from one species and inserting them into another in an attempt to transfer a desired characteristic. Genetic engineering involves using a technology referred to as recombinant DNA (rDNA) to transfer deoxyribonucleic acid (DNA), the molecule that carries a cell's genetic information, from one microorganism, plant or animal, to another. This allows for the creation of plants with characteristics from other plants, or even animals, which would not be possible through traditional plant breeding methods. In 1998, 25 percent of corn, 38 percent of soybeans, 45 percent of cotton, and 42 percent of canola were genetically modified in the United States.

REGULATION

The Food and Drug Administration (FDA) regulates most new foods, new food additives, and animal feed. FDA determines whether genetically engineered foods are safe to eat. Regulatory responsibility for biotechnology in FDA is shared between the Center for Food Safety and Applied Nutrition and the Center for Veterinary Medicine. In 1992 FDA ruled that foods produced through biotechnology would be subject to the same review and approval processes as are other new food products. Federal regulations evaluate the end product, not the process by which a product is made. Therefore, FDA evaluates new food biotechnology products for their individual safety, allergenicity, and toxicity, under the guidelines of the Federal Food, Drug and Cosmetic Act, just as are other new foods. Questions that must be answered during the review period are:

Has there been an increase in any naturally occurring toxins in the plant?

Has an allergen not commonly found in the plant been introduced?

Has there been a change in the levels of any important nutrients?

Have new substances that raise safety questions been introduced into the food?

Are there any negative environmental effects?

Have accepted, established scientific procedures been followed?

Calgene's FlavrSavr tomato, one of the very first food biotechnology products to come under FDA regulation, is a good example. An antibiotic marker used in the genetic engineering of the tomato produced very small amounts of a protein not normally found in tomatoes. FDA viewed this new protein as a food additive since it was a substance new to tomatoes, and regulated it as such. In part because of strong public input from public outreach meetings in 1999, FDA plans to strengthen its pre-market review of genetically engineered foods.

Current U.S. labeling laws require foods produced through biotechnology to have labels stating such if a known food allergen has been introduced, the nutritional content of the food has been changed, or the product's composition has been substantially altered. To protect consumers who have food allergies, products must be labeled if they contain any of the eight most common food allergens—milk, eggs, wheat, fish, shellfish, tree nuts, peanuts, and soy. FDA evaluates all new food products, biotech products, and traditional products for the presence of these allergens.

The primary agency responsible for biotechnology in the U.S. Department of Agriculture is the Animal and Plant Health Inspection Service (APHIS). APHIS governs the field testing of agricultural biotechnology crops. APHIS determines whether genetically engineered plants are safe to grow. The Environmental Protection Agency (EPA), as the federal agency that regulates pesticides, has jurisdiction over biotechnology plants that produce pesticides to protect themselves from insects and other pests. EPA determines whether genetically engineered plants are safe for the environment. In 1996 EPA approved the use of *Bacillus thuringiensis* (Bt), which is regulated as a pesticide since it controls pests.

THE CASE AGAINST FOOD BIOTECHNOLOGY

Opponents of food biotechnology define genetic engineering as altering or disrupting the genetic blueprints of living organisms. They believe that it is inherently unpredictable and dangerous, fraught with uncertainties, and that consumers are now guinea pigs in a vast genetic experiment. As evidence of lax government regulation, they point out that FDA uses the results of industry-sponsored research to determine the safety of GE foods, instead of conducting its own studies. Opponents argue that the current level of knowledge is so low that it is impossible to predict the long-term effects of releasing new organisms into the environment. These new organisms can interact and breed with other forms of life and pass on their newly acquired characteristics to unintended species. Once released, it will be impossible to contain these new organisms, whether they be bacteria, viruses, plants, or animals. Examples abound of humankind altering ecosystems with unintended and disastrous results. Scientists opposed to the new technology claim that academic research departments now receive over 50 percent of their funding from private corporations and that producing results that these corporations don't like isn't likely to result in further funding. Opponents break down the hazards of genetically engineered products into three types—human health, environmental, and socioeconomic.

Human Health Hazards

Most food allergies are due to specific proteins found in foods. Some people are so sensitive to certain proteins that eating that protein could cause sudden death. With up to 6 percent of children and 2 percent of adults suffering from food allergies, if a foreign protein that triggered these allergies were spliced into a food, the results could be catastrophic. The gene transfers in genetic engineering result in the production of novel proteins. Since most of the genes introduced into food products come from sources that have never been part of the human diet, opponents believe that it cannot be known whether the proteins produced by these genes will cause allergic reactions. If a protein were inserted into a food where it doesn't normally occur, it is possible that many people could eat foods to which they might have a reaction. They claim that under current labeling guidelines of GE foods, it would be hard for people to avoid foods that might trigger an attack. As an example of the potential dangers, opponents cite the case of GE soybeans that had a gene from a brazil nut added to its genetic makeup to improve the soybean's protein content. Nuts are one of the most common foods to which people are allergic. When these new soybeans were tested with samples of blood serum taken from individuals with nut allergies, tests indicated that had they consumed the soybeans they would have had an allergic reaction (Anderson 1999).

Those opposed to GE foods claim that they have the potential to produce unexpected compounds. This genetic tinkering could cause a plant to produce higher levels of toxins that it already produces in small amounts, or to switch on genes that could produce an entirely new toxin. They cite Dr. Arpad Pusztai's research with GE potatoes spliced with DNA from the snowdrop plant. The resulting GE-snowdrop potatoes had a different chemical composition than regular potatoes and damaged the vital organs and immune systems of laboratory rats fed the potatoes. Another case cited by opponents of the technology is the case of L-tryptophan, a popular food supplement that was produced by the Showa Denko company in Japan. The company developed a process by which genetically engineered bacteria were used to produce L-tryptophan in greater amounts than usual. More than 1,500 people became ill and 37 died after using the product. Although the exact cause remains controversial, some scientists believe that the supplement produced by the GE bacteria contained small amounts of a highly toxic compound not normally found in conventionally produced L-tryptophan.

Another area of concern is the potential decreased quality and nutrition of GE foods. Opponents mention a study by Dr. Marc Lappe that found the beneficial phytoestrogen compounds, thought to play a role in protecting against heart disease and cancer, were lower in GE soybeans than in traditional soybeans. Antibiotic resistance is another potential danger. In order to tell if gene splicing was successful, gene engineers use a marker gene called an antibiotic resistance marker (ARM) gene. Some researchers warn that these ARM genes might unexpectedly combine with pathogenic bacteria in the environment, and transfer this antibiotic-resistant quality to that bacteria. If animals or humans were then infected with these new bacteria, they could not be cured with the traditional antibiotics now on the market.

Another argument against food biotechnology is that it will lead to increased pesticide use, and therefore of pesticide residues in food. Some scientists point to studies showing that farmers growing GE crops use just as many, if not more, herbicides and pesticides as conventional farmers. One of the main qualities genetically engineered into crops is the ability to be resistant to specific herbicides. This practice is so popular that 71 percent of the GE crops planted world-wide in 1998 were herbicide-resistant crops (Anderson 1999). The companies producing these herbicide-resistant plants make them resistant to herbicides that they manufacture, thereby increasing the amount of herbicide that farmers buy from them. Monsanto produces a GE soybean that is resistant to Roundup, a Monsanto weed killer that is one of the most potent plant killers around. A field planted with Roundup-resistant soybeans can be sprayed with Roundup, which kills everything except the soybeans. As weeds become resistant to Roundup it will be necessary to apply larger amounts to crops.

Environmental Hazards

Opponents worry that wind, rain, insects, and birds will carry pollen from GE foods over to fields planted with traditional or organic crops, thereby "polluting" those fields. This genetic pollution will permanently pollute traditional crops, since once GE crops are released into the environment, it will be virtually impossible to eradicate them. Pollinators such as bees can pick up pollen from GE plants and carry it for several miles, cross-pollinating even distant conventional crops. There is no way to control this type of cross-pollination. A study in 1999 reported that researchers planted a field of sterile oilseed rape plants up to two-and-a-half miles away from a crop of GE oilseed rape. Since the test plot plants were all sterile, any seeds produced must have been the result of cross-pollination from the GE field. The scientists found that 5 percent of the flower buds on the test plants were pollinated.

Related to genetic pollution is the drifting of pesticides sprayed on fields with pesticide resistant crops to fields planted in conventional crops. Products like Roundup can drift to neighboring fields not planted with Roundup-resistant soybeans and kill those soybeans. This forces the farmer not using that technology to switch to it.

Genetic material is often and easily transferred between living organisms. Critics of food biotechnology fear that herbicide-resistant GE crops will eventually pass on those resistance traits to the very weeds and pests to which they were engineered to be superior, creating "superweeds" and "superpests." It will be necessary to use higher and higher doses of chemicals to control these "superweeds." Anti-GE literature cites studies showing that herbicide-resistant rapeseed (canola) spreads resistance properties to wild mustard plants.

As a natural course of events, weeds and insects (and bacteria for that matter) eventually develop resistance to the chemicals used to control them. Because farmers will be using Roundup more and more, weeds will develop resistance to it sooner. Opponents fear that it will be necessary to apply more and more Roundup until finally it won't be effective at all, and farmers will have even fewer choices to combat weeds in their fields. Another example of this danger is the case of *Bacillus thuringiensis* (Bt), a soil bacterium that produces a natural toxin that organic farmers use as a method of biological pest control. The toxin in naturally occurring Bt bacteria are only activated by enzymes in the digestive tract of certain insects, notably caterpillars. Crops have now been produced that have the gene for the Bt toxin, giving them a built-in insecticide. While in the past farmers have only occasionally applied the Bt toxin when they had an infestation, the Bt toxin in the GE crops is produced all the time. Therefore, insects are continually exposed to the Bt toxin, which speeds up the time in which they will develop resistance to Bt. Scientists who believe that some insects have already developed Bt resistance predict that within three to five years most target insects will be resistant to Bt. There is also concern that the Bt toxin in the GE crops is of a slightly different form than the natural toxin, and that it may harm a wider range of insects, including some that are beneficial.

Since the understanding of molecular genetics is still in its infancy, some researchers fear that gene splicing will inevitably result in unanticipated and dangerous surprises. They are exploring whether genetically altering plants to withstand certain viruses and pathogens will cause those viruses and pathogens to mutate into new and/or stronger forms. In the same way that the introduction of exotic species into an environment tends to cause the decline of the native species, introducing GE plants into an environment may eventually overpower the native species. As an example, opponents hypothesize that if GE salmon that are bigger and hardier than the wild varieties are released into habitats, they will out-compete those wild varieties and cause their extinction. This genetic bio-invasion could set off a whole chain of environmental events not yet dreamed of.

Socioeconomic Hazards

Opponents criticize that the promised benefits of increased crop yields from GE crops have not come about. They point to examples of large crop failures from GE crops for evidence that the plants don't function as advertised. Bt cotton planted in the southern United States in 1996 was supposed to be from 90 to 95 percent effective against the bollworm. Instead, it is thought the plants were only 60 percent effective, and the region suffered a major bollworm infestation that had to be combated with emergency insecticide spraying. Opponents cite studies showing that the yields of GE crops are, in fact, lower than those of conventional varieties.

Another example of this is the FlavrSavr tomato, which in 1994 was the first genetically engineered food approved for sale in the United States. It was supposed to ripen longer on the vine and still be hard enough at picking to withstand the rigors of packing and transport. But the tomatoes instead were often soft and bruised, making them unmarketable as fresh (Anderson 1999). The FlavrSavr made a brief appearance in the American marketplace, then quickly disappeared.

Seed companies have started producing seeds that are genetically modified to make them infertile. This means that the seeds produced by the plants can't be saved by farmers to plant the next year's crop. This "terminator technology" forces farmers to buy new seed every year, which many cannot afford to do. Critics suspect that companies will develop crops that won't grow or germinate unless treated with certain chemicals, which again forces farmers to become dependent on the companies producing those chemicals. Opponents claim that farmers will be driven off the land and that consumers' food choices will be dictated by a few multinational corporations.

Finally, opponents state that genetically engineering plants and animals reduces them to just another manufactured product, like a chair or a car, and strips them of their integrity and sacred qualities. They believe that the whole idea of food biotechnology perpetuates the view that nature should be dominated, exploited, and forced to yield more. Citing a consumer's "right to know," these critics want foods with genetically engineered components to be labeled so they can avoid them.

THE CASE IN FAVOR OF FOOD BIOTECHNOLOGY

Proponents of food biotechnology emphasize that altering the genetic makeup of plants and animals is nothing new. It is a technique humankind has practiced for centuries through breeding. The foods we eat today—rice, corn, apples, pigs, chickens, etc.—bear little resemblance to their wild, native varieties. Breeders have selected and promoted desirable traits, while minimizing or eliminating undesirable traits. Nature itself practices genetic engineering, constantly altering and improving organisms to better suit their environment. Today's food biotechnology is nothing more than the evolution of traditional agricultural methods. Since almost all the foods we eat have been genetically modified by nature or by science over the years, proponents claim that today's genetic engineering does not introduce any new safety concerns. In traditional forms of plant and animal breeding the creation of genetic diversity has limits. It may now be possible to insert a gene that allows arctic fish to withstand cold into food crops to make them frost-resistant. To supporters of the technology, genetic modification means genetic enhancement. Proponents break down the benefits of genetically engineered products into three types-human health, environmental, and socioeconomic.

Human Health Benefits

Instead of harming consumers, proponents claim that products recently introduced into the marketplace provide such benefits as enhanced flavor and freshness, increased nutritional value, and reduced saturated fat content. As examples of the benefits food biotechnology can bring to consumers, they cite:

- Tomatoes with increased levels of the antioxidant lycopene, thought to reduce the risk of cancer
- Genetically enhanced soybeans that are lower in saturated fats
- Cooking oils that have a more healthful fat content
- Peanuts and rice with improved protein content
- Fruits that are genetically engineered to produce vaccines for diseases
- Potatoes with a higher starch content, thereby reducing the amount of oil absorbed during production of french fries and potato chips
- Plants with reduced levels of natural toxins
- Fruits and vegetables fortified with higher levels of vitamins such as C and E

Proponents agree that allergenicity is a key issue in food biotechnology. They see food biotechnology as being able to help people with food allergies by minimizing or eliminating proteins in foods that cause allergic reactions. They point to a low-allergen form of rice developed in Japan as an example of how biotechnology can minimize the effects of food allergies. Proponents cite the same example of the discovery that the brazil nut gene inserted into soybeans would cause an allergic reaction in some people as evidence that the system is working. Testing revealed the product was unsafe, so it was discontinued. While opponents of the technology criticize government actions concerning regulation, supporters feel the government is setting stringent food safety standards. Consumers can be confident that GE foods are safe and properly labeled so that those with allergies can avoid eating foods that will cause allergic reactions.

Countering opponents' claims of lack of research into the safety of these products, advocates cite years of research indicating that the benefits of agricultural biotechnology far outweigh any risks. Proponents claim that the scientific consensus is that risks associated with food-biotechnology products are the same as for other foods. They point to years of research and the absence of harmful evidence as indicators that biotech foods are safe. As for the L-tryptophan case, it is now thought that the problems came not from the genetically modified bacteria, but rather from impurities in the growth medium. Those in favor of food biotechnology consider the research by Dr. Arpad Pusztai with GE potatoes to be flawed, poorly designed, and incapable of leading to meaningful conclusions. Supporters state that the chances of unintentionally transferring a naturally occurring toxin or other dangerous substance are greater with conventional plant breeding than with genetic engineering. They claim that modern biotechnology methods that target a single gene are more precise and predictable than traditional breeding techniques that transfer hundreds of genes.

Environmental Benefits

Proponents claim that agricultural biotechnology products will help, not harm, the environment. Benefits include decreased pesticide and herbicide use, more efficient use of pesticides and fertilizer, and water and soil conservation. Crops with the internal ability to resist insects and other pests will require fewer applications of pesticides. This will mean fewer chemical residues will find their way into ground and surface water supplies and onto foods. Less land will have to be converted to agricultural use because of the increased yield of GE crops. Those in favor of biotechnology cite GE corn as a positive example. When fed to hogs, GE corn will reduce the phytic acid in animal waste that contributes to algae growth in water.

Another proposed advantage of genetic engineering is that it would increase the genetic variation in staple crops by breeding into them desirable traits from previously unavailable sources. Researchers aim to use biotechnology to discover which genes of value reside in which plants and then transfer those genes into crops now in use around the globe. It will enable scientists to learn what important genes are actually contained in the millions of plant specimens housed in gene banks around the world.

Scientists favoring genetic engineering claim there is no scientific evidence that "superpests" or "superweeds" could occur through GE foods. Insects and weeds naturally develop resistance to chemicals in their environment. Biotechnology can better manage this evolution in resistance. There are already systems in place—crop rotation, hybrid rotation, and insect resistance management—that help prevent resistance from developing. With regard to insects developing resistance to Bt crops, supporters point to the practice of insect resistance management (IRM). This is a practice in which growers plant non-Bt crops near the genetically modified resistant plants. Pests infecting these non-Bt plants will not develop Bt resistance and will breed with their counterparts in the Bt crop fields, which will lessen the chances of the development of resistance. Proponents argue that research demonstrating the possibility of resistance has been done in the laboratory, and thus may not be applicable to the natural environment.

Socioeconomic Benefits

Citing studies that indicate increasing world population will require the food supply to increase 250 percent from its current level, proponents see biotechnology as helping to alleviate world hunger. Food biotechnology can increase crop yields by several mechanisms. Increasing a plant's ability to withstand environmental factors can expand a product's geographical growth range. By building into plants better tolerance to droughts, floods, salts, metals, heat, and cold, marginal land can be made available for agriculture. Growers will be able to plant crops in areas that are now considered unsuitable for farming. This could improve the economies of developing nations. Globally pests destroy 45 percent of the world's crops. Biotechnology can decrease this amount of waste by building in resistance to pests and weeds. Supporters claim that agricultural biotechnology will reduce the risk of crop failures. In addition, growing animals for food can be made more efficient and feasible for the world by producing animal feed that will help animals to better digest their food through improved protein quality of animal feed crops.

Proponents claim that advantages of food biotechnology that will be noticed in the marketplace are foods that have longer shelf life and better flavor, appearance, and texture. They use as examples peppers modified to be tastier and sweeter; smaller seedless melons for use as single servings; bananas and pineapples with delayed ripening properties; sweeter peas; bananas resistant to fungus; and strawberries with higher crop yields and improved freshness, flavor, and texture. Using biotechnology, familiar food products can be produced more cheaply. For example, before genetic engineering techniques became available, the enzyme used to make cheese, rennet, was obtained from the lining of calves' stomachs. Using biotechnology, researchers have identified and removed the specific gene responsible for rennet production and inserted it in bacteria, which then produce rennet.

Instead of spending between 10 and 12 years breeding plants in the traditional manner and mixing thousands of genes that could have unpredictable outcomes, with genetic engineering modern plant breeders can select a specific genetic trait from any plant or animal and move it into any other plant or animal. This way genetic engineers can design plants with specific beneficial traits and without specific undesirable traits. They point out that this latest development in agricultural breeding is faster and more precise than previous methods of plant and animal breeding, and offers farmers a broader choice of how to improve their crops and manage their farms.

SOURCES

Anderson, Luke. 1999. *Genetic Engineering, Food, and Our Environment.* White River Junction, VT: Chelsea Green.

BioDemocracy and Organic Consumers Association. December 1998. *Quotes from Scientists and Other Folks on the Dangers of Genetically Engineered Foods and Crops.* Little Marais, MN: BioDemocracy and Organic Consumers Association. http://www.purefood.org/ge/sciquotes.htm.

Cummins, Ronnie. Date Unknown. Hazards of Genetically Engineered Food and Crops: Why We Need a Global Moratorium. *GE-Fact Sheet and Guidelines for Grassroots Action.* Little Marais, MN: BioDemocracy and Organic Consumers Association. http://www.purefood.org/.

Food Marketing Institute. Rev. October 1998. *Backgrounder: Biotechnology and Food.* Washington: Food Marketing Institute.

Institute of Food Science and Technology. 1998. *Position Statement: Genetic Modification of Food.* London: Institute of Food Science and Technology. http://www.ifst.org/hottop10.htm.

International Food Information Council (IFIC). August 1999. *Myths and Facts about Food Biotechnology.* Washington: International Food Information Council. http://ificinfo.health.org/foodbiotech/mythsfacts.htm.

International Food Information Council (IFIC). February 2000. *What the Experts Say about Food Biotechnology.* Washington: International Food Information Council. http://ificinfo.health.org/foodbiotech/whatexpertssay.htm.

International Food Information Council (IFIC). Updated April 1999. *Backgrounder—Food Biotechnology.* Washington: International Food Information Council. http://ificinfo.health.org/backgrnd/bkgr14.htm.

Vogt, Donna U., and Mickey Parish. June 2, 1999. *Food Biotechnology in the United States: Science, Regulation, and Issues.* Report no. RL30198. Washington: Congressional Research Service.

Bovine Somatotropin

Somatotropin (ST) is a naturally occurring protein hormone that regulates growth in humans and other animals. Each species of animal has its own version of somatotropin. Human somatotropin (HST) is used to treat dwarfism. Research beginning in the 1930s revealed that administering somatotropin to animals increased milk yield. At that time there was little commercial interest because the only way to obtain somatotropin was to extract and purify it from animal pituitary glands, a process that was prohibitively expensive. The development of modern biotechnology techniques in the 1970s enabled scientists to produce somatotropin, human and otherwise, in the laboratory. This made it economically feasible to study the effects of bovine somatotropin (BST) on milk production in cows, with the first reports appearing in the literature in 1982. Laboratory-produced somatotropin is called recombinant somatotropin. Because BST is a type of growth hormone, it is also referred to as recombinant bovine growth hormone. BST is also referred to as rBST, bST, BGH, and rBGH. The company that produces BST, Monsanto, markets it under the trade name Posilac.

According to proponents of BST, scientists worldwide have conducted more than 2,000 studies on BST. These studies have clearly shown the efficacy, safety, and benefits of BST use in dairy production. Before approving BST, FDA required companies to prove that the products of BST-supplemented animals are safe for human consumption, that BST is safe for the animals, and that BST is safe for the environment. Pro-BST scientists claim that studies show BST does not adversely affect the health of treated cows, does not change the composition of milk, and does not pose any risk to humans. Supporters claim that the public has been deliberately misled by groups who oppose the use of animals for food, want to promote organic foods, or have their own anti-industry, anti-technology agenda. In light of the continuing debate and possible new evidence, in 1999 FDA re-evaluated BST in the most extensive post-approval study ever conducted on any animal product in the United States. The conclusion was the same—that BST is safe for humans and animals.

Opponents of BST claim that there has been a major hijacking of the scientific and regulatory apparatus by Monsanto. By virtue of their size and wealth, big multinational companies such as Monsanto are able to exert their influence on news media, government agencies, and academia to portray their products in a good light. As evidence of this, critics point to the sudden cancellation (and subsequent firing of the producers) of a Fox News documentary that was to reveal negative aspects of BST; Monsanto's threats of lawsuits to school boards if they banned BST from school cafeterias; aggressive lobbying against BST labeling laws in Congress and in individual states; and firing of scientists if they expressed concerns about the safety of BST.

BST critics claim that Monsanto influenced and manipulated rulings from federal agencies responsible for granting BST approval. As an example of the close working relationship between industry and the government, they cite a former Monsanto researcher who worked on BST and also had major responsibility for crafting the official FDA position on BST. Opponents allege that FDA never actually examined data from a Monsanto study, but instead based their safety assessment on Monsanto's summary of the study. Furthermore, it is claimed that Monsanto suppressed unfavorable results from studies, blocked publications from other scientists that showed negative results, selectively emphasized positive points, and compensated farmers who had increased veterinary bills from using BST on their cows. This range of influence extends to Canada too, as one of the experts assigned to review the safety of BST previously worked as a consultant to Monsanto. In Canada, several scientists claim they were pressured by supervisors to approve BST even though they had reservations about its safety. Critics claim that the Canadian government might have been influenced to approve BST because one of the experts assigned to review its safety had previously worked as a consultant to Monsanto. Anti-BST activists allege that Monsanto offered the Canadian government between one and two million dollars if Monsanto received approval to market BST in Canada without having to submit data from any further studies (Anderson 1999). This is an allegation that Monsanto firmly denies. BST opponents believe that, as with other food biotechnology products, BST is an ill-advised experiment with American consumers as the guinea pigs, and that release of such a substance has major potential health risks for the entire U.S. population.

In 1993 FDA approved BST for commercial use. It was the first biotechnology product approved for animal use, and it ushered in the whole era of food biotechnology. Although the United States and 25 other countries have approved the use of BST, it remains banned in Canada. The European Union (EU) has imposed a moratorium on its use. Scientists from the Food and Agriculture Organization of the United Nations could not reach a consensus on BST when they met in 1999. Debate on the safety of BST still remains strong. Issues center on human health, animal health, and socioeconomics.

HUMAN HEALTH ISSUES

Human health issues can be broken down into the possible effects of BST itself, and the possible relationship of insulin-like growth factor I (IGF-I) and cancer. Recombinant BST is indistinguishable from natural BST, as it contains the same amino acids in the identical sequence, with the same shape and properties. BST occurs naturally in cows' milk and meat in very small quantities. Supplemental administration of BST to cows does not increase the amount of BST found in their milk. Because BST and human somatotropin are very different in structure, BST is not active in humans, even if it is injected into the bloodstream. BST does not change the composition of milk in any significant way. Furthermore, BST would not be a human food safety concern because it is digested in the stomach just like any other protein. For these reasons, some scientists say BST itself poses no human health risk.

BST regulates another protein hormone found in milk, insulin-like growth factor I (IGF-I). IGF-I is a normal component in the human gastrointestinal tract, where it occurs in much greater amounts than it does in cows' milk. Normal concentration of IGF-I in the blood of adults and children can be more than 100 times greater than that found in cow's milk, which means that the amount of IGF-I in milk is small compared to what the human body produces. Both sides agree that levels of IGF-I are higher in milk produced from BST-treated cows than from non-treated cows, however it is the interpretation of this that differs.

Bovine IGF-I and human IGF-I are identical in structure, a fact that BST opponents believe poses serious risks for human health. They cite studies showing that women with small increases of IGF-I levels in their blood are up to seven times more likely to develop breast cancer than women with lower levels, and that high levels of IGF-I are also a risk factor for prostate and colon cancer. Proponents of BST claim that higher levels of IGF-I in milk are not a safety risk since it is a protein and therefore is digested and rendered harmless just like all other dietary proteins. These proponents also point out that the person who first published the link between BST and cancer did so in a non-research journal of which he is on the editorial board, and that he is an activist of many years standing in the crusade against use of any chemicals in food. In spite of proponents claiming that IGF-I is fully digested, opponents claim that in the presence of casein, a normal milk protein, IGF-I resists digestion. Opponents allege that contrary to what FDA and Monsanto claim, long-term toxicology studies addressing such possibilities as sterility, infertility, birth defects, and cancer have not been performed for BST.

ANIMAL HEALTH ISSUES

Proponents claim that hundreds of studies have been performed, none of them showing an increased incidence of ill health in BST treated cows. Even in studies where large doses of BST, up to 60 times the commercial dose, were given to cows, the health of the animals was not affected. In answer to the apparent increased incidence of mastitis (inflammation of the udder), they admit there has been a small positive association between milk yield and mastitis. However, proponents believe the interpretation of this should not be that BST supplementation causes mastitis. Other means of increasing milk production, such as selective breeding, also result in increased mastitis, and cows that are naturally high producers also have higher incidence of mastitis. Some BST proponents go so far as to claim that BST may even improve a cow's health since somatotropin plays a key role in maintaining an animal's immune system.

Other scientists disagree with the findings that BST is not harmful to cows. A panel of animal health experts found that cows injected with BST have a higher rate of infertility, increased lameness, increased mastitis, and a shorter life expectancy. Canada refused marketing approval for BST in January 1999 because of concerns about animal welfare. EU scientists, citing health concerns, came to the same conclusion and voted to continue the moratorium on BST. For opponents of BST, more mastitis means more antibiotics administered to cows, which means more drug residues in milk. But the other side counters that when cows are medicated due to an infection or other illness and treated with drugs, FDA requires that farmers wait a specified amount of time (from 72 to 96 hours) to give the drug time to clear the animal's system before products from it are obtained.

SOCIOECONOMIC ISSUES

About the only fact that pro-BST and anti-BST groups agree on is that BST use results in a 10 to 15 percent increase in milk yield when administered to dairy cows. As with other agricultural biotechnology issues, proponents claim that the burgeoning world population will require more efficient methods of food production. BST fits the prescription since it allows for more output, milk in this case, per input of feed. While opponents agree that BST increases milk production by between 10 and 15 percent, they bring up the point that the problem in the dairy industry is an overproduction of milk. With U.S. taxpayers paying a subsidy to dairy farmers to buy surplus milk to prevent the price of milk from plummeting, why is BST even necessary? Proponents counter that since supply is not really a problem, farmers would use BST to improve productivity rather than increase total amount of milk—producing the same volume of milk from fewer cows.

As with other food biotechnology products, proponents claim that the use of BST will benefit the environment. Reducing the amount of feed required to produce milk will reduce the need for fertilizer and other inputs associated with growing, harvesting, processing, and storing animal feed. Increases in productive efficiency also reduce the production of animal waste.

Labeling of milk from BST-treated cows is another hotly contested issue. Those who think it shouldn't be labeled point to FDA claims that there is no difference in milk from BST and non-BST treated cows. Retailers may label milk products as coming from cows that were not treated with BST, but since there is no difference between BST milk and non-BST milk, and since all milk has some BST, FDA has ruled that labeling milk BST-free would be false labeling. Those who believe milk from BST-treated cows poses a risk want labeling so they can avoid feeding milk from BST-treated cows to their families.

SOURCES

Anderson, Luke. 1999. *Genetic Engineering, Food, and Our Environment.* White River Junction, VT: Chelsea Green.

Etherton, Terry D. 1994. *The Efficacy, Safety and Benefits of Bovine Somatotropin and Porcine Somatotropin.* New York: American Council on Science and Health. http://www.acsh.org/publications/booklets/somatotropin.html.

Institute of Food Science and Technology. 1999. *Position Statement: Bovine Somatotropin (BST).* London: Institute of Food Science and Technology. http://www.ifst.org/hottop8a.htm.

Vogt, Donna U., and Mickey Parish. June 2, 1999. *Food Biotechnology in the United States: Science, Regulation, and Issues.* Report no. RL30198. Washington: Congressional Research Service.

FOOD IRRADIATION

Food irradiation is not a new technology. Research began in earnest with President Eisenhower's "Atoms-for-Peace" policy after World War II. Much of the early research was carried out by the U.S. Army and the Atomic Energy Commission. The first commercial use of food irradiation occurred in 1963, when the Food and Drug Administration (FDA) approved its use to control insects in wheat and flour. Large-scale implementation of food irradiation in the United States has been slow due to concerns about its safety. Realization that pathogens are the major concern in food safety has reignited interest in food irradiation.

BACKGROUND

Food irradiation is a method of controlling insect pests and pathogenic or spoilage bacteria in food and agricultural commodities. Instead of using heat or chemicals for processing, irradiation uses gamma energy, electron beams, or X-rays. Sometimes it is referred to as cold pasteurization. Similar technology is used to sterilize medical equipment and devices so they can be used in surgery and implanted without risk of infection.

Food irradiation has different uses depending on the strength of radiation used. It can be used to control mold, inhibit sprouting in vegetables, control insect pests, reduce bacterial pathogens, or, at the strongest dose, sterilize food. At low doses irradiation is an alternative to fumigation with chemicals to eliminate insects. Low doses have been used to inhibit the growth of mold in strawberries and to inhibit sprouting in potatoes, thereby prolonging the shelf life of these products. From 1995 to 1999 approximately 800,000 pounds of tropical fruit from Hawaii have been irradiated before shipping to the mainland. This eliminated the need for fumigating them to destroy fruit flies that could spread to the mainland. Spices are the most widely irradiated product, with about 25 percent of the total world spice trade undergoing irradiation (Derr 1999). The current push for irradiation is to kill bacteria and parasites that would otherwise cause foodborne illness. The dose of irradiation needed to kill *Salmonella* in chicken is about seven million times more than that of a chest X-ray. NASA irradiates food that astronauts eat in space. Their food is irradiated to the level of sterilization.

Three different irradiation technologies exist, which use three different kinds of rays: gamma rays, electron beams, and X-rays (CDC 1999). The first technology uses the radiation given off by a radioactive substance. This can be either a radioactive form of the element cobalt (cobalt 60) or of the element cesium (cesium 137). These substances give off high-energy photons, called gamma rays, which can penetrate foods to a depth of several feet. These particular substances do not make anything around them radioactive. This technology has been used routinely for more than 30 years to sterilize medical, dental, and household products. It is also used for radiation treatment of cancer.

Electron beams, or e beams, are produced in a different way. The e beam is a stream of high-energy electrons, propelled out of an electron gun. This electron gun apparatus is a larger version of the device in the back of a TV tube that propels electrons into the TV screen at the front of the tube, making it light up. The electron beam generator can be simply switched on or off. No radioactivity is involved. The electrons only penetrate food to a depth of a little more than an inch, so the food to be treated must be no thicker than that. Two opposing beams can treat food that is twice as thick. E-beam medical sterilizers have been in use for at least 15 years.

The newest technology is X-ray irradiation. This is an outgrowth of e-beam technology, and is still under development. The X-ray machine is a more powerful version of the machines used in many hospitals and dental offices to take X-rays. To produce the X-rays, a beam of electrons is directed at a thin plate of gold or other metal, which produces a stream of X-rays coming out the other side. Like gamma rays, X-rays can pass through thick objects. However, like e beams, the machine can be switched on and off, and no radioactive substances are involved.

Irradiation kills microbes by damaging their DNA. Because of this, bigger organisms like parasites and insects are more susceptible to irradiation because they have more DNA. A higher dose is necessary to kill bacteria since they have less DNA. Viruses, which are very small and have very little DNA, are generally resistant to irradiation at the doses approved for use in foods. Not all foods are suitable for irradiation. The quality of some foods, such as eggs and shellfish, decreases below the point of consumer acceptability. Irradiation also changes some of the taste and texture qualities of foods. The higher the dose, the more pronounced the changes, just like in conventional cooking.

FDA and USDA are responsible for determining the safety of irradiation, setting the maximum dosage levels and approving packaging materials. When approval is granted by FDA and/or USDA to irradiate a food product, a specific maximum dose for that food is set. Materials used in packaging that will undergo irradiation with the food product must also be approved. The Nuclear Regulatory Commission (NRC) has responsibility for ensuring the safety of the facilities themselves, and the Department of Transportation for the safe transport of radioactive sources. E-beam and X-ray sources are monitored by the part of FDA that regulates medical X-ray devices. State authorities may also have a role in regulation of irradiation.

THE CASE IN FAVOR OF IRRADIATION

The technology to irradiate foods to make them safer has been available for decades, but it languished in legislative limbo brought about by those opposed to it. The current flurry of activity in favor of food irradiation started after the 1994 deaths of four children who died after eating hamburger meat contaminated with *E. coli* O157:H7 from a fast food restaurant. The 1997 recall of 25 million pounds of hamburger meat from a major meat processing plant in Nebraska added fuel to the fire.

Proponents of food irradiation claim that the safety of irradiated foods has been studied by feeding them to animals and to people. These extensive studies include animal feeding studies lasting for several generations in several different species, including mice, rats, and dogs. There is no evidence of adverse health effects in these well-controlled trials. Irradiating foods does produce a very small amount of unique radiation products—about three milligrams per kilogram of food, equivalent to three drops in a swimming pool (Derr 1999). Even something that was toxic, and these substances have not been shown to be, would not be dangerous at that level. NASA astronauts eat foods that have been irradiated to the point of sterilization (substantially higher levels of treatment than those approved for general use) when they fly in space. In addition, proponents of irradiated food cite studies showing that irradiated foods do not differ substantially in nutritional value from non-irradiated food. Levels of the vitamin thiamin are slightly reduced, but not enough to result in vitamin deficiency.

Irradiation proponents emphasize that it is not a substitute for good sanitation. For irradiation to be effective, the food that is to be irradiated already needs to be clean. The more initial contamination there is, the higher dose of irradiation it would take to eliminate possible pathogens, and the greater the change in the taste and quality of the food. So, irradiating poor-quality or spoiled food will result in a product that will be of poorer quality after irradiation, making it impossible to sell. It is in the best interest of industry to irradiate clean, good-quality food. Irradiation adds an extra measure of protection to food, and is only one tool in the arsenal to fight foodborne pathogens.

Medical sterilization facilities have been operating in this country for more than 30 years, without a fatal accident. More than 100 such facilities are currently licensed, along with at least that many medical radiation treatment centers and bone marrow transplant centers. No events have been documented in this country that led to exposure of the population at large to radioactivity. Most irradiation facilities use cobalt 60, which decays by 50 percent in five years. The cobalt is a solid metal that is stored in long cobalt "pencils," which are shipped back to a nuclear reactor to be recharged.

Proponents are convinced that the American public would accept irradiation if they understood it better. They have done surveys demonstrating that if people are educated about the process first, they will be in favor of it.

> Food is placed into a shielded chamber, an energy source is provided, the food absorbs the amount of energy necessary to accomplish the desired effect, the food is removed from the chamber, and is immediately ready to be further processed or consumed. (Derr 1998)

While the above description sounds like it could be describing high-tech food irradiation, it could also describe conventional cooking in an oven. The "chamber" would be a typical kitchen oven and the "energy source" gas or electric heat. It only appears to be a "high-technology" process because of the description given.

THE CASE AGAINST IRRADIATION

Opponents of food irradiation claim it is being pushed on consumers by agri-business, food processors, and the nuclear industry. Citing a 1997 CBS poll that found 73 percent of Americans opposed food irradiation and 77 percent said they wouldn't eat irradiated food, opponents say it is just a big public relations ploy by the Department of Energy, the Nuclear Regulatory Commission, and the International Atomic Energy Agency to put a positive face on nuclear power. As with other biotechnology issues, the food industry is heavily involved in lobbying Congress to pass laws in its favor. From 1995 to 1998 food industry political action committees gave $1,736,112 to the Democratic Party and $6,154,749 to the Republican Party (Hauter 1999). The food industry also contributes heavily to individual members of Congress who they lobby to support its pro-irradiation views. Critics remain convinced that the risks involved with food irradiation far outweigh the presumed benefits.

Health concerns of those opposed to irradiation center around the unique radiation products formed during the irradiation process. They fear that these completely new chemicals have not even been identified, much less tested for toxicity. Critics claim that irradiation destroys essential minerals and the vitamins A, B, C, E, and K, with a 20 to 80 percent loss not uncommon. Furthermore, viruses and bacterial spores not killed by irradiation could mutate into "superbugs." Evidence of this possibility is a non-pathogenic bacterium, D. *radiodurans*, which can survive very high levels of irradiation. Irradiation opponents claim to know of radiation-resistant strains of *Salmonella* have been developed in the laboratory (Meeker-Lowry 1998).

Irradiation foes claim that no long-term studies have been performed to examine the health effects of eating irradiated foods, and that some of the studies that have been done show harmful effects. They allege that even FDA admits studies used to prove the method is safe were flawed. Critics cite the following studies to bolster their views:

- In one study animals fed a diet of irradiated food experienced weight loss and miscarriage, almost certainly due to irradiation-induced vitamin E deficiency.
- Raltech Scientific Services, Inc., fed irradiated chicken to several different animal species. The studies indicated the possibility of chromosome damage, immunotoxicity, greater incidence of kidney disease, cardiac thrombus, and fibroplasia.
- In another study rats fed irradiated food may have developed kidney and testicular tumors.
- A study from India found that four out of five children fed irradiated wheat developed a chromosomal abnormality that may be related to future cancer development.
- In one experiment, cooked irradiated beef had seven times more benzene, a known carcinogen, than did cooked non-irradiated beef.

Opponents point out that many of the studies proving irradiation is safe have been conducted in the test tube or on animals. Human studies have not been done, but we are about to embark on a very large human study by offering irradiated products in the marketplace.

Some of the consumer groups who previously opposed food irradiation on health grounds are focusing on the danger to workers in irradiation plants. They quote the Nuclear Regulatory Commission as reporting 54 accidents at 132 irradiation facilities since 1974. They claim that the nuclear industry wants to shift the burden of nuclear waste from weapons production to consumers. They recognize that right now cobalt 60 is used, but claim that since it is in short supply, industry will use cesium 137, which is a waste product from nuclear power plants.

Another reason some groups oppose irradiation is because they believe food processors will rely on irradiation to sterilize food processed under unsanitary conditions. They point to the real causes of unsafe food as filthy farms and slaughterhouses and imported food produced under lax sanitation standards. Current large-scale production practices of crowding animals together in unsanitary conditions throughout the growing, transportation, and slaughter periods makes it impossible to keep fecal material out of meat products. The groups feel that these problems should be cleaned up rather than covered up with irradiation.

SOURCES

Centers for Disease Control and Prevention (CDC). 1999. *Frequently Asked Questions about Food Irradiation.* Washington: Centers for Disease Control and Prevention. http://www.cdc.gov/ncidod/dbmd/diseaseinfo/foodirradiation.htm

Derr, Donald D. 1999. *You Asked . . . ?* Foundation for Food Irradiation Education. http://www.food-irradiation.com/you_asked.htm.

Derr, Donald D. 1998. *Food Irradiation—The Basics.* Foundation for Food Irradiation Education. http://www.food-irradiation.com/basics.htm.

Hauter, Wenonah. 1999. *Food Irradiation: Do You Know Where Your Dinner Has Been?* Washington: Public Citizen's Critical Mass Energy Project.

Meeker-Lowry, Susan, and Jennifer Ferrara. 1998. *Meat Monopolies: Dirty Meat and the False Promises of Irradiation.* Walden, VT: Food and Water.

PESTICIDE RESIDUES IN FOODS

This section examines the topic of pesticide residues in foods. It does not take into account environmental issues, nor the health of those involved in the application of pesticide residues to crops. It is concerned with the health effects from dietary exposure to pesticide residues. Chapter 1 contains general information on pesticides.

INTRODUCTION

Public concern about pesticide residues in foods peaked in 1989 when a national television broadcast highlighted a report linking Alar, a chemical used to control ripening in apples, to cancer in children. At the height of the Alar controversy in 1989, 82 percent of consumers in the annual *Trends: Consumer Attitudes and the Super-*

market survey rated pesticides as a serious hazard. Since then the percentage has dropped steadily to 66 percent in 1997 (see table 2-1).

Other reports linking pesticides to cancer in laboratory animals, and allegations of poor government regulation of pesticides, further inflamed public anxiety and ultimately led to reform in pesticide regulation under the 1996 Food Quality and Protection Act. Of particular note was the 1993 National Research Council (NRC) report, *Pesticides in the Diets of Infants and Children*. The U.S. Congress requested that NRC study the scientific and policy issues regarding pesticides in the diets of infants and children. The 14-member panel composed of experts in pediatrics, toxicology, statistics, food science, nutrition, child growth and development, and epidemiology criticized the federal government's ability to assess risks and protect infants and children from potentially harmful pesticide residues in their diets (NRC 1993).

One of the main criticisms was that the government ignores differences between infants and children relative to adults, especially in the areas of sensitivity and exposure to pesticides. Children are not just "small adults"; physiological differences make them more susceptible to some pesticides, while less sensitive to others. In some cases the less-developed immune system of a child makes the child more susceptible to certain chemicals. But, in other cases, a child may not absorb a chemical as rapidly as an adult, which means the child is less susceptible to the chemical (Winter 1996). The report recommended more laboratory toxicology studies to look at the effects of chemicals in immature animals. Also, children tend to eat fewer foods than adults. Thus if a major food item in a child's diet contains relatively high levels of a pesticide residue, the child could have greater exposure to that pesticide than would an adult, who eats a smaller part of that food in his or her total diet. The report recommended better identification of what foods different ages of infants and children eat (NRC 1993).

Pesticide residues in the American diet come from four sources: pesticides applied on the farm; pesticides applied post-harvest, pesticides applied on imported foods, and discontinued pesticides that persist in the environment. Of the fresh fruit and vegetable consumption in the United States, approximately 80 percent by weight is grown in the United States. While some residues may be higher on imported produce, our main sources of pesticide residues are still from domestic produce, since we

Table 2-1
Consumers Rating Residues from Pesticides and Herbicides as a Serious Hazard (%)

Year	Percentage	Year	Percentage
1984	77	1991	80
1985	73	1992	76
1986	75	1993	79
1987	76	1994	72
1988	75	1995	74
1989	82	1996	66
1990	80	1997	66

Source: Food Marketing Institute, *Trends: Consumer Attitudes and the Supermarket*, yearly reports 1984–1997.

consume a greater amount of it. Even though legal use of DDT ended in 1972, degradation products of DDT are still detected in apples and green beans, possibly from DDT applied as long ago as 50 years.

A survey of pesticide residues on fruits and vegetables by Kuchler et al. pointed to pesticides applied post-harvest as contributing more to pesticide residue intake than from other sources. The primary classes of post-harvest pesticides are fungicides and plant growth regulators applied to reduce shipping losses and to enhance shelf life. As these pesticides are applied after the produce is picked, they are not exposed to the rain, wind, sunlight, and other environmental factors that tend to break down pesticides. Additionally, they are applied directly to edible products, often in wax to ensure that they remain on the produce. On the basis of this data, Kuchler et al. argue that most pesticides applied on-farm do not lead to detectable pesticide residues, and that targeting programs to reduce on-farm pesticides will not have an effect on the other sources of pesticide residues, especially post-harvest pesticides. For potatoes (the most consumed vegetable in the United States), residues from chemicals that persist in the environment accounted for 12 percent of detected residues, on-farm use of pesticides accounted for 15 percent, and post-harvest chemicals 73 percent. Since almost all potatoes consumed in the United States are domestically grown, residues on imported sources were negligible (Kuchler et al. 1996).

Pesticide residues in food and water are expressed as parts per million (ppm), parts per billion (ppb), or parts per trillion (ppt). The following comparisons may help put these quantities into perspective.

1 ppm = 1 gram (g) of residue in 1,000,000 g of food; 1 inch in 16 miles; 1 minute in 2 years; 1 cent in $10,000; or 1 pancake in a stack 4 miles high.

1 ppb = 1 g of residue in 1,000,000,000 g of food; 1 inch in 16,000 miles; 1 second in 32 years; or 1 cent in $10 million.

1 ppt = 1 g of residue in 1,000,000,000,000 g of food; 1 inch in 16 million miles; 1 second in 32,000 years; 1 square foot of floor tile on a floor the size of the state of Indiana.

Source: Reprinted from the International Food Information Council Foundation, 1995.

For pesticides, and other potentially dangerous substances, "The dose makes the poison." In other words, the amount of a substance a person is exposed to is as important as how toxic the chemical might be. For example, small doses of aspirin can be beneficial to people, but at very high doses, this common medicine can be deadly. In some individuals, even at very low doses, aspirin may have adverse health effects. The following formula is important when determining risk from a substance:

$$\text{RISK} = \text{TOXICITY} \times \text{EXPOSURE}$$

This means that the risk to human health from pesticide exposure depends on both the toxicity of the pesticide and the likelihood of people coming into contact with it. At least *some* exposure and *some* toxicity are required to result in a risk. For example, if the pesticide is very poisonous, but no people are exposed to it, there is no risk. Likewise, if there is ample exposure but the chemical is nontoxic, there is no risk. However, usually when pesticides are used, some toxicity and some exposure exist, which results in a potential risk (EPA January 1999).

PESTICIDE REGULATION

Three federal agencies share responsibility for ensuring that pesticide residues in foods are not present at levels that will pose a danger to health.

Environmental Protection Agency (EPA)

Before a pesticide can be used, it must be granted a registration by EPA, which regulates its distribution, sale, and use. EPA examines the ingredients of the pesticide; the particular site or crop on which it is to be used; the amount, frequency, and timing of its use; and storage and disposal practices. Manufacturers must test their products for short-term (acute) and long-term (chronic) health consequences, including carcinogenicity, chronic toxicity, reproductive and developmental toxicity; environmental consequences; effects on wildlife; and possible contamination of surface water or groundwater. The degree to which a pesticide is harmful depends on how toxic it is, the amount likely to be ingested from residues remaining on food and in drinking water, and the level of exposure through other uses (such as occupational and residential exposure). Before registering a pesticide, EPA conducts a risk assessment of the proposed uses by evaluating the available toxicity studies along with pesticide residue data, food consumption data, and related information (EPA January 2000). EPA also approves the language that appears on each pesticide label. A pesticide product can only be used according to the directions on its accompanying label. Through the label, EPA restricts when pesticides may be applied during the growing season, how much may be applied, and on which crops.

If a product is for use on food crops, EPA establishes a tolerance, called the maximum residue level, which is the maximum level of a residue permitted in a food, feed, or food ingredient. Tolerances are specific for each pesticide and for each food. To set tolerances, EPA needs to know the maximum levels of pesticides likely to be found in foods. This is determined through studies of residues found on crops grown when pesticides are applied at the highest rate allowed. The tolerances apply to imported foods, as well as to those grown in the United States. The maximum residue levels are based on the assumptions that:

1. Residue level at the time of consumption is at the maximum allowable level.
2. All of the crop in question has been treated with the pesticide.
3. Crops are treated with the maximum allowable amount of a pesticide.

These worst case assumptions lead to an overestimate of dietary intake of pesticide residues because:

1. Levels at the time of consumption may be only 20 to 40 percent of the permitted levels established at harvest, largely due to the effects of processing, washing, and cooking.
2. Not all crops are treated.
3. Often much less pesticide is used than what is allowed. Many farmers have reduced pesticide application by using integrated pest management programs.

EPA also determines the amount of a chemical that, if ingested on a daily basis over a lifetime, is not expected to cause any adverse health effects in any part of the population, from infants to adults. This is the Reference Dose (RfD). It is calculated by first finding the highest dose of a chemical to which test animals can be exposed without developing any observable adverse biological effects. This is called the no observable effect level (NOEL). To obtain the RfD, the NOEL is then divided by a factor of between 10 and 1,000 to provide an extra margin of safety to account for the uncertainty of applying animal studies to humans, and for individual human differences in sensitivity. For cancer risks, EPA evaluates multiyear studies of animals to determine levels unlikely to pose more than a negligible risk of cancer, which has been defined as one cancer for every million persons over a 70-year lifetime. EPA may also require studies designed specifically to assess risks to infants and children. These include developmental toxicity studies, which examine risks to developing fetuses that result from exposure of the mother to pesticides during pregnancy; developmental neurotoxicity studies, which specifically examine the risks to the developing nervous system; and two-generation reproduction studies, which provide information about the possible effects on the health of both the individual and its offspring (EPA November 1999).

Food and Drug Administration (FDA)

FDA is responsible for enforcing EPA tolerances on all foods except meat, poultry, and certain egg products, which USDA monitors. FDA collects and analyzes domestically produced and imported foods for pesticide residues to see if pesticide residues in any samples exceed EPA tolerances. If FDA detects residues that exceed EPA tolerances, it can take regulatory action, such as seizing the product or stopping shipments of foreign produce at ports of entry. In addition to monitoring foods for human consumption, FDA also samples and analyzes domestic and imported animal feed for pesticide residues.

As part of its regulatory pesticide residue monitoring program FDA tests between 8,000 and 10,000 domestic and imported food items for pesticide residues every year. Samples are collected as close as possible to the point of production to maximize residue levels. Fresh produce is tested unwashed and unpeeled, even bananas. Because food processors, and most consumers, wash or peel produce before eating or using it in food products, many of the violative samples reported in the FDA studies show higher residues than would be expected in real life. The goal of the FDA monitoring activities is to detect residues in excess of the tolerance, not to estimate the amount of residues on foods. Results from the 1998 monitoring efforts in table 2-2 show that pesticides seldom appear in food at levels above EPA tolerances.

Table 2-2
FDA 1998 Pesticide Residue Monitoring Program (1998)

Source	Samples Tested	No Violative* Residues Detected	No Residues Detected
Domestic	3,625	99.2%	64.9%
Imported	4,969	97%	68.1%

*A violative residue is defined as a residue that exceeds a tolerance, or a residue at a level of regulatory significance for which no tolerance has been established in the sampled food.
Source: Food and Drug Administration Pesticide Program, Residue Monitoring 1998

Toxicity and amount consumed, i.e., exposure, determine how harmful a pesticide is. One way to determine exposure to pesticide residues is to look at what foods Americans eat and how much pesticide residue they would consume in that diet. To do this FDA conducts the Total Diet Study, sometimes called the Market Basket Study. FDA staffers shop in supermarket or grocery stores four times a year, once in each of four geographical regions of the country. Shopping in three cities from each region, they buy the same approximately 260 foods selected from nationwide dietary survey data to typify the American diet. Staffers then prepare the foods as a consumer would prepare them. For example, staffers make beef and vegetable stew from the collected ingredients using a standardized recipe. FDA analyzes the prepared foods for pesticide residues and uses the results to estimate the dietary intakes of pesticide residues for Americans, ranging from infants to senior citizens. As the study is designed to measure the total dietary intake of pesticide residues, it does not show which foods have which residues. This estimated dietary intake of pesticide residues can then be compared to the EPA Reference Dose.

U.S. Department of Agriculture (USDA)

The USDA Food Safety and Inspection Service (FSIS) enforces EPA pesticide tolerances for meat, poultry, and processed eggs through its National Residue Program (NRP). Any meat tissues or egg products that contain pesticide residues in excess of EPA tolerances are considered adulterated and violative. FSIS tests for residues in both domestic and imported products.

Since 1991 the USDA Agricultural Marketing Service (AMS) has conducted a non-regulatory operation, the Pesticide Data Program (PDP), to collect data on pesticide residues in food. In order to obtain the most realistic estimates possible, samples are collected as close to the point of consumption as possible. This takes into account consumer practices such as peeling produce before consuming and pesticide degradation during storing, cooking, and processing. PDP tests about 40 different commodities in the raw and processed state for more than 160 pesticides from both domestic and imported products. As part of a federal-state partnership, ten participating states collect the samples and analyze them in a combination of state and federal laboratories. The focus of the PDP is on detecting residues, no matter how small, rather than detecting only those that exceed the tolerances.

From the results below it can be seen that while many samples have detectable residues, very few are above the EPA tolerances.

1998 PDP Results from Produce, Milk, and Soybean Samples

Total samples collected: 8,500 (84 percent domestic, 15 percent imported, 1 percent unknown)

Detectable pesticide residues from produce (domestic and imported): 61 percent

Detectable pesticide residues from milk: 15 percent

Detectable pesticide residues from soybeans: 51 percent

Residue detection from all samples exceeding EPA tolerances: 0.15 percent

Pesticide residues were significantly lower in processed products than in fresh products. This could be because products grown for processing receive different pesticide applications than do products grown for fresh sale, and because processing procedures involving heat and time degrade pesticides. For example, diphenylamine was detected in 7.1 percent of processed apple juice, and in 86 percent of raw apples. Some imported produce had higher levels of certain residues, while domestic produce had higher levels of other residues (USDA 1998).

FOOD QUALITY PROTECTION ACT (FQPA)

In 1996, Congress strengthened pesticide laws by enacting the Food Quality Protection Act. The FQPA amended the laws under which EPA regulates pesticides. It required that EPA consider:

A New Safety Standard: FQPA strengthened the safety standard that pesticides must meet before being approved for use. EPA must ensure with a reasonable certainty that no harm will result from the legal uses of the pesticide.

Exposure from All Sources: In evaluating a pesticide, EPA must estimate the combined risk from that pesticide from all non-occupational sources, such as food, drinking water, and residential use.

Cumulative Risk: EPA is required to evaluate pesticides in light of similar toxic effects that different pesticides may share. EPA is currently developing a methodology for this type of assessment.

Special Sensitivity of Children to Pesticides: EPA must ascertain whether there is an increased susceptibility to infants and children from pesticide exposure.

In addition, EPA is reassessing all pesticide tolerances that were in effect as of August 3, 1996, when the FQPA was signed. This effort is designed to ensure that existing tolerances and exemptions meet the new safety standard. Reassessment of tolerances and exemptions is to be completed by 2006, with the first third to be completed by August 1999. This reassessment is a large task: approximately 9,700 tolerances were in effect at the passage of FQPA. EPA is giving highest priority to pesticides that appear to pose the greatest risk.

ARE PESTICIDE RESIDUES DANGEROUS?

Many health professionals believe the danger from pesticide residues to be minimal, and much less of a concern than other food safety problems such as microbial contamination of foods, environmental contaminants, and naturally occurring toxins (Winter 1996). They point out that a diet rich in fruits and vegetables is associated with a reduced risk of chronic disease, including many cancers. The benefits from eating fruits and vegetables significantly outweigh the theoretical risks posed by pesticide residues.

Human data on the cancer-causing properties of pesticides come from studies showing that farmers and others who use and apply pesticides have an increased rate of certain cancers. Studies have not shown a cause and effect relationship between *dietary exposure* to pesticides and cancer. However, showing such a relationship would be very difficult because exposure occurs over decades and how cancer develops is not well understood. Pesticide-related deaths have been caused by accidents or misuse where workers are exposed due to improper or inadequate care in handling and use, such as not wearing protective clothing or masks. A large proportion of deaths attributed to pesticides are accidental poisonings of children.

EPA tolerances are established for raw foods. However, most pesticides break down with exposure to sunlight, rain, and other elements, so that they are usually below tolerance levels even before leaving the farm. Processing methods such as washing, canning, freezing, pasteurizing, and cooking further decrease the amount of pesticide residues in foods as eaten. Surveys of actual dietary exposure in the United States have demonstrated that typical intake averaged less than 1 percent of the Reference Dose, in itself a very conservative measure of safety (Ritter 1997). The majority of illegal residues are considered illegal because they are not registered for the product on which they are found, although they are registered on other commodities. Exposure to these illegal residues does not necessarily represent any toxicologic danger.

The general public, most of whom are poorly qualified to determine risks, is easily swayed by media hype and the story of the day. Risk perception is often based on emotions, rather than science. Pesticides are a sensitive issue because we perceive the risks as out of our control. The risk is involuntary versus voluntary. People think nothing of driving a car out onto a busy highway and the risk it involves, yet are concerned about the risk of pesticide residues in their food. A study conducted in the late 1980s highlights the wide gulf between perceived risks and established risks. Three groups, college students, League of Women Voters, and business people, were asked to rate various risks on a scale from 1 to 30, with 1 being the highest and 30 the lowest. College students ranked pesticides at a risk level of 4, women voters ranked them at 9, and business people at 15. But placement of the risk from pesticides based on factual mortality data resulted in a risk level of 28, lower than motor vehicles, swimming, bicycles, home appliances, power lawn mowers, and skiing. It is estimated that approximately 30 people die each year from pesticides, mostly children from accidental poisonings. In comparison, about 50,000 people die annually in motor vehicle accidents, 3,000 die while swimming, and 1,000 die in bicycle accidents. Yet people perceive that they have a choice and at least some control over the outcome in these other risks, whereas they have no control over the presence, amount, or type of pesticides in their food.

Those involved in the crusade against pesticides argue that the risks from pesticide residues on foods are more than merely theoretical. EPA's Non-Occupational Pesticide Exposure Study (NOPES) examined 32 pesticides and pesticide residues and found that the route of most exposure for the general population was via dietary exposure. A small amount of this was due to pesticide residues in drinking water, and an even smaller amount from inhalation or other pathways, but most was from dietary exposure via foods. Many of the older pesticides still in use were approved before more stringent controls and better laboratory methods were put in place. In its report, *Overexposed: Organophosphate Insectides in Children's Food*, the Environmental Working Group (EWG) claims that every day, one million American children age five and under consume unsafe levels of organophosphate pesticides that can harm the developing brain and nervous system (Wiles 1998). In addition, EWG criticizes FDA for shortcomings in its pesticide monitoring program, proposing that U.S.-grown produce is more than twice as contaminated with illegal pesticides than the FDA reports (Elderkin 1995).

The big unknown factor with chemicals, including pesticides, is that not a lot is known about their long-term effects on the human body. Scientists can only conduct long-term studies in animal models; little research exists on long-term effects of pesticides accumulated in humans. The medical community does not fully understand how and why cancer develops, but carcinogens appear to be cumulative, and pesticides probably impair the immune system over a lifetime.

Some scientists argue that EPA's pesticide residue tolerances do not represent safe levels. Tolerances are established as enforcement tools for monitoring to ensure that pesticides are used according to regulations. The enforced tolerances are not based on human health risk, and so these maximum residue levels have very little to do with safety. Because of this, it is difficult to determine whether illegal residues are unsafe, or, conversely, whether residue levels below the tolerances are safe (Winter 1992; Groth 1999). After analyzing USDA data, Consumers Union scientists determined that safety margins established by EPA are not adequate to protect children from the harmful effects of pesticides (Groth 1999).

Critics of the EPA's efforts to regulate pesticides point to the system for approving pesticide registrations as rife with fraud and manipulated by pesticide manufacturers. The tests that EPA relies on to determine tolerances and reference doses are designed and conducted by manufacturers or by laboratories that they have hired. Twice, in the mid-1970s and again in the early 1990s, major testing labs were found to have faked vital safety tests on pesticides. Congress does not fund EPA with sufficient resources to carry out its own research, which forces EPA to rely on data from manufacturers. With 70,000 chemicals in commerce and hundreds under active review at any given time, it isn't realistic to expect that the EPA can take over the job of testing all of them for safety.

Many consumer and health advocates claim that chemical companies subtly slant scientific research as part of their campaigns to keep dangerous products on the market. Looking at the source of a study's funding can be an accurate means of predicting its results. Critics claim that when chemical companies finance studies, the results tend to show that the chemicals are not dangerous to human health or the environment. But when independent scientists from governments, universities, and medical and charitable organizations conduct studies, they tend to show the chemicals in an unfavorable light. When manufacturers don't like the results of their own studies, they have sometimes withheld them from EPA. In 1991 and 1992 EPA offered amnesty to manufacturers who turned in unpublished studies that should have been submitted earlier. Chemical companies suddenly produced more than 10,000 studies showing that products from all classes of chemicals (not just pesticides) already on the market could pose "substantial risk of injury to health or to the environment." These are the kinds of never-published data that the law says must be presented to the government immediately (Fagin 1999).

Finally, critics point to the revolving door phenomenon. An analysis by EWG on the employment of former top EPA pesticide regulators after they left the agency revealed that two-thirds of the highest ranking officials since the pesticide program was established had received at least part of their paycheck from pesticide interests. This includes four out of six former assistant administrators for Pesticides and Toxic Substances, and two out of four former directors of the Office of Pesticide Programs. An additional dozen former EPA staffers who occupied positions important to the evaluation of pesticide moved to private-sector careers representing pesticide interests (Headen 1999). Fagin and Lavelle estimate that nearly half of EPA officials who leave top-level jobs in toxic substances and pesticides go to work for chemical companies, chemical trade associations, or as lobbyists for the chemical industry (Fagin 1999).

SOURCES

Bohmont, Bert L. 1997. *The Standard Pesticide User's Guide*. 4th ed. Upper Saddle River, NJ: Prentice-Hall, Inc.

Elderkin, Susan, Richard Wiles, and Christopher Campbell. 1995. *Forbidden Fruit: Illegal Pesticides in the U.S. Food Supply.* Washington: Environmental Working Group. http://www.ewg.org/pub/home/reports/Fruit/forbid_short.html.

Environmental Protection Agency (EPA). Updated April 12, 2000. *The Food Quality Protection Act (FQPA) Background.* Washington: Environmental Protection Agency. http://www.epa.gov/oppfead1/fqpa/backgrnd.htm.

Environmental Protection Agency (EPA). Updated January 20, 2000. *Pesticide Registration.* Washington: Environmental Protection Agency. http://www.epa.gov/pesticides/citizens/registration.htm.

Environmental Protection Agency (EPA). November 17, 1999. *Protecting the Public from Pesticide Residues in Food.* Washington: Environmental Protection Agency. http://www.epa.gov/opp00001/citizens/protect.htm.

Environmental Protection Agency (EPA). January 1999. *Assessing Health Risks from Pesticides.* Washington: Environmental Protection Agency. http://www.epa.gov/pesticides/citizens/riskassess.htm.

Fagin, Dan, and Marianne Lavelleby.1999. *Toxic Deception: How the Chemical Industry Manipulates Science, Bends the Law, and Endangers Your Health.* Monroe, ME: Common Courage Press.

Food Marketing Institute (FMI). February 1999. *Backgrounder: Pesticides in the Food Supply.* Washington: Food Marketing Institute. http://www.fmi.org/media/bg/pests.html.

Groth, Edward, III, Charles M. Benbrook, and Karen Lutz. 1999. *Do You Know What You Are Eating?* New York: Consumers Union. http:// www.ecologic-ipm.com/Do_You_Know.pdf.

Headen, Emily. 1999. *From Bureaucrats to Fat Cats: EPA Pesticide Program Is a "Farm Team" for the Pesticide Lobby.* Washington: Environmental Working Group. http://www.ewg.org/pub/home/reports/fatcats/fatcats.html.

International Food Information Council (IFIC). January 1995. *IFIC Review: On Pesticides and Food Safety.* Washington: International Food Information Council. http://ificinfo.health.org/review/ir-pest.htm.

National Research Council (NRC) Committee on Pesticides in the Diets of Infants and Children. 1993. *Pesticides in the Diets of Infants and Children.* Washington: National Academy Press.

Ritter, Len. 1997. Ad Hoc Panel on Pesticides and Cancer, Canadian Network of Toxicology Centres, Guelph, Ontario, Canada. *Cancer* 80: 1887–1888. http://www.pmac.net/canadian.htm.

United States Department of Agriculture (USDA), Agricultural Marketing Service. 1998. *Pesticide Data Program Annual Summary 1998.* Washington: United States Department of Agriculture. http://www.ams.usda.gov/science/pdp/.

U.S. Food and Drug Administration. March 1999. *Residue Monitoring 1998.* Washington: U.S. Food and Drug Administration. http:// vm.cfsan.fda.gov/~dms/pes98rep.html.

Wiles, Richard, Kert Davies, and Christopher Campbell. 1998. *Overexposed: Organophosphate Insectides in Children's Food.* Washington: Environmental Working Group. http://www.ewg.org/pub/home/reports/ops/oppress.html.

Winter, Carl K. 1996. Pesticide Residues in Foods: Recent Events and Emerging Issues. *Weed Technology.* 10: 969–973.

Winter, Carl K. 1992. Pesticide Tolerances Are Their Relevance as Safety Standards. *Regulatory Toxicology and Pharmacology.* 15: 137–150.

Drinking Water Quality

This section explores one of earth's most plentiful, most valuable resources—water, and our attempts to make it safe to drink. Following examples of the antiquity of water treatment practices, the reader is introduced to the U.S. public water supply. Hazards to the water supply and regulations to counter those hazards are examined. Statistics relating to waterborne disease outbreaks are in chapter 5.

HISTORY

Ancient civilizations, as well as more modern ones, established themselves around water—the liquid of life. Water makes up two-thirds of our bodies and is a necessity of life, all life. It appears that an understanding that some water sources caused disease, while other water sources did not, evolved long before an understanding of potential hazards in food. Sanskrit medical lore from around 2000 B.C.E. mentions boiling foul water, exposing it to sunlight, and filtering it through charcoal. Walls from Egyptian tombs from the fifteenth and thirteenth centuries B.C.E. depict an apparatus for clarifying liquids, either wine or water, by siphoning off settled liquid. Cyrus the Great, King of Persia in the sixth century B.C.E., took vessels of boiled water with his troops when they traveled to do battle. Residents of Alexandria, Egypt, around 50 B.C.E. drank Nile River water brought to the city through a series of underground aqueducts to cisterns where it was clarified by sedimentation, while other parts of the city used single, double, and even triple filtration to purify water. Sextus Julius Frontinus, water commissioner of Rome in the year 97, wrote the first detailed description of a public water system in his *Two Books on the Water Supply of Rome*. Granted, these early water engineers had no understanding of bacteria and were probably treating water to decrease its cloudiness and improve its looks and taste; nevertheless, they developed the earliest water treatment systems (Baker 1948).

Dr. John Snow linked drinking water to disease through his epidemiologic detective work during the great cholera outbreak of 1854 in London. At the time, 13 pumps provided free water to residents of the city. After a number of deaths from cholera in the city, Dr. Snow obtained a list of where those who died of cholera lived and plotted them on a map of the city. He noticed that most of the deaths occurred in people living and drawing their water from the Broad Street pump. Presenting this evidence to city officials, he persuaded them to remove the pump handle from the Broad Street pump, thereby halting the epidemic, but not before it claimed more than 600 lives. All of this happened almost 30 years before Robert Koch in 1883 finally identified *Vibrio cholerae* as the causative agent of cholera (Frerichs 1999).

Philadelphia in 1799 was the first U.S. city with a public water system that pumped water from a surface source and distributed it through a series of pipes to residents. By 1900 there were more than 3,000 public water systems in the United States. Although this greatly increased the readily available supply of water to residents, it did not necessarily guarantee a safe water supply. Some of those systems actually contributed to major disease outbreaks in the early 1900s. If the water supplies were contaminated, the pumped and widely distributed water provided a means for spreading bacterial disease throughout communities (EPA 1999). Federal regulation of the nation's drinking water began in 1914 when the U.S. Public Health Service (PHS) imposed bacteriological standards for drinking water. These standards were revised in 1925, 1946, and 1962, and eventually adopted by all 50 states. After World War II, industrialization and use of fertilizers on crops began to have a negative impact on the environment and public health. It became increasingly clear in the late 1960s and early 1970s that water quality problems were broader than those outlined by the Public Health Service. A 1969 survey showed that only 60 percent of water systems delivered water that met PHS standards. A study in 1972 detected 36 chemicals present in already treated water taken from the Mississippi River. This increased awareness of the problems with the water supply led to the passage of federal environmental and health laws dealing with polluted water, hazardous waste, and pesticides. The 1974 Safe Drinking Water Act, discussed below, was also a part of this increased awareness of the vulnerability of the nation's water supply.

THE U.S. WATER SUPPLY

Water use in the United States averages about 100 gallons of drinking water per person per day, more than just about any other country. A very small proportion of this water per person, approximately two gallons, is actually used for drinking and cooking. We use the majority of the water that comes into our homes for bathing, flushing toilets, doing laundry, watering lawns, filling swimming pools, and washing cars. Drinking water comes from either surface water or groundwater. Surface water includes rivers, lakes, and reservoirs, while groundwater is pumped up from wells drilled into aquifers. Aquifers are underground geologic formations that contain water. Groundwater is the source for a little over half the nation's drinking water supply.

The more than 170,000 water systems in the United States are either private or public. Private water systems do not draw water from a public water supply, and serve only one or a few homes. Public water systems include community water systems, and those at schools, factories, campgrounds, and restaurants if they have their own water supply. Community water systems deliver water to people year-round in their homes. In most community water systems, a network of underground pipes transports water under pressure to smaller pipes, called house service lines, which then enter individual homes.

Depending on the conditions and types of contaminants likely to be found in a particular water source, water suppliers use a variety of treatment methods. Most water systems use a combination of two or more treatment processes. Major water treatment processes are:

- *Flocculation/sedimentation*—Flocculation is the process of getting small particles to combine into heavier particles called floc. The heavier particles can then be removed by letting them settle out as sediment. Once settled, the particles combine to form a sludge that is later removed.
- *Filtration*—Filtration removes particles from water by passing the water through a permeable fabric or porous bed of materials. Groundwater is naturally filtered as it flows through porous layers of soil. Some filtration processes can remove very small particles, including microorganisms.
- *Ion exchange*—Ion exchange processes are used to remove inorganic constituents such as arsenic, chromium, excess fluoride, nitrates, radium, and uranium if they cannot be removed adequately by filtration or sedimentation. Electric current is used to attract negative and/or positive ions to one side of a treatment chamber for removal.
- *Adsorption*—Adsorption involves having organic contaminants that cause undesirable color, taste, or odor stick to the surface of granular or powdered activated carbon.

- *Disinfection*—Disinfection refers to killing harmful microorganisms. The three most commonly used methods of disinfection are chlorination, ozonation, and ultraviolet treatment. Chlorination is most often used in the United States, while ozonation is very common in Europe.
- *Chlorination*—Chlorine kills bacteria by forming hypochlorus acid, which attacks the respiratory, transport, and nucleic acid activity of bacteria. Most bacteria are very susceptible to chlorine, while viruses are less so. Cysts from *Giardia lamblia* are very resistant to chlorine, and *Cryptosporidium* cannot be readily killed by chlorination. Of concern with this method of disinfection is the disinfection by-products (DBPs), particularly trihalomethanes (THMs), formed when chlorine reacts with organic matter that is in the water. Long-term exposure to some DBPs may increase the risk of cancer or have other adverse health effects. THMs are cancer group B carcinogens, i.e., shown to cause cancer in laboratory animals. EPA regulations limit the amount of these by-products allowed in drinking water.
- *Ozonation*—Ozone is created by passing air through an electric current. The ozone gas is then dissolved in water, where it acts as an oxidant to destroy microorganisms. The ozone must then be removed before the water is used. As there is no residual antimicrobial effect, it is still necessary to chlorinate the water after ozone treatment. Ozone has received increased attention because it appears to be the only disinfectant that is very effective against *Cryptosporidium.*
- *Ultraviolet light*—Ultraviolet (UV) light does not actually kill bacteria. Instead it effectively sterilizes them, making it impossible for them to reproduce. Ultraviolet systems are only practical for small systems due to the need for the microorganisms to be close to the radiation source. UV does not inactivate *Giardia* or *Cryptosporidium* cysts.

With so many different bacteria that can cause illness, it is not possible to test the water supply for each of these separately. Instead, indicator organisms are used. Coliform bacteria are the most popular indicator organisms for drinking water as they are easily detected in water. Coliforms are a group of bacteria common in the environment and in the digestive tracts of humans and animals. While these organisms are themselves harmless, their presence indicates possible contamination with human and/or animal waste. The effectiveness of disinfection is judged by analyzing water supplies for total coliform bacteria. Presence of coliform bacteria is not acceptable in public water supplies and is a sign that disinfection is required.

HAZARDS TO THE WATER SUPPLY

Because water is the universal solvent, many chemicals and other materials easily dissolve in it. Water supplies become contaminated through many different channels—chemicals can migrate from disposal sites; animal wastes and pesticides may be carried to lakes and streams by rainfall runoff; human wastes may be discharged to receiving water that ultimately flows to water used for drinking. Other sources of contamination include discharge from industry, erosion of natural deposits, corrosion of household plumbing systems, and leaching from septic tanks. Nitrates, inorganic compounds that can enter water supplies from fertilizer runoff and sanitary wastewater discharges, are especially harmful to young children. Excessive levels can result in a condition known as “blue baby syndrome,” which limits the ability of blood to carry oxygen from the lungs to the rest of the body. If untreated, the condition can be fatal. Naturally occurring contaminants also are found in drinking water. For example, the radioactive gas radon-222 occurs in certain types of rock and can seep into groundwater. People can be exposed to radon in water by drinking it while showering or when washing dishes. As is the case with food, it would be impossible to remove all contaminants from our water supply. At very low levels, many contaminants are generally not harmful.

Most outbreaks of waterborne disease are due to contamination by bacteria and viruses, probably from human or animal waste. Two pathogens commonly associated with drinking water are *Cryptosporidium parvum* and *Giardia lamblia*. Both are protozoa that cause gastrointestinal illness and whose cysts are difficult to destroy. *Cryptosporidium* in particular may pass through water treatment filtration and disinfection processes in sufficient numbers to cause health problems. A 1993 outbreak of cryptosporidiosis in Milwaukee, Wisconsin, is the largest outbreak of waterborne disease to date in the United States. Milwaukee's water supply, which comes from Lake Michigan, is treated by filtration and disinfection. Due to an unusual combination of circumstances during a period of heavy rainfall and runoff, the treatment plant was ineffective, resulting in an increase in the turbidity of the treated water. This increased turbidity also contributed to the ineffectiveness of the filtration and disinfection methods. More than 400,000 persons were affected by the disease, more than 4,000 were hospitalized, and more than 50 deaths (some counts are as high as 100) have been attributed to the disease. The original source of contamination is uncertain.

Runoff from farms is another source of hazards to the nation's drinking water. In 1994 the Environmental Working Group released *Tap Water Blues*, a report in which they identified more than 10 million individuals exposed to five herbicides at levels above the Environmental Protection Agency's (EPA) negligible cancer risk standard of one additional case per million individuals. A second report in 1995, *Weed Killers by the Glass*, analyzed herbicides in the tap water of 29 midwestern cities. Again, their results show Americans are exposed to harmful pesticides in their drinking water at levels high above federal health standards.

REGULATION

Local governments, public water systems, the states, and the EPA work together towards the goal of ensuring that all public water supplies are safe. Local governments have a direct interest in protecting the quality of their drinking water source, be it groundwater or surface water. Part of their job in protecting the water supply is to oversee land uses that can affect the quality of untreated source water. State public health and environmental agencies have the primary responsibility for ensuring that federal drinking water quality standards, or more stringent ones required by the state, are met by each public water supplier. Municipal water systems test their own water systems for residues, but do not regulate or test private wells. For households on private wells, state and local health departments usually have some standards for the drinking water, but it is generally up to the homeowner to maintain the quality of the drinking water.

The EPA Office of Water sets standards for pesticides and other chemicals in drinking water. EPA issues Maximum Contaminant Levels (MCLs), which limit the amount of each substance that can be present in drinking water, for more than 80 contaminants. Scientists use a process called risk assessment to set drinking water quality standards. When assessing the cancer and non-cancer risks from exposure to a chemical in drinking water, the first step is to measure how much of the chemical could be in the water. Next, scientists estimate how much of the chemical the average person is likely to drink. This amount is called the exposure. In developing drinking water standards, EPA assumes that the average adult drinks two liters of water each day throughout a 70-year life span. MCLs are set at levels that will limit an individual's risk of cancer from that contaminant to between 1 in 10,000 and 1 in 1,000,000 over a lifetime. For non-cancer effects, risk assessment provides an estimate of an exposure level below which no adverse effects are expected to occur. EPA also takes into account the ability of various technologies to remove the contaminant, their effectiveness, and cost of treatment.

To comply with MCLs, public water systems may use any state-approved treatment. When it is not economically or technologically feasible to set an MCL for a contaminant—for example, when the contaminant cannot be easily measured—EPA may require use of a particular treatment technique instead. EPA requires that the nation's approximately 55,000 community water systems test for more than 80 contaminants. According to 1996 statistics, 7 percent or 4,151 systems, reported one or more MCL violations, and less than 2 percent (681 systems) reported violations of treatment technique standards.

If a system does not have water quality problems, it can apply to the state for permission to test less frequently for certain contaminants. If, after scientific analysis, state regulators believe it is unlikely that human or natural activities will affect the system's water quality in the future, they may grant the request to avoid unnecessary testing. Testing continues, but at a reduced frequency. At the first indication of any problem—or likelihood of a problem—the system must notify the state and the state may instruct the system to return to a more rigorous monitoring schedule. Table 2-3 shows the major groups of contaminants and minimum frequency that water systems must test for them.

Table 2-3
Sample Monitoring Schedule

Contaminant	Minimum Monitoring Frequency
Acute Contaminants	
Bacteria	Monthly or quarterly, depending on system size and type
Protozoa and Viruses	Continuous monitoring for turbidity, monthly for total coliforms, as indicators
Nitrate	Annually
Chronic Contaminants	
Volatile Organics (e.g., benzene)	Ground water systems, annually for 2 consecutive years; surface water systems, annually
Synthetic Organics (e.g. pesticides)	Larger systems, twice in 3 years; smaller systems, once in 3 years
Inorganics/Metals	Ground water systems, once every 3 years; surface water systems, annually
Lead and Copper	Annually
Radionuclides	Once every 4 years

Note: General requirements may differ slightly based on the size or type of drinking water system.

Source: Environmental Protection Agency (EPA). July 1997. *Water on Tap: A Consumer's Guide to the Nation's Drinking Water.* Washington: Environmental Protection Agency. http://www.epa.gov/OGWDW/wot/ontap.html.

Safe Drinking Water Act

The 1974 Safe Drinking Water Act (SDWA) authorized EPA to establish national, enforceable health standards for contaminants in drinking water. Prior to 1974 each state ran its own drinking water program and set local standards. As a result, drinking water protection standards differed from state to state. In 1986 the act was strengthened through the Surface Water Treatment Rule, which requires public water systems to filter and disinfect all surface water supplies. The act was amended again in 1996 to extend protection of drinking water from source to tap. Provisions in the 1996 amendment include:

- The requirement that consumers receive more information about the quality of their drinking water supplies. Water suppliers must notify customers within 24 hours of violations of EPA standards "that have the potential to have serious adverse effects on human health as a result of short-term exposure." If such a violation occurs, the system must announce it through the media and provide information about potential adverse effects on human health, steps taken to correct the violation, and the need to use alternative water supplies (such as boiled or bottled water) until the problem is corrected. When microorganisms such as those that indicate fecal contamination are found in drinking water, water suppliers may be required to issue "boil water notices." Boiling water kills the organisms that can cause disease. At least 725 communities, including New York City and the District of Columbia, have issued boil water notices affecting more than 10 million people.
- The SDWA amendments also require public water systems to prepare Consumer Confidence Reports. These are to inform consumers about the source of their water supply, contaminant levels detected in their water, and the health effects of contaminants detected above the established safety limit. Beginning in 1999, systems are to prepare and distribute the reports annually.
- Under the new amendments, each state must develop a program to identify potential contamination threats and determine the susceptibility of drinking water sources to activities that may harm the source water.
- The new law also requires that water systems be operated by qualified professionals. Each state must carry out an "operator certification program," including training and certification for individuals responsible for operating the drinking water plant. Most states required operator certification before it was mandated by federal law.
- The 1996 SDWA Amendments provide up to $9.6 billion over the next six years for improving the drinking water infrastructure. Water systems can apply for low and no-interest loans to upgrade their facilities and ensure compliance with drinking water standards. Other sources of funding also are available to water systems through the U.S. Department of Agricultures Rural Utility Service (RUS). As part of the Water 2000 initiative, which is aimed at providing clean, safe, and affordable drinking water to all rural homes, RUS administers a water and wastewater loan and grant program. Under the RUS programs, rural areas and small cities and towns can receive loans or grants to restore a deteriorating water supply, upgrade a water or wastewater facility, or develop new systems.
- Substantial federal funding is provided to states for assessments and for source water protection programs if states choose to operate such a program. EPA is encouraging states and communities to undertake source water protection programs.

Finally, Healthy People 2010, a national health promotion and disease prevention initiative, has two goals for water quality:

1. Increase the proportion of persons served by community water systems who receive a supply of drinking water that meets the regulations of the Safe Drinking Water Act. The current baseline is 73 percent; the 2010 goals aim to increase that to 95 percent.
2. Reduce waterborne disease outbreaks from drinking water among persons served by community water systems. Currently an estimated six outbreaks per year originate from community water systems. The goal is to decrease that to two outbreaks per year.

SOURCES

Baker, M. N. 1948. *The Quest for Pure Water: The History of Water Purification from the Earliest Records to the Twentieth Century.* New York: American Water Works Association.

Environmental Protection Agency (EPA). December 1999. *25 Years of the Safe Drinking Water Act: History and Trends.* Washington: Environmental Protection Agency. http://www.epa.gov/safewater/sdwa25/sdwa.html.

Environmental Protection Agency (EPA). July 1997. *Water on Tap: A Consumer's Guide to the Nation's Drinking Water.* Washington: Environmental Protection Agency. http://www.epa.gov/OGWDW/wot/ontap.html.

Environmental Working Group (EWG). May 1996. *Just Add Water.* Washington: Environmental Working Group. http://www.ewg.org/pub/home/reports/JustAddWater/jaw_short.html.

Frerichs, Ralph R. 1999. *Snow on Cholera. Part 2: Broad Street Pump Outbreak.* Los Angeles: UCLA School of Public Health. Internet slide show. http:// www.ph.ucla.edu/epi/snow/Snowpart2_files/frame.htm.

National Drinking Water Clearinghouse. 1996–1999. *Tech Briefs.* Morgantown, WV: National Drinking Water Clearinghouse. http://www.estd.wvu.edu/ndwc/EduprodFrame.html.

RESTAURANT FOOD SAFETY

In 1998 two out of three people ate their main meal away from home at least once a week, with the typical consumer eating food away from home at least four times per week (Collins 1997). Americans spend 50 cents of every food dollar on food prepared outside the home, which contributes to restaurant industry sales of $376 billion per year. Almost half of all adults were restaurant patrons on a typical day during 1998, and ate almost 50 billion meals in restaurants and school and work cafeterias (NRA 2000). A lot of people are eating out these days, which also means a lot of people are employed in the restaurant industry.

According to Bureau of Labor Statistics (BLS) data from 1998, the restaurant industry employs 8 percent of the U.S. workforce, or 11 million people. This makes the restaurant industry the nation's largest employer outside of government. Teenagers account for 27 percent of workers in the industry. Partly because of the young age of workers in the industry, and partly because of the nature of the jobs, 38 percent of persons in food service have less than a high school diploma. Many are part-time employees, working an average of 25.5 hours per week. BLS projects that the number of workers in the restaurant industry will reach 12.5 million by the year 2008 (Obenauer 2000).

The restaurant industry has typically been seen as a starting place for those entering the workforce. One-third of all adults in the United States have worked in the restaurant industry at some time during their lives, often as a first or early job. Pay for most of the jobs is low, benefits are few, usually with no retirement or health insurance and little or no paid vacation or sick leave. Without sick leave, workers who are sick must nevertheless come to work. They can ill afford to lose pay. Sick workers and poor hygiene have been the beginnings of numerous foodborne illness outbreaks. Turnover at restaurants is very high and training very low. Training is expensive, and owners cannot afford to train an employee who might not even last a year. Many of the workers are relatively inexperienced or unskilled, and many do not speak or read English well.

Ideally new employees would come into an establishment with a good background in how to handle food properly. But this is not the case. In fact, just the opposite is happening. Young people today do not learn kitchen skills as their parents did. Home economics classes in schools, where cooking and food safety would be learned, are on the decline. With the fast pace of life these days, less and less cooking is done at home, so many teenagers have little experience handling anything but convenience foods. These are the same young adults that are employed in kitchens around the country.

REGULATING THE INDUSTRY

Restaurants, supermarkets, convenience stores, fast food restaurants, fairs and other temporary events, hospitals, schools, nursing homes, prisons, caterers, vending machine operations, and other institutions that serve food are regulated by local governments. Most jurisdictions rely on the regulations set forth by their state agencies. Cities and counties can enforce their own health and food codes, which must be at least as stringent as those set by their state government. In most states adoption of a new food code requires the bill to go through the legislative process, which can be lengthy. Many states adopt all or part of the Food and Drug Administration's (FDA) Food Code. The FDA Food Code, updated every two years, provides model requirements for the safe preparation of food. After a new Food Code is issued, it takes from three to five years before a significant number of jurisdictions adopt it. Examination of the status of Food Code adoptions on the FDA Web site reveals that many jurisdictions are still using the 1993 Food Code. While many are in the process of updating their regulations to be more in line with newer versions of the Food Code (FDA 2000), even more cities, counties, and states are still using all or parts of the 1976 Food Code.

Local inspectors are responsible for inspecting food service establishments in their jurisdiction. A typical staffing situation might be 12 inspectors responsible for inspecting 3,000 food service operations. They may also have other duties, such as inspecting wells, pools, schools, health care facilities, day care facilities, and other institutions for environmental and health conditions. The number of times a facility is inspected per year varies from jurisdiction to jurisdiction. It could be anywhere from once a year to six times a year, with an average of about every six months. Operations serving high-risk foods or clientele might be inspected more often.

Most inspectors use some sort of check-off form to inspect and grade a facility. Many places use a scale of 0 to 100, and may also issue letter grades of A, B, or C. In spite of attempts over the years to standardize the process, it can still be subjective. Inspection procedures and grading may not be consistent from one inspector to another, even in the same jurisdiction. Also, it should be emphasized that an inspection is only a snapshot of what is going on in a facility at that time.

PUBLIC POSTING OF INSPECTION SCORES

We live in an information age. People want more and more information. Couple that with food safety, and it means people want more information about the food they eat. They want to know that restaurants are preparing and serving food safely and that they won't become ill when they eat out. This desire for knowledge has translated into the public posting of restaurant inspection scores. Scores may be posted in the window, the newspaper, or even on the Internet. Public officials are walking a tightrope, trying to balance the public's right to know about the food they eat with the industry's demands for fairness. Many questions remain about the wisdom of posting restaurant scores.

First, what do the scores really mean and will the public know how to interpret them? Do inspections and subsequent scores really reflect food safety practices that could make someone ill; are they really critical? It is difficult to separate real from imaginary risks—dried food on silverware, lipstick on glasses, garbage improperly stored in an alley are not critical hazards that will cause foodborne illness. Many involved in food safety claim that inspections are not based enough on critical issues that have a high association with causing foodborne illness. This is because many current health codes force inspectors to focus on "floor, wall, and ceiling" issues, instead of critical factors such as improper holding temperatures of cold and/or hot foods, or improper cooking temperatures. For example, in one inspection a restaurant lost 10 points due to a dented can in the kitchen and an unmarked spray bottle for olive oil. Another restaurant scored a B instead of an A on their inspection due to a missing ceiling tile. There is a need to assess the real risks and go after those problems, which is not easily done in a regulatory environment.

A good grade does not mean that a restaurant is safe at the time a patron eats there; it only implies that the establishment was in compliance with the food codes at the time the inspection occurred. Some say that there is the same likelihood that an establishment with an A rating will have a foodborne illness outbreak as an establishment with a C rating. Yet there is definitely a perception among the general public that food from a restaurant with an A rating is safe. This is not necessarily so.

Owners of eating establishments question the fairness of requiring them to publicly post inspection results. Once the corrections to the violations have been made, which is usually done immediately, what need is there to publicize the establishment's name and thus harm its reputation and business? Even though the problem is usually corrected immediately, the lower grade could stay posted until the next inspection, which could be six months away. The impact on business is disproportionate to the offense. Some argue that making names public does away with the "innocent until proven guilty" credo of the United States. While the operator may eventually be exonerated, the damage is already done, with the restaurant considered guilty in the public mind. What if an inspector is biased, or a restaurant is just having a bad day when the inspector comes? And what about the potential for blackmail? In Los Angeles an inspector was arrested and pleaded no contest to demanding $200 from a restaurant owner in exchange for an A rating.

Yet in spite of all the above objections, consumers do want to know their food is safe. They claim that publicly posting inspection scores will force restaurant operators to serve safer food. Much of the debate on this topic will be carried out in the media and the courtroom.

EDUCATION

With doubts about the effectiveness of inspections to prevent foodborne illness, education and training appear to be on the menu. In most states it is not necessary for food workers to have any particular certification or training before being allowed to handle food. Compared to some professions, such as hair styling, in which operators must have a license to practice their craft, this seems rather lax. Slowly the tide is turning. Each state sets its own criteria for training and certification for food service employees. It is voluntary in most states. In a few states all those who handle food must have some sort of food handler's card. More states require that there be one food service manager on duty. Counties, and even cities, may set stricter standards than state requirements. Indeed, this is the case in many cities. The National Restaurant Association Educational Foundation maintains a list of requirements for states and other jurisdictions throughout the country at: http://www.edfound.org/NewASP/training/research/jurisdict/servjurisdict.asp. Examples of requirements found in jurisdictions around the United States include:

- All food handlers working in full food service, limited food service, or day care must obtain a food handler's card. Requirements for obtaining such a card vary from just passing an exam to taking a course of several hours.
- Each food service establishment must have an owner or employee who has completed an approved food protection course (these vary from one to six hours) and successfully passed an examination. Information about these exams is listed in chapter 6. In some places there must be an accredited person on duty at all times, in other places not. In some jurisdictions managers must be recertified every three to five years, in others there is no recertification requirement.
- A manager must be able to demonstrate knowledge of food safety. How one demonstrates such knowledge varies, and is often unclear. Several states have proposed bills in their legislatures requiring food service establishments to have a certified manager trained in food safety in all restaurants.

Another response to the need for food safety education is to teach it in schools so everyone can learn how to handle food properly. Many organizations, notably the Food and Drug Administration, the USDA Food Safety and Inspection Service, and the USDA Cooperative State Research, Education, and Extension Service, have developed or funded development of food safety curricula for use in schools. The only state to require food safety education for all students is Arkansas. This lack of basic food safety education in the United States could lead one to reason that food prepared in restaurants could be safer than food cooked in many homes. At least most restaurant employees have some minimal training in properly handling food, have procedures to follow, and have a manager looking over their shoulder.

SOURCES

Collins, J. E. 1997. Impact of Changing Consumer Lifestyles on the Emergence/Reemergence of Foodborne Pathogens. *Emerging Infectious Diseases* 3(4): 471–479.

Food and Drug Administration (FDA). December 27, 2000. *Status of Food Code Adoptions.* Washington: Food and Drug Administration. http://vm.cfsan.fda.gov/~ear/fcadopt.html.

Foodsafe discussion group postings. 1997–2000. http://www.nal.usda.gov/foodborne/.

Kuchler, Fred, Ram Chandran, and Katherine Ralston. 1996. The Linkage between Pesticide Use and Pesticide Residues. *American Journal of Alternative Agriculture.* 11(4): 161–167.

National Restaurant Association (NRA). 2000. *Restaurant Industry Pocket Factbook.* Washington: National Restaurant Association. http://www.restaurant.org/research/pocket/.

Obenauer, Irina. March 2000. Foodservice Trends: Who's Who in the Restaurant Industry. *Restaurants USA* (20) 2:38–42. http://www.restaurant.org/RUSA/.

Restaurantsafety.com. June 3, 2000. *Producing Profitable Results: The Restaurant Management Resources Network.* http://www.restaurantsafety.com/inspections.html.

Chapter 3

Chronology of Food Safety-Related Events

Any chronological depiction of a topic as diverse as food safety involves a look at an array of eclectic, seemingly unrelated events. This chronology weaves together those events from a wide range of subject areas including basic biology, bacteriology, and microbiology; inventions such as refrigeration, freezing, canning, and irradiation; major foodborne illness outbreaks; and government regulations.

6000 B.C.E.	Techniques for drying and smoking foods are developed in Europe and elsewhere.
2600 B.C.E.	Egyptians preserve fish and poultry by drying in the sun.
1000 B.C.E.	Chinese cut ice and use it for refrigeration. They also preserve food through drying and pickling.
500 B.C.E.	Mediterranean people develop marinating. They soak fish guts in salty solution, then leave them in the sun until they ferment, producing a strong smelling liquid. At about the same time, people across Europe master the preservative technique of salting, which leads to the development of curing and pickling. Salt thus becomes a major commodity in international trade.
312 B.C.E.	Roman engineers complete an aqueduct into Rome, providing the city with its first pure drinking water.
Early 700s	Tea gains in popularity in China, possibly because drinking a hot beverage was safer than drinking water, which may be contaminated.
857	The first recorded major outbreak of ergotism occurs in the Rhine Valley. Thousands die after eating bread made from rye contaminated with the fungus *Claviceps purpurea*, which contains the alkaloid drug ergot amine. Ergot amine is transformed into a hallucinogen during baking, causing a form of madness. The cause of the disease would not be realized until almost the 17th century.
943	40,000 die in France from ergot poisoning after eating bread made from rye contaminated with *Claviceps purpurea*.

1266 Assize of Bread and Assize of Beer laws are passed in England to prevent the adulteration of bread and beer with cheaper ingredients.

1500s Acidic cooking techniques—fermenting foods, then spicing and salting them—come to the fore, leading to the development of such foods as sauerkraut and yogurt.

1587 Ergotism becomes endemic in parts of Germany, France, and Spain, bringing insanity and death to thousands.

1597 The faculty of medicine at Marbourg, France, associates ergotism with eating rye.

1641 Massachusetts passes Meat and Fish Inspection Law to ensure that meat exported from the colony to Europe is of high quality and not adulterated.

1668 Italian physician and poet Francisco Redi experiments with maggots and meat, proving that maggots are not the result of spontaneous generation.

1673 Anthony van Leeuwenhook improves the microscope, allowing magnification up to nearly 200 times, permitting him to see what no other man in his century could.

1679 French physicist Denis Papin develops a steam digester, boiling water in a vessel with a tight fitting lid. The accumulating steam creates pressure that allows the temperature inside to rise above the boiling point of water. This is the basis of the modern pressure cooker, which is used to cook and pressure can meats and vegetables.

1692 Salem witch trials. A number of women are accused of being bewitched. They exhibit signs of psychosis, hallucinations, visions, and strange sensations, many of the same symptoms of ergotism. Later scholars suspect a link between the "bewitchings" and ergot poisoning.

1709 German physicist Gabriel Fahrenheit invents the Fahrenheit alcohol thermometer (replaced with mercury in 1714). It will take two centuries before ovens have thermometers, requiring cooks to rely on experience and guesswork to determine temperatures and cooking times.

1735 The first case of botulism food poisoning appears in Germany from sausage.

1768 Italian biologist Lazzaro Spallanzani disproves the widely believed theory of spontaneous generation of microorganisms. (Redi earlier disproved spontaneous generation of maggots.)

1774 Captain Cook almost dies from blowfish (fugu) poisoning after merely tasting the Japanese delicacy, which contains tetrodotoxin—275 times more powerful than cyanide and not destroyed by cooking.

1785 Massachusetts enacts the first general food adulteration law in the United States, penalizing those who sold diseased, corrupted, contagious, or unwholesome food.

1794 Napoleon Bonaparte offers a prize of 12,000 francs for the invention of a process to preserve foods for long periods of time to supply France's long military campaigns.

1810 Nicolas Appert develops the modern canning process, winning Napoleon Bonaparte's prize.

1820 Colonel Robert Gibbon Johnson, Salem County, New Jersey, Horticultural Society President, eats a raw tomato in front of a crowd, thus disproving the conventional wisdom of the day that they are poisonous. Frederic Accum, an English chemist, publishes *A Treatise on Adulteration of Food and Culinary Poisons.*

1823 English chemist and physicist Michael Faraday discovers that when certain gases are kept under constant pressure they will condense until they cool. This discovery will form the basis of mechanical refrigeration. The first mechanical refrigerators are sold in 1862.

1835 James Paget and Richard Owen describe the parasite *Trichinella spiralis* for the first time.

1847 Hungarian physician Ignaz Semmelweiss discovers that lack of hand washing on the part of physicians causes high mortality of women in childbirth.

1848 Dr. John Snow demonstrates that cholera spread throughout London from an infected well.

1851 Dr. John Gorrie is granted the first ice machine patent in the United States. Its first public demonstration is in 1950 at a Bastille Day party in Florida, during which it is used to win a wager that there would be iced champagne in spite of the delayed arrival of the ice shipment from the North.

1855 The non-pathogenic form of *Escherichia coli* bacterium is discovered. It later becomes a major research, development, and production tool for biotechnology.

1857 Englishman William Taylor shows that milk can transmit typhoid fever.

1860 German pathologists Friedrich Albert von Zenker and Rudolph Virchow note the clinical symptoms of trichinosis for the first time. The association between trichinosis and the parasite *Trichinella spiralis* will not be realized until later.

1862 President Abraham Lincoln founds the U.S. Department of Agriculture, calling it the "people's department." He appoints Charles M. Wetherill to serve as the first chemist in the new Department of Agriculture's Bureau of Chemistry, which much later becomes the Food and Drug Administration (FDA) in the Department of Health and Human Services.

1863 Louis Pasteur introduces the process of heating wine to prevent souring. He develops a similar process using lower temperatures, later coined pasteurization to be used to sterilize milk. Public fears about the process of pasteurization and myths of its dangers delay implementation for milk on a commercial level for 30 years.

1870 Louis Pasteur firmly establishes the link between spoilage, disease, and microorganisms. He publishes a classic paper showing that microorganisms cause fermentation.

1872 German scientist Ferdinand Julius Cohn founds the science of bacteriology.

1875 British Parliament passes Britain's first food law, the Sale of Food and Drugs Act, designed mainly to prevent adulteration and economic fraud in the food supply.

1877	English researchers A. Downes and T. P. Blunt discover that ultraviolet rays kill germs.
1878	First use of the term "microbe."
1879	Peter Collier, chief chemist of the USDA, begins investigating food adulteration. The following year he recommends a national food and drug law. In the next 25 years more than 100 food and drug bills will be introduced in Congress, but the country does not get a national food law until 1906. A student researcher at Johns Hopkins University discovers saccharin, a synthetic compound derived from coal tar that is 300 times sweeter than sugar. In 1901, Monsanto Chemical Works is founded to produce it. In 1903 and 1905 the entire saccharin output is shipped to a growing soft-drink company in Georgia called Coca-Cola.
1880s	Robert Koch perfects the process of growing pure strains of bacteria in the laboratory and devises Koch's Postulates.
1883	Dr. Harvey W. Wiley becomes chief chemist of the USDA. He immediately assigns members of his staff to expand the studies of food adulteration. Campaigning for a federal law, Dr. Wiley is called the "Crusading Chemist" and "Father of the Pure Food and Drugs Act." He retires from government service in 1912 and dies in 1930. The Impure Tea Act of 1883 goes into effect to prohibit the importation of adulterated tea into the United States.
1885	USDA veterinarian Daniel Salmon works with bacteria that cause foodborne illness, later to be named *Salmonellae.*
1888	August Gärtner, a German scientist, becomes the first to isolate a pathogenic microorganism, *Bacillus enteritidis*, from a case of food poisoning.
1891	Meat Inspection Act passed to provide federal inspection of meats to be exported.
1895	Emilie Pierre-Mare van Ermengem, a Belgian bacteriologist, is the first to isolate the bacterium that causes botulism, *Clostridium botulinum.*
1898	More U.S. soldiers die from eating contaminated meat than do of battle wounds in the Spanish-American War. Called "embalmed beef," it is preserved with harmful chemicals. This incident hastens the appointment of the first veterinarian to the army, whose duty it is to inspect meats supplied to troops.
1900	Six thousand people become ill and 70 die from arsenic poisoning in England after drinking beer that contained small quantities of it. Arsenic is a common ingredient of insecticides in the early part of the century.
1902	Congress appropriates $5,000 to the Bureau of Chemistry to study chemical preservatives and colors and their effects on digestion and health. Dr. Wiley forms the "Poison Squad" to study the health effects of preservatives used in foods. The squad's work continues for five years and draws widespread attention to the problem of food adulteration. *A Popular Treatise on the Extent and Character of Food Adulterations* is published, informing the public that almost everything they purchase is adulterated or mislabeled.

1904 German entrepreneur Reinhold Burger introduces the thermos bottle, which is based on James Dewar's 1892 vacuum flask.

An epidemic of typhoid fever in New York is traced to Mary Mallon, a cook employed in each of the stricken households. She is found to be a carrier of the disease in spite of her lack of symptoms. She refuses medical care, disappears, but continues employment as a cook. Eventually she is tracked down during another typhoid epidemic and is quarantined for life at the New York City Riverside Hospital for Communicable Diseases in 1915. She remains there until her death in 1938.

1906 The original Food and Drugs Act of 1906 is passed by Congress on June 30 and signed by President Theodore Roosevelt. It prohibits interstate commerce in misbranded and adulterated foods, drinks, and drugs.

The Meat Inspection Act is passed the same day to ensure that meat and meat products are wholesome, not adulterated, and properly labeled and packaged.

Upton Sinclair publishes *The Jungle*, which details adulteration and filth common in the Chicago meatpacking industry. Domestic meat sales decline by half within weeks.

1907 First certified color regulations, requested by manufacturers and users, list seven colors found suitable for use in foods.

1908 Chicago becomes first city in the United States to require that milk sold in the city be pasteurized. Unpasteurized milk can spread tuberculosis, undulant fever, brucellosis, dysentery, typhoid fever, and other diseases. By 1917 46 of the 52 largest cities in the United States require pasteurization, and by 1920 almost every city in America requires the pasteurization of milk.

1914 In *U.S. v. Lexington Mill and Elevator Company*, the Supreme Court issues its first ruling on food additives. It rules that in order for bleached flour with nitrite residues to be banned from foods, the government must show a relationship between the chemical additive and the harm it allegedly causes in humans. The court notes that the mere presence of such an ingredient was not sufficient to render the food illegal.

M. A. Barber shows that *Staphylococcus aureus* causes food poisoning.

1916 A mechanical home refrigerator is marketed for the first time in the United States, but it costs $900, about the same price as a motorcar, and few can afford to buy it.

Sweden begins experiments on irradiating strawberries.

1919 A Hungarian agricultural engineer first uses the term "biotechnology."

1920 Botulism sickens 36 Americans, 23 die. The culprit is commercially canned food. The canning industry imposes new production safety standards in the face of decreasing sales.

American Charles Birdseye invents the process of deep freezing foods.

1924 Grade A Pasteurized Milk Ordinance developed.

1925 In a rare instance of food safety making it into popular literature, in *The Painted Veil* by W. Somerset Maugham, a distraught microbiologist commits suicide by eating a fresh salad during a cholera epidemic.

1926 Thousands die in the Soviet Union from ergotism after eating bread made from infected rye.

1927 The USDA Bureau of Chemistry is reorganized to form the Food, Drug, and Insecticide Administration, which in 1930 is renamed the Food and Drug Administration (FDA).

1929 France issues patent for high-energy pasteurization of foods.

1930s Refrigerators finally become affordable enough to purchase for home use.

1933 *100,000,000 Guinea Pigs: Dangers in Everyday Foods, Drugs and Cosmetics* is published, causing a public outcry over the condition of the food supply.

1934 Seafood Inspection Act passed.

1936 Ruth DeForest Lamb, FDA's Chief Educational Officer, writes *The American Chamber of Horrors*, which details abuses in the U.S. food industry.

1938 Congress passes the Food, Drug and Cosmetic Act (FDCA) of 1938, strengthening the 1906 act by broadening the scope of federal regulation and plugging loopholes.

1939 First food standards of identity are issued (for canned tomatoes, tomato puree, and tomato paste).

1940 FDA is transferred from the USDA to the Federal Security Agency (predecessor to the Department of Health and Human Services), with Walter G. Campbell appointed as the first commissioner of Food and Drugs.
Controlled atmosphere storage is used for the first time to slow the ripening of McIntosh apples. The apples are stored in air-tight rooms in which oxygen is removed and replaced with natural gas.
Dr. Percy Spencer, an engineer with the Raytheon Corporation, notices a candy bar in his pocket melting as he tests a new vacuum tube called a magnetron. Intrigued, he places popcorn kernels near the tube and watches as they pop. This leads him to develop the idea of microwave technology—using microwaves to make food molecules vibrate, create friction, and heat, and thus cook food.

1941 The term "genetic engineering" is first used by Danish microbiologist A. Jost in a lecture on sexual reproduction in yeast at the Technical Institute in Poland.

1945 *Clostridium perfringens* first recognized as a cause of foodborne illness.
Formation of the Food and Agriculture Organization (FAO) as part of the United Nations.

1947 Federal Insecticide, Fungicide and Rodenticide Act is enacted to regulate pesticide usage in food production.
Raytheon Corporation introduces the first commercial microwave oven. Weighing in at 750 pounds with a price tag of $5,000, it stands five-and-a-half feet tall. Raytheon calls this new gizmo a "Radarange," the winning name in an employee contest. By the late 1980s it will become a common feature in American households and workplaces, starting a whole new industry of microwaveable foods that will require new food safety technologies.
Joshua Lederberg and Edward Lawrie Tatum discover that bacteria reproduce sexually. This will open up a whole new field of bacterial genetics.

1948 World Health Organization is founded to improve health for all.

1950s Iceless freezers first become available for home use.

1951 Ergotism breaks out again in France after some 300 people eat bread containing illegal amounts of rye. Some go mad, plunging off rooftops in the belief that they can fly.

1952 FDA consumer consultants are appointed in each field district to maintain communications with consumers and ensure that FDA considers their needs and problems.

1953 Factory Inspection Amendment clarifies the 1938 Food, Drug and Cosmetic Act, giving FDA authority to inspect a plant, after written notice to the owner, without a warrant and without permission of the owner. FDA is required to give manufacturers written reports of conditions observed during inspections and analyses of factory samples.
President Eisenhower proposes the "Atoms-for-Peace" policy to the United Nations. The U.S. government forms the National Food Irradiation Program, under which the U.S. Army and the Atomic Energy Commission carry out research projects between 1953 and 1980 on food irradiation.

1954 The Pesticide Residue Amendment to the Food, Drug and Cosmetic Act, also known as the Miller Act, spells out procedures for setting safety limits for pesticide residues on raw agricultural commodities.
FDA carries out the first large-scale radiological examination of food when it receives reports that tuna suspected of being radioactive is imported from Japan following atomic blasts in the Pacific. FDA begins monitoring around the clock to meet the emergency.
The FDA approves use of BHT (butylated hydroxytoluene), a synthetic antioxidant used to delay rancidity and the breakdown of fatty acids and vitamin C.

1955 A committee of 14 citizens is appointed to study the adequacy of FDA's facilities and programs. The committee recommends a substantial expansion of FDA staff and facilities, a new headquarters building, and more use of educational and informational programs.

1957 Congress passes the Poultry Products Inspection Act, requiring poultry to be inspected before and after slaughter.

1958 Under the Food Additives Amendment manufacturers are required to establish the safety of new food additives. The Delaney proviso prohibits the approval of any food additive shown to induce cancer in humans or animals.
FDA publishes the first list of substances generally recognized as safe (GRAS) in the Federal Register. The list contains nearly 200 substances.

1959 U.S. cranberry crop is recalled three weeks before Thanksgiving for FDA tests to check for alleged contamination by aminotriazole, a weed killer found to cause cancer in laboratory animals. Cleared berries are allowed a label stating that they have been tested and have passed FDA inspection, the only such endorsement ever allowed by FDA on a food product.

1960s The National Aeronautics and Space Administration (NASA), the U.S. Army Natick Laboratories, and the Pillsbury Company begin to develop foods for the manned space program. They work on a new system to come as close as possible to 100 percent assurance that food for the astronauts would be free of pathogens. In 1971 they introduce that system, later to be called the Hazard Analysis and Critical Control Points (HACCP) system.

1960	Color Additive Amendment to the Food, Drug and Cosmetic Act is enacted, requiring manufacturers to establish the safety of color additives in foods, drugs, and cosmetics. FDA approves provisional use of Red No. 2 food dye in spite of concern that it causes defects in some animals. In 1976 FDA will ban the use of Red No. 2, citing concern that it may be carcinogenic.
1961	Establishment of the Codex Alimentarius Commission to create an international food standards program—the Codex Alimentarius.
1962	U.S. biologist Rachel Carson writes *Silent Spring*, warning of the dangers of persistent pesticide use.
1963	FDA approves irradiation for white and wheat flour.
1964	FDA approves irradiation for potatoes to control excess sprouting.
1967	Wholesome Meat Act is enacted to amend the 1906 Meat Inspection Act.
1968	Wholesome Poultry Act sets same provisions for poultry products as the Wholesome Meat Act provides for meats.
1969	FDA begins administering sanitation programs for milk, shellfish, food service, and interstate travel facilities.
1970	Environmental Protection Agency is established; takes over FDA program for setting pesticide tolerances. Egg Products Inspection Act gives USDA jurisdiction over egg safety.
1972	Guidelines for unavoidable natural defects ("filth guidelines") first released to the public. These are now called Food Defect Action Levels. NASA feeds irradiated foods to American astronauts for the first time.
1973	Low-acid food processing regulations are issued to ensure that low-acid packaged foods have adequate heat treatment and are not hazardous.
1974	Congress enacts the Safe Drinking Water Act. Aflatoxin, a powerful toxin produced by the fungus *Aspergillus flavus*, in contaminated corn sickens almost 400 people in 150 villages in India; 108 die.
1975 to 1985	Recognition of new foodborne pathogens: *Campylobacter jejuni*, *Yersinia enterocolitica*, *Escherichia coli* O157:H7, *Vibrio cholerae*, *Listeria monocytogenes*.
1977	Congress passes the Saccharin Study and Labeling Act to stop FDA from banning the chemical sweetener, but requires a label warning that it has been found to cause cancer in laboratory animals. Aflatoxin contaminates corn crops in the southeastern United States. Thousands of turkeys, hogs, and cattle die as a result of being fed contaminated corn. Aflatoxin also affects the peanut crop. USDA begins efforts to limit the amount of nitrites meat processors use in bacon and other meat products. The meat industry uses nitrites for col-

oring and to prevent botulinum toxin, but studies report that fried bacon contains nitrosamines, which are carcinogenic.

1978 First documented foodborne outbreak caused by Norwalk virus.

1980 Infant Formula Act establishes special FDA controls to ensure necessary nutritional content and safety of this product.

1981 Contaminated rapeseed oil kills or maims 20,000 people in Spain.
First documented foodborne outbreak of listeriosis in the United States.

1982 First documented foodborne outbreak caused by *E. coli* O157:H7 in the United States.

1985 FDA approves irradiation of pork to prevent trichinosis.
Raw milk contaminates already pasteurized milk in one of the largest dairy processing plants in the Midwest. Almost 200,000 people become ill with a strain of *Salmonella typhimurium* that is resistant to antimicrobial drugs.
FDA approves the use of aspartame, a low-calorie intense sweetener.

1986 FDA approves irradiation for fruits, vegetables, spices, and fungi to inhibit maturation, retard spoilage, and kill insects that infest produce.
The Safe Drinking Water Act is amended.
The Chernobyl nuclear power plant disaster sends a cloud of radioactivity over most of Europe, contaminating field crops and milk.
British cows first come down with bovine spongiform encephalopathy (BSE), also known as mad cow disease, a progressive neurological disorder that causes cows to become aggressive, disoriented, lose body weight, and stagger.
FDA reevaluates the safety of sulfites, estimating that one out of 100 people is sulfite-sensitive. FDA therefore bans the use of sulfites on fresh foods and requires labels to state if a food contains sulfites.
Genetically engineered plants resistant to insects, viruses, and bacteria are field tested for the first time.

1987 Frostban, a genetically altered bacterium that inhibits frost formation on crop plants, is field tested on strawberry and potato plants in California, which are the first authorized outdoor tests of an engineered bacterium.

1988 Aflatoxin again contaminates corn in Illinois, Indiana, and Iowa. The Quaker Oats cereal mill in Cedar Rapids finds 20 percent of the corn it receives is contaminated with aflatoxin and rejects further shipments of corn from the area. Other countries refuse entry of entire shiploads of corn from the United States.
FDA, the Illinois Institute of Technology, the IIT Research Institute, and the University of Illinois create the National Center for Food Safety and Technology (NCFST), a research consortium intended to develop food safety technologies.

1989 Alar (daninozide), a chemical used to improve the quality and appearance of apples, is banned by the EPA, initiating the "Great Alar Scare." Scientists now believe the dangers of alar were overstated, and that the chemical was the victim of politics, bad science, and media-initiated hysteria.
The U.S. Embassy receives an anonymous phone call claiming that grapes from Chile have been injected with cyanide. U.S. Customs officials impound more than two million crates of Chilean fruit, including berries, apples, melons, peaches, pears, and plums as well as grapes. During the embargo, which lasts 11 days, only three suspicious-looking grapes are

	found. More than 20,000 Chilean workers lose their jobs and the impact is felt throughout Chile. Consumers stop eating grapes from any country, including the United States. The FDA allows the import of Japanese fugu fish for the first time. Cooks who prepare the fish must be specially trained to avoid the dangerous tetrodotoxin produced by the fish.
1990	FDA approves the irradiation of poultry, stating that irradiation is a safe and effective means of controlling *Salmonella* and other foodborne bacteria in poultry. USDA will issue rules for irradiating poultry in 1992. The United Kingdom approves the first food product modified by biotechnology—a yeast used in baking. Chy-Max, an artificially produced form of rennet—an enzyme for cheese making, is introduced. It is the first product of recombinant DNA technology in the U.S. food supply.
1992	The first food irradiation facility for treating foods in the United States opens in Florida.
1993	First use of DNA "fingerprinting" by pulsed-field gel electrophoresis (PFGE) to trace a foodborne outbreak. FDA declares that genetically engineered foods are "not inherently dangerous" and do not require special regulation.
April 1993	*Cryptosporidium parvum* traced to the municipal water supply sickens an estimated 403,000 people in Milwaukee, Wisconsin. This is the largest foodborne or waterborne outbreak in U.S. history.
July 1993	An outbreak of *E. coli* O157:H7 in Washington State is traced to undercooked hamburgers purchased at a fast-food restaurant. More than 700 people become ill, and four children die. This incident galvanizes the public, food industry, and government around the issue of food safety.
November 1993	FDA approves use of bovine somatotropin (BST), a genetically engineered growth hormone developed by Monsanto Company that increases the amount of milk dairy cows produce by 10 to 15 percent.
1994	An estimated 224,000 people across the nation become ill with *Salmonella* poisoning traced back to an ice cream processing facility in Minnesota. FDA approves the first genetically engineered whole food product—the FlavrSavr tomato, designed to resist rotting. The claims are overstated and it soon disappears from the American marketplace. The USDA/FDA Foodborne Illness Education Information Center at the USDA National Agricultural Library is formed through a cooperative agreement among the USDA Food Safety and Inspection Service, the FDA Center for Food Safety and Applied Nutrition, and the University of Maryland.
1995	FDA issues the Seafood HACCP Regulation, requiring the seafood industry to implement HACCP-based food safety systems in seafood processing facilities by the end of 1997. The restaurant and food service industry launches National Food Safety Education Month.
July 1995	The Foodborne Diseases Active Surveillance Network (FoodNet) is initiated jointly by the USDA, FDA, and CDC. FoodNet aims to collect more precise information on the extent of foodborne illness in the United States.

1996	British doctors begin to notice an unusual cluster of patients with Creutzfeldt-Jacob disease (CJD). But unlike classical CJD, which affects the elderly, these victims are young. Later this new variant of CJD (nvCJD) would be linked to bovine spongiform encephalopathy (BSE) in cows. FDA and the University of Maryland create the Joint Institute for Food Safety and Applied Nutrition (JIFSAN) to research broad food safety issues.
July 1996	USDA publishes the Pathogen Reduction: Hazard Analysis and Critical Control Points (HACCP) System rule.
August 1996	Food Quality Protection Act of 1996 amends the Food, Drug and Cosmetic Act, streamlining regulation of pesticides by FDA and EPA. President Clinton signs the Safe Drinking Water Act of 1996. The law requires drinking water systems to protect against dangerous contaminants like *Cryptosporidium*, and gives people the right to know about contaminants in their tap water.
January 1997	President Clinton announces the President's Food Safety Initiative.
April 1997	An outbreak of Hepatitis A virus caused by contaminated strawberries imported from Mexico and served in the school lunch program sickens more than 250 teachers and children in Michigan.
August 1997	After an *E. coli* O157:H7 outbreak in Colorado in which 20 people are sickened, 25 million pounds of suspected contaminated hamburger meat is recalled—the largest recall in U.S. history.
October 1997	President Clinton announces the Produce Safety Initiative to improve the safety of imported produce and to develop guidelines for good agricultural practices for domestic produce. The Partnership for Food Safety Education launches the Fight BAC! campaign to educate consumers on the problem of foodborne illness and motivate them to adopt safe food handling practices. Stanley B. Prusiner from the University of California San Francisco wins Nobel Prize for his work on prions and bovine spongiform encephalopathy (BSE).
November 1997	More than 700 people become ill and two die from *Salmonella* poisoning after eating ham stuffed with greens and spices at a church supper in Maryland.
December 1997	FDA bans the import of raspberries from Guatemala for the 1998 season after they are linked to outbreaks of *Cyclospora* in 1996 and 1997, sickening more than 2,400 people. FDA approves the irradiation of red meat.
May 1998	PulseNet is established to link food safety investigators at CDC, FDA, USDA, state health departments, and public health laboratories. Scientists are now able to fingerprint pathogens in contaminated foods to trace foodborne illnesses. Food Outbreak Response Coordinating Group (FORC-G) is formed to strengthen coordination and improve efficiency among USDA, CDC, FDA, and EPA in responding to foodborne illness outbreaks.
June 1998	Potato salad contaminated with *E. coli* enterotoxigenic sickens more than 4,000 people in Illinois.
July 1998	The Joint Institute for Food Safety Research is created to develop a coordinated strategy for federal food safety research in conjunction with the private sector and academia.

July 1998	FDA publishes a rule requiring labels on unpasteurized cider and juices warning of the possible danger of contamination with *E. coli* and other microbial pathogens.
August 1998	President Clinton establishes the President's Council on Food Safety, whose mission it is to recommend changes needed to accomplish food safety goals, coordinate federal food safety budgets, and prioritize food safety research.
September 1998	USDA issues rule requiring that shell eggs be kept refrigerated at 45°F while being processed, shipped, and displayed for sale.
February 1999	USDA proposes a rule governing the use of irradiation in red meats to control disease-causing microorganisms and to extend shelf life. FDA approved irradiation for red meat in 1997.
March 1999	An outbreak of *Listeria monocytogenes* in 22 states traced to hot dogs and deli meats causes approximately 100 illnesses and 21 deaths. USDA announces that rates of *Salmonella* contamination decreased by half in chickens and by a third in ground beef after the first year of HACCP implementation in meat and poultry processing plants.
July 1999	In July the FDA warns that children, pregnant women, the elderly, or persons with weakened immune systems should not eat raw sprouts such as alfalfa, clover, or radish. Over 270 persons have become ill since 1997 from eating sprouts contaminated with *Salmonella* or *E. coli* O157:H7.
September 1999	CDC releases new estimates of foodborne disease illnesses and deaths—approximately 76 million illnesses and 5,000 deaths.
December 1999	The President's Council on Food Safety identifies egg safety as a food safety issue that warrants immediate federal, interagency action. The Egg Safety Action Plan is developed in response to this need. The goal of the Egg Safety Action Plan is to reduce foodborne illnesses associated with *Salmonella enteritidis* in eggs by 50 percent by 2005, and eliminate egg-associated *Salmonella enteritidis* illnesses by 2010.
2000	The USDA Food Safety Research Office is established at the National Agricultural Library to collect government-funded and private food safety research information and make it accessible through the Web and by other means. The President's Council on Food Safety develops the National Food Safety Strategic Plan, a comprehensive plan to protect public health by setting priorities, improving coordination and efficiency, identifying gaps in the current system and ways to fill those gaps, enhancing and strengthening prevention and intervention strategies, and identifying reliable measures to indicate progress.
January 2000	U.S. Agriculture Secretary Dan Glickman names 38 members to a newly formed USDA Advisory Committee on Agricultural Biotechnology. The Committee will advise the Secretary on policy related to the creation, application, marketability, trade, and use of agricultural biotechnology.
February 2000	USDA finalizes rule governing the irradiation of red meats (FDA earlier approved irradiation for red meats). Several meat-processing companies say they will soon begin irradiating ground beef.
May 2000	Saccharin is taken off the National Institute of Health's carcinogen list. FDA announces it will develop new pre-market guidelines for reviewing genetically engineered foods.

June 2000	A food safety recommendation is included in the Dietary Guidelines for Americans for the first time. Two USDA compliance officers and an investigator from the California Department of Food and Agriculture (CDFA) were shot and killed while trying to serve notice of violation at a California sausage factory. A fourth person, a CDFA meat inspector, escaped unhurt.
September 2000	FDA releases the report of the FDA Retail Food Program Database of Foodborne Illness Risk Factors. The data establish a baseline to measure how effective industry and regulatory efforts are in changing behaviors and practices that directly relate to foodborne illness in the retail food industry.
November 2000	FDA approves ultraviolet irradiation for juice products.
December 2000	FDA publishes final rule on egg labeling and refrigeration, which sets 45°F for holding and requires a safe-handling label for egg cartons.
January 2001	FDA publishes rule requiring juice processors to use a HACCP system. EPA proposes revising the current drinking water standard for arsenic from 50 parts per billion (ppb) to 10 ppb. The Bush administration withdraws the proposal.

SOURCES

Andress, Elizabeth L. 1998. *A New National Plan for Food Safety Action.* Athens, GA: University of Georgia Cooperative Extension Service. http://www.fcs.uga.edu/pubs/current/HS07.html.

Asimov, Isaac. 1972. *Asimov's Biographical Encyclopedia of Science and Technology*, rev. ed. Garden City, NY: Doubleday.

Biotechnology Industry Organization. Date unknown. Biotechnology Timeline. Washington: Biotechnology Industry Organization. http://216.33.110.200/timeline/timeline.html. Accessed 4/2/00.

Gallawa, J. Carlton. 1996–2000. *Who Invented Microwaves?* http://www.gallawa.com/microtech/history.html.

Gillis, Anne L. Updated August 24, 1999. *Food Safety: A Chronology of Selected Recent Events, 1992–1998.* Report no. 98-119 C. Washington: Congressional Research Service.

International Food Information Council. 1998. History of Food Development. *Food Insight* July/August 1998. http://ificinfo.health.org/insight/foodhist.htm.

Latta, Sara. 1999. *Food Poisoning and Foodborne Diseases.* Berkeley Heights, NJ: Enslow.

North Carolina Biotechnology Center. 1997. *About Biotechnology—Historical Timeline.* Research Triangle Park, NC: North Carolina Biotechnology Center. http://www.ncbiotech.org/aboutbt/timeline.cfm.

Schultz, Harold William. 1981. *Food Law Handbook.* Westport, CT: AVI.

Tauxe, R., H. Kruse, C. Hedberg, M. Potter, J. Madden, and K. Waschsmuth. 1997. Microbial Hazards and Emerging Issues Associated with Produce. A preliminary report to the National Advisory Committee on Microbiologic Criteria for Foods. *Journal of Food Protection* 60(11): 1400–1408.

Trager, James. 1995. *The Food Chronology.* New York: Henry Holt and Company.

U.S. Food and Drug Administration. May 3, 1999. *Milestones in U.S. Food and Drug Law History.* http://vm.cfsan.fda.gov/mileston.html.

CHAPTER 4

FOOD SAFETY REGULATION

This chapter starts off with an overview of early attempts to regulate food safety, focusing mainly on the United States since there is very little in the historical record from other parts of the world on how, or if, food safety was regulated. After the historical review, the development of food safety regulation in the United States is followed in a chronological progression from the earliest laws to modern regulations, covering:

Massachusetts Meat and Fish Inspection Law of 1641
An Act Against Selling Unwholesome Provisions, 1785
Impure Tea Act of 1883
1891 Meat Inspection Act
Food and Drugs Act of 1906
Federal Meat Inspection Act of 1906
Seafood Inspection Act of 1934
Federal Food, Drug and Cosmetic Act of 1938
Federal Insecticide, Fungicide and Rodenticide Act of 1947
The Pesticide Residue Amendment of 1954
Food Additives Amendment of 1958 and the Color Additive Amendment of 1960
Poultry Products Inspection Act of 1957
Wholesome Meat Act of 1967
Egg Products Inspection Act of 1970
Safe Drinking Water Act of 1974 and Amendments of 1986 and 1996
Infant Formula Act of 1980
Food Quality Protection Act of 1996

The Hazard Analysis and Critical Control Points (HACCP) system phase of food safety regulation is covered, beginning with the FDA's 1995 Procedures for the Safe and Sanitary Processing and Importing of Fish and Fishery Products. This is followed by the USDA's 1996 Pathogen Reduction: Hazard Analysis and Critical Control Points (HACCP) System rule.

The question of who regulates food safety in the United States is answered by reviewing all the federal agencies and state and local groups involved:

Food and Drug Administration
United States Department of Agriculture
Environmental Protection Agency
Centers for Disease Control and Prevention
National Marine Fisheries Service
Federal Trade Commission
U.S. Customs Service
Bureau of Alcohol, Tobacco and Firearms
National Institutes of Health

An overview of international food safety regulation is also included. The chapter closes with a look at what the federal government is doing about food safety now, and examines the President's Food Safety Initiative of 1997, the Healthy People 2010 goals, and the Dietary Guidelines for Americans.

HISTORY OF FOOD SAFETY REGULATION

Early food laws in the Western world dealt mainly with preventing economic deception and adulteration of foods rather than with food safety. Food adulteration includes:

- Adding spices or color to disguise rotted or deteriorated products, especially to meats.
- Diluting a product, as in adding water to wine.
- Removing valuable parts of a food, such as the essential oils from spices.
- Substituting an inferior product or part in a food, for example, using apple cores and skin instead of the fruit in apple jelly.

Foods are adulterated intentionally for economic gain, but also sometimes carelessly or unintentionally, for example, by insect parts, bacteria, or soil.

As cities such as Rome increased in size and armies traveled to distant lands, food became very important to the Roman Empire; so much so that Roman civil law included provisions to protect the populace against adulterated foods. In 200 B.C.E. Cato described a method for determining whether merchants watered down their wine. Several centuries later Pliny the Elder described how unscrupulous Roman merchants adulterated foods such as olive oil, cereal grains, herbs, spices, and wine (Hutt 1984). The English passed their first food law, the Assize of Bread, around 1266 to prevent the adulteration of bread with cheaper, inferior ingredients. As beer was an equally important and adulterated food product, there was also an Assize of Beer to regulate its price and quality. (Assize was a term for a type of legal procedure.) The Judgment of the Pillory, from the same era, was a law spelling out procedures to investigate and punish offenders by fines or, for repeat offenders, the pillory or other bodily punishment. In addition to violations of the Assizes of Bread and Beer, it covered meat and fish:

And if any butcher sells contagious flesh, or that died of pestilence or plague. Also they shall inquire of Cooks that boil flesh or fish with bread or water, or any otherwise, that is not wholesome for man's body, or after that they have kept it so long that it loses its natural wholesomeness, and then boil it again, and sell it. (Halsall 1988, text modernized by author)

Adulteration of foods continued century after century, and became more sophisticated and harder to detect. Flour mixed with chalk, spices diluted with every manner of non-edible ingredients, spoiled grain mixed into good grain to mask its deterioration, bread made with ground peas and beans, and wine and alcoholic spirits watered down with everything from water to oil of turpentine were common. In 1820 Frederick C. Marcus, a chemist whose pen name was Accum, published *A Treatise on Adulteration of Food and Culinary Poisons,* which exposed many of the common food adulterations of the day. The food adulteration situation changed little as illustrated by a 1939 publication, *Deadly Adulteration and Slow Poisoning Unmasked or Disease and Death in the Pot and the Bottle*, which described how "artistes au lait" could approximate cream by skillfully blending just the right amounts of the dye annatto, water, and milk. Those less skilled would add flour, starch, rice powder, or arrow-root. Noting how lax the laws were to punish food adulterators, the author observed that, "a man who robs a fellow subject of a few shillings on the highway should be sentenced to death, while he who distributes a slow poison to a whole community should escape unpunished" (Anonymous 1939). Finally, in 1875 the British Parliament passed the Sale of Foods and Drug Act, which endured as Britain's basic food law for many years. By the end of the century most other European countries also had general laws preventing the adulteration of foods.

Early Food Safety Regulation in the United States

Rules regarding proper weights and measures, purity of ingredients, and fair pricing were at the center of the earliest regulations in the new colonies too. The early settlers passed the first laws not to protect citizens, but to ensure the quality and wholesomeness of foods exported from the colonies to Europe. Trade, not safety, was the motivating factor in establishing early food regulations. Massachusetts was a forerunner in the food safety realm with several notable laws. The Massachusetts Meat and Fish Inspection Law of 1641 dealt with meat destined for export to show that the colony produced and exported high-quality food products. In 1646 Massachusetts passed a law that regulated the quality and price of bread, and required bakers to mark each loaf of bread so that its origin would be traceable. To detect economic deception, the law gave inspectors the authority to enter bakeries and weigh the loaves. Massachusetts also passed the first comprehensive food adulteration law in 1785, penalizing those who sold diseased, corrupted, contagious, or unwholesome food. Previous laws regulated only specific commodities, but this law applied to foods overall. The law, entitled An Act Against Selling Unwholesome Provisions, was short but to the point:

Whereas some evilly disposed persons from motives of avarice and filthy lucre, have been induced to sell diseased, corrupted, contagious or unwholesome provisions to the great nuisance of public health and peace:
Be it therefore enacted by the Senate and House of Representatives in General Court assembled, and by the authorities of the same, that if any person shall sell any such diseased, corrupted, contagious, or unwholesome provisions, whether for meat or drink, knowing the same without making it known to the buyer, and being thereof convicted before the Justices

of the General Sessions of the Peace in the county where such offense shall be committed, or the Justices of the Supreme General Court, he shall be punished by fine, imprisonment, standing in the pillory and binding to the good behavior of one or more of these punishments to be inflicted according to the degree and aggravation of the offense.

Many other states, notably Virginia, Iowa, Oregon, New York, and California, passed food laws throughout the early 1800s.

State and local governments were responsible for food safety regulation until the late 1800s. Food early in the country's history was grown and produced locally, so local laws were adequate to deal with problems. Most people knew the farmer or baker down the road. That being the case, they also knew whether they were honest and whether their products were of good quality.

As the population increased and changed from rural to urban, the food supply became more national in scope and distribution. People no longer had a personal connection with the producers of their food, as much of it came from outside the community. There were many who thought that according to the United States Constitution, Congress did not have the authority to regulate in matters of health and safety. The tide began to turn in the late nineteenth and early twentieth centuries with passage of some of the first federal food safety laws.

The first federal food law was the Impure Tea Act of 1883, passed to prohibit the importation of adulterated tea into the United States. In the early 1890s rumors, often true, of the diseased state of food-producing animals in the United States were circulating in Europe. American meat products earned a reputation as unfit to eat (Schultz 1981). To save the export meat market, which was a major source of revenue at the time, Congress passed the 1891 Meat Inspection Act, requiring the inspection of all live cattle intended for export. In addition, the act required the inspection of all cattle, sheep, and hogs prior to slaughter if they were to be sold in interstate commerce. Post mortem inspections of meat could also be made if deemed necessary. This was the first time Congress authorized the use of the "Inspected and Passed" labeling of meat. Unfortunately, no money was allotted for the program, so its full implementation did not take immediate effect.

Twentieth Century Food Safety Regulation in the United States

Chemists from the U.S. Department of Agriculture (USDA) first suggested a general food law for the United States in 1879, but it took 27 years before the climate was right for it. From 1887 to 1901 the department published the 10–volume *Bulletin 13, Foods and Food Adulterants*, which detailed mass adulteration in all sectors of the food supply. These rather technical treatises were republished into an understandable form for the general public entitled, *A Popular Treatise on the Extent and Character of Food Adulterations*. The media of the day widely publicized this work. In it consumers read that almost every food they purchased was adulterated or mislabeled.

Added to this brew of public dismay of and increased intolerance for food adulteration was the notoriety of the man many consider the father of the Food and Drugs Act of 1906, Dr. Harvey W. Wiley. (His grave in Arlington cemetery bears that inscription.) Dr. Wiley became the chief chemist of the USDA Division of Chemistry in 1883. An accomplished public speaker and respected scientist, Dr. Wiley worked on several fronts to help gain passage of the 1906 act. He ignited public interest through his many speeches and writings in popular newspapers and magazines, lobbied Congress for 20 years for passage of food safety legislation, and spearheaded the publication of *Bulletin 13* and the Poison Squad.

The Poison Squad was a group of 12 chemists from the USDA, which was formed in 1902 to study preservatives used in food products. The group's job was to consume food made with chemical preservatives and then to note the effects on their health. They ate all their food at a USDA kitchen. Department scientists analyzed everything they ate and everything they excreted. During these studies they ingested boric acid, sulfurous acid, sulfites, benzoic acid, copper sulfate, saltpeter, and formaldehyde. While none of the Poison Squad succumbed to their job, they did find that many of these chemicals were harmful to human health. This was the start of the federal government's role in approving chemicals used in food production, a process that is still one of the main duties of the federal government (Janssen 1981). The work of the Poison Squad captured the public's attention, further flaming the desire for regulation of the food industry. Even the minstrel shows of the time had songs about the squad—designated the "Hygienic Table."

O, they may get over it but they'll never look the same,
That kind of bill of fare would drive most men insane.
Next week he'll give them mothballs, a la Newburgh or else plain;
O, they may get over it but they'll never look the same.
(Chorus from "Song of the Poison Squad," Lew Dockstader's Minstrels, October 1903 [FDA 1981])

The publication of the novel, *The Jungle* by Upton Sinclair, in 1906 also helped shape the force of public opinion. Sinclair's book described in lurid detail the filthy conditions and adulteration of meat that was common in the Chicago meat industry. Widely read magazines such as *Collier's* and *The Ladies Home Journal* fueled the public's indignation over the state of the food they were eating. *The New York Evening Post* contributed this to the fray (Janssen 1982):

> Mary had a little lamb,
> And when she saw it sicken,
> She shipped it off to Packingtown,
> And now it's labeled chicken.

Finally, on June 30, 1906, President Theodore Roosevelt signed into law both the Food and Drugs Act and the Federal Meat Inspection Act.

The Food and Drugs Act

The Food and Drugs Act defined food as "all articles used for food, drink, confectionery, or condiment by man or other animals, whether simple, mixed, or compound." It forbade adulteration of foods, drinks, and drugs in interstate commerce specifically "preventing the manufacture, sale, or transportation of adulterated or misbranded or poisonous or deleterious foods, drugs, medicines, and liquors, and for regulating traffic therein, and for other purposes." The act considered foods misbranded if they were labeled so as to deceive the public, if the contents in terms of weights and measures were either incorrect or not present on the package, or if the label contained any false or misleading statement concerning the ingredients of a food. The federal government had the authority to seize adulterated or misbranded foods. Violators were guilty of a misdemeanor and subject to fines of up to $500 and/or imprisonment of up to one year for the first offense.

Capitalizing on the Food and Drugs Act, Dr. Wiley and his chemists looked at the 80 food colorants that were in use in 1907. Of those, 30 had never been tested for safety, 26 had been tested but the results were contradictory, experts considered eight to be harmful, and the remaining 16 were thought to be more or less harmless. From that list of 16, only seven passed final scrutiny to be certified under the Food Inspection Division 77, issued September 25, 1907. This legislation certified those seven colorants and established procedures for colorants to be certified in the future. Of those original seven certified colorants only three, erythrosine (FD&C Red No. 3), Naphthol Yellow S (Ext. D&C Yellow No. 7), and Indigo Disulfo Acid, Sodium Salt (FD&C Blue No. 2), are now allowed in foods, drugs, or cosmetics (Marmion 1991).

The Federal Meat Inspection Act

The situation with the meatpacking industry was different from the rest of the food suppliers. The meat industry favored government regulation. They felt that a federal meat inspection program could reopen markets for American meats in Europe, as most major European countries banned the import of American meats in the 1880s. Having federal inspection would add legitimacy to their products. Already Congress started the process with the Meat Inspection Act of 1891. This earlier act was successful in that several European nations did remove their bans on American meat products in 1892. However, in the 1891 act Congress did not allocate money for the cost of the federal inspection program, weakening its effect.

The Jungle had a great impact on the meat industry. Upton Sinclair's novel meant to highlight the horrible working conditions of the nation's working class. The fact that the novel took place in a meatpacking plant was secondary. The nation, though, was more horrified at the thought of rats and other undesirables mixed in with their sausage than of the poor treatment of workers. Sinclair later wrote, "I aimed at the public's heart and by accident hit it in the stomach" (Shumsky 1997). Domestic meat sales declined by half within weeks after publication of *The Jungle*, which further fueled industry's desire for regulation. Earlier draft versions of the 1906 Meat Inspection Act placed the burden of cost on the packers by charging an inspection fee for every animal. The meatpacking industry lobbied hard against this and in the end Congress appropriated federal money for meat inspection. This is still a contentious issue today, with the USDA regularly requesting inspection fees and industry trying to persuade Congress not to grant them. The Federal Meat Inspection Act of 1906 protected consumers by "assuring that meat and meat food products distributed to them are wholesome, not adulterated, and properly marked, labeled, and packaged." The act mandated inspection of cattle, sheep, goats, and equines, both before and after slaughter. It required continuous USDA inspection of slaughter and processing operations and established sanitary standards for the industry. What the act didn't do was cover poultry products or meat that was not intended for interstate commerce. That would come much later. The quality of food overall, sanitation in food plants, and the shipment and handling of foods improved under the Federal Meat Inspection Act and the Food and Drugs Act.

The Food, Drug and Cosmetic Act (FDCA)

Although it was a good start and accomplished much, from the beginning the Food and Drugs Act had some very large flaws. It did not set standards as to what exactly should be in a particular food, so it was almost impossible to prove adulteration of a food. For example, without knowing the amount of strawberries that was supposed to be in strawberry jam, the federal lawyers could not prove that a product with almost no strawberries in it was not strawberry jam. Furthermore, the act required the government to prove that alleged offenders of the law *intended* to deceive or poison consumers with their product. When brought to court defendants pleaded ignorance of the results of their actions. While the law prohibited false labeling, producers did not have to list ingredients in their products. Nevertheless, the act endured as the major law regulating the food supply with only a few minor amendments until the early 1930s when the movement for reform started anew.

In 1933 Arthur Kallet and F.J. Schlink published the immensely popular book *100,000,000 Guinea Pigs: Dangers in Everyday Foods, Drugs and Cosmetics.* The book was biased and contained many inaccuracies, but it also contained a good deal of truth. Written in true muckraking style, it once again stirred the public's ire at the condition of the food they were eating. The basic premise of the book was that the federal government was unable to protect consumers from bad food and drugs, both due to incompetence and to the lack of adequate laws.

In 1930 the USDA's Division of Chemistry was renamed the Food and Drug Administration (FDA), later to be transferred out of the USDA altogether. In 1933 the FDA chief, Walter Campbell, presented a bill to replace the 1906 act. It would take many battles and five years of legislative maneuvering before Congress passed the new bill.

As with passage of the 1906 act, public opinion played a strong role in sending the message to Congress that reform was needed. Since much of the media sided with the food manufacturing industry against reform, the FDA took its message directly to the people, speaking at women's clubs, to civic organizations, and on the radio. At one point, while preparing for Senate hearings on the bill, Walter Campbell collected hundreds of products (both food and drug) that had injured or cheated consumers. He emphasized that the 1906 act did not regulate these products enough to prevent such occurrences. The exhibits were photographed and converted into posters to illustrate the need for new laws. They were displayed at FDA talks and at a museum in FDA headquarters. The exhibit was christened the "Chamber of Horrors," and led to the publication of *The American Chamber of Horrors* by the FDA's chief educational officer, Ruth deForest Lamb, in 1936. Written from inside the government, it was more detailed and accurate than was the earlier *100,000,000 Guinea Pigs.* Ms. Lamb recounted some of the little-known behind-the-scenes details of the food industry. When discussing a new method that an FDA scientist invented for analyzing butter for contamination, she wrote:

> Examination of only a few samples by this new method was enough to fill regulatory officials with dismay and incredulity. Butter that looked perfectly clean and wholesome to the naked eye disclosed a history of filth leading all the way back to the farm. Hay; fragments of chicken feathers; maggots; clumps of mold—blue, green, white and black; grasshoppers; straw chaff; beetles; cow, dog, cat and rodent hairs; moths; grass and other vegetable matter; cockroaches; dust; ants; fly legs; broken fly wings; metallic filings; remains of rats, mice and other animals were revealed to the astonished eye—all impregnated with yellow dye from the butter. (deForest Lamb 1936)

In arguing the need for a new food and drug law, she noted that the 1906 laws were outdated due to new modes of living, new kinds of products, new methods of manufacturing and selling, new tricks of sophistication, and new scientific discoveries, all demanding a more modern method of control.

Finally, in 1938, Congress passed the federal Food, Drug and Cosmetic Act (FDCA), which President Franklin Roosevelt signed into law as part of the New Deal's crusade for a stronger food and drug law. This act, with a number of adjustments and amendments, is still the major force regulating foods. It continued with many of the intentions of the 1906 act, but broadened the scope of federal regulation and plugged many of the loopholes. The new act covered all kinds of foods sold across state lines (except meat and poultry) and all substances found naturally in foods and those added intentionally or unintentionally. It included imported and exported foods. The original bill also gave FDA regulatory power over advertising of food and drugs, but this was dropped from the final bill. However, the Federal Trade Commission received this authority. For the first time the law

- defined adulteration to include bacteria or chemicals that are potentially harmful; insect parts, rodent hairs, and other unintentional substances; and deceptive degrading of the quality of a product from its perceived content
- allowed the FDA to inspect food manufacturing and processing facilities
- required ingredients of non-standard foods to be listed on labels
- prohibited the sale of food prepared under unsanitary conditions
- gave FDA the authority to monitor animal drugs, feed, and veterinary devices
- authorized mandatory food standards for identity, quality, and fill of container. Standards of identity tell the name of the product, the definition of the product, necessary ingredients (sometimes with amounts), optional ingredients and, if applicable, the packaging and processing requirements. Full-fat ice cream, for example, must have a minimum of 10 percent milk-fat content. Standards of quality establish the minimum quality allowed for a product. Standards of fill establish the minimum weight or volume that a specific package of food must hold.

Few, if any, laws have as great an impact on the life and health of Americans as does the Food, Drug and Cosmetic Act. The overall function of the law was to prevent the distribution of harmful or deceptive food and drug products.

Originally the Food, Drug and Cosmetic Act did not provide for seafood inspection. This is because the Seafood Inspection Act enacted in 1934 was already in place. Unlike other food items regulated by the FDA, seafood regulation came about on a voluntary basis. In the early 1930s, canned shrimp processors found that increasingly large amounts of their product were being seized by the FDA because of decomposition. Poor fishing practices and poorly supervised packing operations contributed greatly to the spoilage of shrimp products. As the canners could not themselves influence fishermen and packers to improve their handling of the product, they requested that Congress enact an inspection law. Packers of any seafood product could request an inspector to examine the premises, equipment, methods, containers, and materials they used. If the inspection was favorable, they could use that information on their label. The new seafood inspection program had an almost immediate favorable effect on the canned seafood, especially shrimp, industry. Product quality improved and the industry was able to regain consumer confidence in their product. The Seafood Inspection Act was added to the FDCA in 1943.

The Federal Insecticide, Fungicide and Rodenticide Act (FIFRA)

The Federal Insecticide, Fungicide and Rodenticide Act of 1947 (FIFRA) regulates pesticide usage in food production. While the FDCA is concerned with pesticide residues, FIFRA deals with pesticide registration, protection of the environment, use of pesticides, and the safety of those using them. Pesticides were then called "economic poisons" and were required to be registered, and any claims made in respect to the efficacy of the product were to be substantiated. FIFRA required stricter labeling, including ingredients, directions for use, and a warning statement. Originally USDA administered FIFRA, but after the Environmental Protection Agency (EPA) was formed in 1970, it took responsibility for FIFRA. Approximately 25,000 pesticide products are registered under FIFRA.

Amendments to the Food, Drug and Cosmetic Act (FDCA)

Three amendments to the Food, Drug and Cosmetic Act further increased FDA's regulatory responsibility. The Pesticide Residue Amendment of 1954 spelled out procedures for setting safety limits for pesticide residues on raw agricultural products. The original 1938 Food, Drug and Cosmetic Act considered as adulterated any food to which a poisonous substance was added. However, some substances cannot be avoided in the production of food and are not dangerous at low levels. The 1954 amendment allowed a food to be exempted from being considered adulterated if the added substance was within tolerance levels. The Food Additives Amendment of 1958 and the Color Additive Amendment of 1960 required manufacturers of new food and color additives to establish the safety of additives before they could be used in a food. For the first time it was illegal to introduce any substance into the food supply without assurances of its safety first. The law stipulated that additives in use prior to January 1958, and thought to be safe due to a substantial history of safe use, be declared generally recognized as safe (GRAS) and exempted from the provisions in the Additives and Color Amendments. The Delaney Clause of the Additives and Color Amendments prohibited the approval of any food additive or substance shown to cause cancer in humans or animals.

Additional Regulation of Poultry, Meat, and Eggs

Congress passed the Poultry Products Inspection Act in 1957, declaring, "It is essential in the public interest that the health and welfare of consumers be protected by assuring that poultry products distributed to them are wholesome, not adulterated, and properly marked, labeled, and packaged." Earlier in the century local butchers slaughtered most poultry in plain sight of the consumer, thereby providing consumers some power to avoid poultry slaughtered under unsanitary conditions. After World War II there was explosive growth in the poultry industry. As the poultry industry became more centralized and meat was shipped greater and greater distances, the need for some sort of national legislation became apparent. The act required that poultry and poultry products be inspected before and after slaughter if they were to be sold in interstate or foreign commerce. Many states already inspected poultry in intrastate commerce. The act was revised in 1962 to extend to products in intrastate commerce if the state did not have its own inspection program.

Congressional investigation of meat inspection programs in the early 1960s revealed that 15 percent of all commercially slaughtered animals and 25 percent of all commercially prepared meat products were not subject to inspection because they were intended only for intrastate commerce, since the Meat Inspection Act only covered meat intended for interstate commerce. Furthermore, only 29 states imposed mandatory inspection during slaughter of animals intended for sale as food in intrastate commerce. To correct these deficiencies in the original Meat Inspection Act, Congress enacted the Wholesome Meat Act of 1967. It extended the federal inspection program to states that did not have inspection programs comparable to those of the USDA. States could still have their own inspection programs if their requirements were "at least equal to" federal requirements, but if their programs were inadequate, consumers would still be protected. In addition, it incorporated provisions against adulteration and misbranding of food products almost identical to Food, Drug and Cosmetic Act provisions. The Wholesome Poultry Act of 1968 amended the 1957 poultry act, modeling it after the Wholesome Meat Act to provide for continuous inspection of poultry operations and federal coverage if a state did not have an adequate poultry inspection program.

The Egg Products Inspection Act of 1970 required USDA to ensure that egg products are safe, wholesome, and accurately labeled. It defined adulterated and misbranded egg products in terms similar to the Food, Drug and Cosmetic Act. At that time the USDA Agricultural Marketing Service was responsible for egg inspection; those duties were transferred to the USDA Food Safety and Inspection Service in 1995.

The Safe Drinking Water Act (SDWA)

The 1974 Safe Drinking Water Act authorized EPA to establish national, enforceable health standards for contaminants in drinking water. It encouraged federal-state partnerships in protecting the nation's water supply, and required notification to alert customers to water system violations. In 1986, the act was strengthened to require all water systems to be disinfected and all surface water supplies to be filtered, expanding the number of regulated contaminants (now more than 90) and establishing a monitoring program for unregulated contaminants. The 1996 amendments to the act extended the protection of drinking water from source to tap. Water systems can apply for low- and no-interest loans to upgrade their facilities and ensure compliance with drinking water standards. Under the act local water systems must issue annual Consumer Confidence Reports to customers to inform them about the source of their water supply, contaminant levels detected in their water, and the health effects of contaminants detected above the established safety limit. The act also requires states to examine all drinking water sources, identify contaminant threats, and determine susceptibility to contamination.

Saccharin Study and Labeling Act

In 1977 a Canadian researcher reported that saccharin fed in very high doses to rats caused those rats to develop bladder cancer. Under the Delaney Clause of the Food, Drug and Cosmetic Act, any additive that was found to cause cancer at any dose in any animal was to be banned. It didn't matter that researchers fed the rats the equivalent of 800 cans of diet soda a day. Accordingly, FDA proposed a ban on saccharin. As it was the only artificial sweetener in use at the time, a great public outcry ensued. Congress quickly passed the Saccharin Study and Labeling Act, which placed a two-year moratorium on any ban of the sweetener while additional safety studies were conducted. The law also required that any foods containing saccharin must carry a label that reads "Use of this product may be hazardous to your health. This product contains saccharin which has been determined to cause cancer in laboratory animals." Although the act was originally to last only 18 months, Congress has extended the moratorium several times, most recently renewing it until 2002. Saccharin was not new to controversy. In 1907 when a top food safety official tried to ban it, President Theodore Roosevelt proclaimed him to be "an idiot." Editorial cartoonists lampooned the Canadian study's 800-cans-a-day figure by showing bloated rats staggering around holding cans of diet soda. One congressman suggested saccharin products carry a warning label saying, "The Canadians have determined saccharin is dangerous to your rat's health." Later research showed that saccharin caused bladder cancer in rats through a mechanism that was not present in human beings. Nevertheless, in 1991 saccharin was added to the National Institute of Health's carcinogen list. Although removed from the list in May 2000, debate still lingers, as some scientists maintain that saccharin's safety has not yet been proven.

The Infant Formula Act

Although not strictly a food safety issue, the Food, Drug and Cosmetic Act was amended again in 1980 with the Infant Formula Act. Because formulas are usually the sole source of nutrients for infants, it is critical that they provide all of the necessary nutrients. In 1979 a soy-based infant formula caused 120 infants to become ill from chloride deficiency. The act required infant formulas to contain specified levels of nutrients and to be processed under good manufacturing practices.

The Food Quality Protection Act (FQPA)

In August 1996 Congress signed into law the Food Quality Protection Act (FQPA). The new law amended the Federal Insecticide, Fungicide and Rodenticide Act (FIFRA) and the Food Drug and Cosmetic Act, fundamentally changing the way EPA regulates pesticides. Highlights of the FQPA are:

- Special Provisions for Infants and Children. EPA must make an explicit determination that tolerances are safe for children. Because little data exist on pesticide intake for children, an additional safety factor of up to 10-fold, if necessary, is to be used. In addition, consideration of children's special sensitivity and exposure to pesticide chemicals must be taken into account when setting tolerance levels.
- Tolerance Reevaluation. Requires that all existing tolerances be reviewed within 10 years to make sure they meet the requirements of the new health-based safety standard.
- Enforcement. Includes enhanced enforcement of pesticide residue standards by allowing FDA to impose civil penalties for tolerance violations.
- Pesticide Registration Renewal. Requires EPA to periodically review pesticide registrations, with a goal of establishing a 15-year cycle, to ensure that all pesticides meet updated safety standards.
- Health-Based Safety Standard for Pesticide Residues in Food. Most important, the new law establishes a health-based safety standard for pesticide residues in all foods. It uses "a reasonable certainty that no harm" will result from all combined sources of exposure, including drinking water, as the general safety standard.

This last facet of the FQPA is perhaps the most important because it eliminates the Delaney Clause of the Food, Drug and Cosmetic Act, which prohibited the addition of any cancer-causing substance, no matter how small the amount, to be added to foods.

Although the Delaney Clause appeared to be a reasonable law when it was proposed in 1958, advances in science and technology have made it obsolete. At the time it was written, laboratory methods could detect substances in parts per million. Analytical methods have improved to the extent that substances can be measured in parts per trillion or even parts per quadrillion. This means that it is now possible to detect amounts that are so small as to present no significant risk of human cancer. In addition to providing safe food, federal regulations aim to ensure that the United States has an abundant, varied, nutritious, and affordable food supply. If every chemical that caused cancer in test animals at one part per trillion were prohibited, our choice of foods would be severely limited (Pape 1982).

Hazard Analysis and Critical Control Points (HACCP)

The original Meat Inspection Act of 1906 relied on inspectors to use their eyes and nose to determine whether meat was safe. It has become obvious that this system is no longer effective with today's pathogens, bacteria so small that they can't be seen or smelled. An outbreak of *E. coli* 0157:H7 in hamburgers in the northwest United States in 1993 supplied a major impetus to change the current meat inspection system. In 1996 USDA issued its Pathogen Reduction: Hazard Analysis and Critical Control Points (HACCP) System rule. This rule requires that all 6,500 meat and poultry processing plants in the United States operate under an HACCP system.

HACCP started from a National Aeronautic and Space Administration (NASA) food safety program in the 1960s. NASA needed to ensure that the food astronauts consumed in space was safe and would not cause any ill effects. The U.S. Army Natick Laboratories, in conjunction with NASA, began to develop the foods needed for manned space exploration. They contracted with the Pillsbury Company to design and produce these first space foods. While Pillsbury struggled with certain problems, such as how to keep food from crumbling in zero gravity, it also undertook the task of coming as close as possible to 100 percent assurance that the foods they produced would be free of bacterial or viral pathogens. Traditional food quality control programs did not provide the degree of safety desired. Pillsbury discarded its standard quality control methods and began an extensive evaluation, in conjunction with NASA and Natick Labs, to evaluate food safety. They soon realized that to be successful they needed to have control over their process, raw materials, environment, and people. In 1971, they introduced HACCP as a preventive system that enables manufacturers to produce foods with a high degree of assurance that the foods were produced safely.

FDA began its own HACCP regulations in 1995 with the seafood industry by publishing the *Procedures for the Safe and Sanitary Processing and Importing of Fish and Fishery Products*, which mandated seafood processing facilities have in place an HACCP plan by 1997. Since then the agency has been expanding its use of HACCP. The FDA Food Code incorporates HACCP principles, and in 1998 FDA proposed HACCP controls for fruit and vegetable juices after several high-profile foodborne illness outbreaks from juice. FDA is experimenting with HACCP in other sectors of the food industry, working with companies who volunteer to develop pilot HACCP programs. The dairy industry is also moving towards an HACCP system.

The HACCP system identifies critical points during food processing where contamination is likely to occur. This allows food industry personnel to focus on these critical areas and put in place controls to prevent contamination. HACCP places primary responsibility for the safety of food on the food processing industry. The government's role is to verify that industry is carrying out its responsibility, and to initiate appropriate regulatory action if necessary. Meat, poultry, and seafood production and processing facilities must have an HACCP plan in place. Other parts of the food processing and retail food industry are also beginning to implement HACCP programs.

One of the key advantages of the HACCP concept is that it focuses on identifying and preventing hazards from contaminating food, thereby allowing for control in the manufacturing environment rather than after production. HACCP is a preventive, systematic approach to food safety, rather than a reactive method. It is a system based on sound science, and as such will evolve as science advances. It permits more efficient and effective government oversight, primarily because record keeping allows investigators to see how well a firm is complying with food safety laws over a given period, rather than how well it is doing on any given day. HACCP has international recognition as the most effective means of controlling foodborne disease. The joint Food and Agriculture Organization/World Health Organization Codex Alimentarius Commission and the U.S. National Advisory Committee on Microbiological Criteria for Foods (NACMCF) endorse its use.

HACCP involves seven principles:

- Analyze hazards. Identify potential hazards associated with a food and determine measures to control those hazards. The hazard could be biological, such as a microbe; chemical, such as a toxin; or physical, such as ground glass or metal fragments.
- Identify critical control points. These are points in a food's production—from its raw state through processing and shipping to consumption—at which it is possible to control or eliminate the potential hazard. Examples are cooking, cooling, packaging, and metal detection.
- Establish preventive measures with critical limits for each control point. For a cooked food, for example, this might include setting the minimum cooking temperature and time required to ensure the elimination of any harmful microbes.
- Establish procedures to monitor the critical control points. Such procedures might include determining how and by whom cooking time and temperature should be monitored.
- Establish corrective actions to be taken when monitoring shows that a critical limit has not been met. For example, reprocessing or disposing of food if the minimum cooking temperature is not met.
- Establish procedures to verify that the system is working properly. This could involve testing time and temperature recording devices to verify that a cooking unit is working properly.
- Establish effective record keeping to document the HACCP system. This includes maintaining records of hazards and their control methods, monitoring safety requirements, and taking action to correct potential problems. Each of these principles must be backed by sound scientific knowledge; for example, published microbiological studies on time and temperature factors for controlling foodborne pathogens.

WHO REGULATES FOOD SAFETY TODAY?

Regulating the entire food system is no easy task. Our food system has evolved from providing consumers with the basic ingredients that they use to prepare meals at home, to one that provides foods that are highly processed and require minimal preparation, are ready-to-eat, or come from abroad. It extends from farm to table starting with feed suppliers and producers on the farm; continuing to the shippers, processors, wholesalers, importers, and distributors in the middle; and ending with retailers, food preparers, and consumers. International in nature, it encompasses the food systems of other countries too. It is a complex, competitive, multilevel system involving legal, political, social, and economic forces.

The current system for regulating the safety of the food supply involves federal, state, and local governments with many interactions among them. These agencies set rules, standards, and processes to control risks to the food supply; guide or conduct research to apply modern science and technology to food safety problems and decisions; monitor risks in the food supply; conduct surveillance to monitor the effectiveness of food safety measures; and provide education to all those involved in the production, distribution, and handling of food (NRC 1998). Food inspectors, microbiologists, epidemiologists, and other food scientists working for city and county health departments, state public health agencies, and various federal departments and agencies continually monitor the food supply. Their precise duties are dictated by a complex and continually evolving set of local, state, and national laws; guidelines; and other directives.

Food Safety at the Federal Level

The federal part of the food safety system consists of a dozen departments and agencies implementing more that 35 statutes. Providing oversight on these statutes are 28 House and Senate committees. The main congressional committees responsible for food safety are the Agriculture Committee in the House of Representatives and the Agriculture, Nutrition, and Forestry Committee in the Senate. These committees aid Congress in passing legislation by interviewing agency personnel, holding public hearings to gather information and views from experts, and providing written reports to Congress summarizing the issues. The principal federal regulatory players are the Food and Drug Administration (FDA) of the Department of Health and Human Services (DHHS) and the Food Safety and Inspection Service (FSIS) of the U.S. Department of Agriculture (USDA). Together, FDA and FSIS receive more than 90 percent of the total funding and staffing in the federal food safety regulatory arena. However, other agencies do have important responsibilities in safeguarding the food we eat. Federal agencies are not engaged solely in the regulation of food safety. Most also have education and research components. All are vital links in the large network necessary to provide a safe and wholesome food supply.

Food and Drug Administration (FDA)

As part of the Department of Health and Human Services, FDA ensures that domestic and imported food products (except for most egg products and meat and poultry products) are safe, sanitary, nutritious, wholesome, and honestly labeled. It does this by monitoring the manufacture, importation, transport, storage, and sale of these products. While USDA regulates most meat and poultry products, FDA has responsibility for rabbit, dear, moose, buffalo, quail, and ratites (ostriches, emus, and rheas). Altogether FDA regulates about $570 billion worth of food products per year. The Food, Drug and Cosmetic Act; the Public Health Service Act; and the Egg Products Inspection Act govern FDA's food safety activities. Three main offices carry out FDA's food safety and quality activities—the Center for Food Safety and Applied Nutrition (CFSAN), the Center for Veterinary Medicine (CVM), and the Office of Regulatory Affairs (ORA). These offices share many of their duties. Although FDA carries out many food safety activities, some of the most important are:

- Inspect food processing plants and warehouses for compliance with regulations concerning sanitation, labeling, good manufacturing practices, and food standards. Inspectors collect and analyze food samples for physical, chemical, and microbial contamination. With 53,000 food establishments to inspect and only 800 inspectors, FDA inspects plants under its jurisdiction on average once every eight years. Some state agencies have cooperative agreements with FDA, bringing inspections of food processing plants in those states up to once every five years in 1995 (GAO March 1996). Manufacturers, who have a self-interest in producing safe food, are primarily responsible for the safety of their products. It is FDA's role to work with the food industry and to monitor it to see that it is meeting its responsibility. Manufacturers that produce foods that are potentially more hazardous are visited more frequently than those whose products are less likely to cause harm. For example, a plant that produces cheese would be visited more frequently than one producing pretzels.
- Inspect imported foods at airports, seaports, and other locations to make sure that this food meets U.S. standards.
- Review animal drugs for safety to animals that receive them, and to humans who eat food produced from the animals. Monitor the safety of animal feed (including pet food), making sure they are safe, effective, and properly labeled and manufactured.
- Work with state government agencies to provide technical assistance, conduct training programs for state and local inspectors, and evaluate state food safety programs. FDA produces the U.S. Food Code, a reference manual that provides food safety guidance for retail food establishments such as restaurants, cafeterias, vending machine operators, stores that sell food, hospitals, prisons, nursing homes, and other institutions. While it does not carry the weight of a law or regulation, it does promote a uniform system of regulation among the several thousand federal, state, and local agencies responsible for protecting the food supply.
- Collect and analyze samples of domestic and imported foods under its jurisdiction to ensure that they meet EPA pesticide residue tolerances.
- Regulate the bottled drinking water industry by requiring that bottled water be processed, packaged, transported, and stored under safe and sanitary conditions.
- Provide recommendations for establishing good food manufacturing practices and HACCP programs, through documents such as the *Guide to Minimize Microbial Food Safety Hazards for Fresh Fruits and Vegetables.*
- Approve all new food additives and review earlier decisions to ensure that those additives are still safe. This includes anything that might become part of food, such as coloring agents, preservatives, food packaging, and sanitizers.
- Monitor all domestic and imported seafood products to make sure they are wholesome, fit for human consumption, and processed and stored properly.
- In addition to its regulatory role, FDA carries out food safety research to improve the detection and prevention of contamination.
- Educate consumers and industry on safe food preparation practices.

U.S. Department of Agriculture (USDA)

The USDA Food Safety and Inspection Service (FSIS) regulates all raw beef, pork, lamb, goat, horse meat, chicken, turkey, duck, and goose, as well as approximately 250,000 different processed meat and poultry products, ensuring that they are safe, wholesome, and accurately labeled. In addition, FSIS is responsible for the safety of liquid, frozen, and dried egg products, while the FDA is responsible for whole eggs. FSIS regulates about $120 billion worth of food products a year. The main laws under which FSIS operates are the Federal Meat Inspection Act, the Poultry Products Inspection Act, and the Egg Products Inspection Act. Among duties performed by FSIS are:

- Inspect meat and poultry slaughter and processing plants. Approximately 8,000 FSIS inspectors inspect some 6,500 meat and poultry plants on a continuous basis. They visually examine more than six billion poultry carcasses and 125 million livestock carcasses each year for diseases that can affect safety and quality.
- Develop food safety guidance on food safety procedures for the meat and poultry industry by publishing documents such as generic HACCP models, Sanitation Standard Operating Procedures (SSOPs), and the HACCP Based Inspection Reference Guide; and by operating a microbiological baseline data collection program, a technical service center, and an HACCP hotline for inspectors.
- Certify that all foreign meat and poultry processing plants exporting products to the United States operate under an inspection system that is equivalent to the U.S. system.
- Ensure that state meat and poultry inspection programs are at least equal to the federal program.
- Work with the animal production community to develop science-based food safety practices that will reduce the risk of chemical, microbiological, and physical hazards in the food supply.
- Educate consumers and industry on safe food preparation practices.

Several other agencies within USDA play a role in food safety. Although the Animal and Plant Health Inspection Service (APHIS) has no regulatory food safety authority, some of its programs do affect food safety. It is responsible for the health of animals and plants from diseases and pests, some of which, such as brucellosis and bovine spongiform encephalopathy (BSE), could affect human health. The Agricultural Marketing Service (AMS) is responsible for establishing standards of quality (as opposed to safety) and for the grading of egg, dairy, fruit, vegetable, meat, and poultry products. AMS also inspects egg product processing plants to ensure that egg products are wholesome, unadulterated, and truthfully labeled. The Grain Inspection, Packer and Stockyard Administration (GIPSA) inspects rice and grains for quality and aflatoxin contamination. It also develops and shares information with other agencies about chemical residue levels in grains. Another agency that plays an important role, although not a regulatory one, is the Agricultural Research Service (ARS). As the principal research agency for USDA, ARS conducts food safety research in support of FSIS's inspection and education programs. As an example, FSIS relied on research conducted by ARS scientists to determine whether it is safe to recommend cooking hamburgers until they are no longer pink. As it turns out, due to premature browning, some hamburgers turn brown before they reach a safe temperature. The Cooperative State Research, Education, and Extension Service (CSREES) works with U.S. colleges and universities to develop research and education programs on food safety for farmers, industry, retail, and consumers.

Environmental Protection Agency (EPA)

The Environmental Protection Agency's main food safety regulatory actions are in the area of pesticides and drinking water. Two offices are responsible for these areas—the Office of Pesticide Programs and the Office of Water. EPA's regulatory functions are guided by the Federal Food, Drug and Cosmetic Act; the Federal Insecticide, Fungicide and Rodenticide Act; the Safe Drinking Water Act; and the Food Quality Protection Act. EPA activities include:

- Determining safety of new pesticides, establishing maximum allowable pesticide residue levels on food for human and animal consumption, and publishing directions on safe use of pesticides.
- Regulating toxic substances and wastes to prevent their entry into the environment and food chain.
- Establishing safe drinking water standards.
- Assisting the more than 170,000 public water systems in the United States with monitoring the quality of drinking water and finding ways to prevent its contamination.

Centers for Disease Control and Prevention (CDC)

The Centers for Disease Control and Prevention, as part of the Department of Health and Human Services, is charged with protecting the nation's public health. Most of CDC's food safety work is in the area of surveillance of foodborne disease rather than in the regulatory arena. CDC is guided by the Public Health Service Act. CDC's food safety activities include:

- Investigating sources of foodborne disease outbreaks with local, state, and other federal officials to determine contributing factors.
- Maintaining a nationwide system for reporting foodborne disease outbreaks and working with other federal and state agencies to monitor rates of and trends in outbreaks. This includes designing and putting in place rapid, electronic systems for reporting foodborne illnesses.
- Developing and advocating public health policies to prevent foodborne disease.
- Conducting research to help prevent foodborne illness.
- Training local and state food safety personnel.

National Marine Fisheries Service (NMFS)

The National Marine Fisheries Service is part of the Department of Commerce. Although FDA is primarily responsible for ensuring the safety of seafood products, NMFS conducts a voluntary seafood inspection and grading program that focuses on marketing and quality attributes of fish and shellfish. Unlike other federal inspection programs, industry pays for this inspection system since it is voluntary. The program covers about 20 percent of the seafood consumed annually in the United States. The primary legislative authority for NMFS's inspection program comes from the Agricultural Marketing Act of 1946 and the Fish and Wildlife Act of 1956. If contracted to provide services, NMFS can:

- Inspect and certify fishing vessels, seafood processing plants, and retail facilities for federal sanitation standards.
- Evaluate seafood products for general condition, wholesomeness, and proper grading and labeling.
- Test products for species identification, contamination, and decomposition.

Federal Trade Commission (FTC)

The Federal Trade Commission enforces the Federal Trade Commission Act, which prohibits unfair or deceptive practices in advertising. Examples of cases that have come under FTC jurisdiction are false advertising claims for devices that test fresh produce for pesticide residues, and claims for a home test kit for food impurities.

U.S. Customs Service

The Customs Service of the U.S. Treasury Department administers the Tariff Act of 1930 and other related laws, ensuring that all goods entering and exiting the United States do so according to U.S. laws and regulations. In this role it assists FSIS and FDA in their regulatory responsibilities.

Bureau of Alcohol, Tobacco and Firearms (ATF)

The Bureau of Alcohol, Tobacco and Firearms, also a part of the U.S. Treasury Department, enforces food safety laws governing production, labeling, and distribution of alcoholic beverages. It has primary federal responsibility for ensuring the safety of alcoholic beverages and also investigates cases of adulterated alcoholic products, sometimes with help from the FDA.

National Institutes of Health (NIH)

NIH has no regulatory function, but it does contribute to food safety research. Although it does not have a research program specifically for food safety, it does conduct research on foodborne diseases as part of its overall mission to understand disease processes in humans and to improve human health. Much of the research relating to how microorganisms cause foodborne diseases has resulted from NIH-sponsored research.

Food Safety at the State and Local Levels

State and local government agencies are also vital players on the nation's food safety team. They include more than 3,000 city, county, tribal and state health, agriculture, and environmental protection agencies (NRC 1998). They inspect and issue licenses to restaurants, grocery stores, and other retail food establishments, as well as dairy farms, milk processing plants, grain mills, and food manufacturing plants within their local jurisdictions. In many states the regulatory authority is split between the state agriculture and health departments. State and local governments investigate foodborne illnesses within their jurisdictions in conjunction with the CDC.

The federal government aids state and local agencies to ensure the safety of food produced and sold within local jurisdictions. States may choose to operate their own interstate meat and/or poultry inspection programs instead of using federal inspection, and are responsible for meat and poultry inspection for products sold within state boundaries. FSIS monitors the process to be sure that state inspection programs are at least equal to federal programs. If states do not have their own inspection programs, FSIS handles meat and poultry inspection. Many states have their own fish inspection programs. States may adopt all or part of the FDA Food Code as part of their state regulations for retail food establishments. Some states and tribal authorities have adopted some parts of different editions of the Food Code, but uniformity in Food Code adoption is lacking. Each state has its own set of regulations, which vary from state to state. Unlike the Food Code, all 50 states, the District of

Columbia, and United States trust territories have adopted the Grade A Pasteurized Milk Ordinance. This ordinance, created by public and private entities in 1924 to develop effective programs for preventing milkborne disease, is the national standard for milk sanitation.

Food Safety at the International Level

Several international organizations interact to improve the safety of the world's food supply. The Food and Agricultural Organization (FAO) was founded as part of the United Nations in 1945 to raise levels of nutrition and standards of living, to improve agricultural productivity, and to better the condition of people in rural areas. Food safety is an important part of FAO's mission since foodborne disease is one of the most widespread threats to human health, as well as an important cause of reduced economic productivity. The World Health Organization (WHO), founded in 1948, has as its mission to set global standards of health and to aid governments in strengthening national health programs. WHO recognizes that protecting consumers from contaminants and preventing foodborne diseases are two of the most important strategies for overcoming malnutrition in the world. WHO's activity in food safety issues centers around development of national food safety policies and infrastructures, food legislation and enforcement, food safety education, promotion of food technologies, food safety in urban settings and in tourism, surveillance of foodborne diseases, and monitoring of chemical contaminants in food. FAO and WHO collaborate on many food safety issues as joint FAO/WHO committees and conferences.

One of the most important joint FAO/WHO commissions is the Codex Alimentarius Commission. This body's task is the development of uniform food standards that can be used by governments throughout the world. This food code is known as the Codex Alimentarius. The name comes from a collection of standards and product descriptions developed by the Austro-Hungarian Empire between 1897 and 1911 that was called the Codex Alimentarius Austriacus. The present-day Codex Alimentarius consists of food standards for commodities, codes of practice for hygiene and technology, pesticide evaluations and limits for pesticide residues, evaluations of food additives, guidelines for contaminants, and evaluations of veterinary drugs. Although the main goal of the Codex is to set uniform regulatory standards in the interests of international trade, it has also served to raise food safety standards in many countries. One hundred forty member nations accept its standards and follow its codes of practice. The Codex is the preferred international reference for ensuring fair practices in the sale of food and for facilitating international trade in food. The Codex Alimentarius Commission also generates scientific texts, convenes numerous expert committees and consultations, and holds international meetings. The U.S. Codex office is at the USDA Food Safety and Inspection Service in Washington, D.C.

The World Trade Organization (WTO), created in 1995, also plays a role in food safety, as it is the main body that deals with rules of trade between nations. WTO replaced the General Agreement of Tariffs and Trade (GATT), which has since been incorporated into WTO agreements. Much of international trade involves food. WTO recognizes the Codex as the international standard of reference, and uses it to establish much of its legal ground rules for international commerce and trade policy. Other trade agreements such as the North American Free Trade Agreement (NAFTA) also work to harmonize food safety standards and regulations as a way of promoting international trade.

WHAT IS THE FEDERAL GOVERNMENT DOING ABOUT FOOD SAFETY NOW?

President's Food Safety Initiative

In January 1997 President Clinton announced a national Food Safety Initiative (FSI) designed to reduce the incidence of foodborne illness to the greatest extent possible. He directed three of his Cabinet members—the Secretary of Agriculture, the Secretary of Health and Human Services, and the Administrator of the Environmental Protection Agency—to consult with consumers, producers, industry, states, universities, and the public, and to report back to him in 90 days. The resulting report, *Food Safety from Farm to Table: A National Food Safety Initiative*, while recognizing that our food supply is among the safest in the world, acknowledges that changes in consumers and their lifestyles, the food system itself, and pathogens require a change in methods to protect the food supply. It addresses food safety hazards that present the greatest risk, how to make the best of limited resources, how to increase coordination between public and private organizations, and how to improve coordination within and between government agencies. (NRC 1998) Areas of emphasis in the President's Food Safety Initiative are:

- Improve inspections and expand preventive safety measures. The main activities under this area relate to mandating the HACCP system for the seafood industry and for meat and poultry processing plants. FDA's Food Code also incorporates HACCP principles to give guidance to state and local inspectors of retail food service establishments. In addition, FDA is proposing HACCP regulations for other parts of the food industry, especially for fruit and vegetable juices.
- Increase research to develop new tests to detect foodborne pathogens and to assess risks in the food supply. Some pathogens, like the hepatitis A virus and *Cyclospora cayetanensis*, cannot now be detected in many foods because of the lack of laboratory methods to do so. Two new entities were created to ensure that sound science is the basis for regulatory decisions the Joint Institute for Food Safety and Applied Nutrition (JIFSAN) and the Joint Institute for Food Safety Research (JIFSR).
- JIFSAN, created in 1996, is a cooperative program between FDA and the University of Maryland. Scientists at JIFSAN will research a wide range of food safety issues, including food composition, toxins and microbial pathogens, animal drug residues, and animal health. JIFSAN is also home to the Food Safety Risk Analysis Clearinghouse, which provides data and information on aspects of risk analysis as it pertains to food safety. This institute joins a similar FDA cooperative program developed in 1988, the National Center for Food Safety and Technology (NCFST), in Summit-Argo, Illinois. This consortium of government, industry, and academia is financially supported by FDA and the Illinois Institute of Technology, the IIT Research Institute, and the University of Illinois. It focuses on the safety of food processing and packaging technologies, applied microbiology, and Hazard Analysis and Critical Control Points (HACCP) food safety programs.
- The second newly created entity under the President's Food Safety Initiative, JIFSR, was created in 1999 to coordinate federally funded food safety research and to foster effective translation of research results into practice along the farm-to-table continuum. The Department of Health and Human Services and the U.S. Department of Agriculture will have joint leadership of the institute.
- Build a national early warning system to detect and respond to outbreaks of foodborne illness earlier, and to obtain data needed to prevent future outbreaks. FoodNet and PulseNet are the main components of this food safety surveillance system. The FoodNet surveillance program tracks cases of foodborne disease to determine the frequency and severity of

foodborne illness and to determine which foods are most responsible. FoodNet is discussed in chapter 5 of this book.

- PulseNet is a national electronic network of public health laboratories and the CDC that performs DNA "fingerprinting" on bacteria suspected of causing a foodborne outbreak. This technology uses pulsed-field gel electrophoresis (PFGE) to subtype isolates so they can be compared. Samples from ill persons and from food are compared to determine if they are from the same source. State laboratories can quickly compare local samples with samples from the national database via the Internet. PulseNet helps public health authorities recognize when cases of foodborne illness occurring at the same time in different locations are caused by the same strain of bacteria, and may be due to a common food item. This information is then communicated rapidly nationwide to help trace outbreaks in order to remove contaminated foods from the marketplace. In 1996 epidemiologists traced an outbreak of *E. coli* O157:H7 infections in patients from four states and one Canadian province to commercial unpasteurized apple juice. DNA "fingerprinting" by the Washington State public health laboratory showed that isolates from patients and the apple juice were the same strain. Prompt recognition of the commercial apple juice as the source of this outbreak allowed rapid recall of the widely distributed product, and, as a result, fewer people became ill from it.
- Establish national education campaigns that will improve food handling in homes, schools, and retail outlets. Federal agencies are partnering with the private and other public sectors on a number of projects to raise public awareness of safe food practices. FDA, USDA, and the National Science Teachers Association produced a new food science supplemental curriculum aimed at middle and high school students. Students learn the significance of bacteria in foodborne illness and methods to reduce related health risks. FDA and the American Association of Retired Persons (AARP) developed information for seniors on food safety. Federal agencies joined the restaurant and food service industry in celebrating National Food Safety Education Month (NFSEM). Each September NFSEM focuses public attention on foodborne illness and safe food handling practices that consumers and commercial food workers can follow to stay healthy. The National Food Safety Information Network, formed in 1998 by FDA and USDA, brings together the USDA Meat and Poultry Hotline, FDA Outreach and Information Center, USDA/FDA Foodborne Illness Education Information Center, FoodSafety.gov Web site, National Food Safety Educator's Network (EdNet), and Foodsafe discussion group as the federal government's primary mechanisms for providing food safety information to the public. The federal agencies combined to form public awareness campaigns alerting consumers to the risk that raw sprouts and unpasteurized or untreated juices may present to vulnerable populations. Federal agencies, industry associations, academia, state/local regulatory associations, and consumer representatives established the Food Safety Training and Education Alliance (FSTEA) for Retail, Food Service, Vending, Institutions and Regulators. This group is working to promote training of government and industry employees in retail food service.
- The most visible education component of the Food Safety Initiative is the Fight BAC! campaign, a public-private partnership consisting of industry, producer and consumer groups, federal and state agencies, and academia. Fight BAC! combines the resources of all these groups to conduct a broad-based food safety education program designed to reach men, women, and children of all ages. The Partnership for Food Safety Education uses public opinion research, professional advertising and marketing strategies, and expert scientific and technical review to develop campaign concepts, messages and graphics that are accurate, understandable, and persuasive. The campaign centers on BAC!, a big, mean, green bacteria character who serves as the official "spokescum" to put a "face" on invisible foodborne bacteria. The partnership has developed food safety curricula, games, calendars, T-shirts, mugs, aprons, patches, magnets, and a BAC! puppet to get its message out.
- Strengthen coordination and improve efficiency among USDA, CDC, FDA, and EPA to improve responses to foodborne illness outbreaks. One of this area's major programs be-

gan in May 1998 with the creation of the Food Outbreak Response Coordinating Group (FORC-G). FORC-G links federal, state, and local government agencies to improve coordination, use resources more efficiently, prepare for new and emerging threats to the food supply, and measure progress towards the common goal of reducing foodborne illness.

- Ensure the safety of domestic and imported fruits and vegetables. FDA and USDA have developed guidance on good agricultural and manufacturing practices for use by both domestic and foreign growers to improve the safety of produce sold to American consumers. FDA is increasing its international food inspection force to inspect food safety conditions abroad and at points where foreign produce enters the U.S. market. Produce that is not produced under standards that are comparable to those in the United States will not be allowed to enter the country.

Healthy People 2010

Healthy People is a national health promotion and disease prevention initiative that brings together national, state, and local government agencies; nonprofit, voluntary, and professional organizations; businesses; communities; and individuals to improve the health of all Americans, eliminate disparities in health, and improve quality of life. It is a statement of national health objectives designed to identify the most significant preventable threats to health and to establish national goals to reduce these threats. Healthy People provides objectives in a format that enables diverse groups to combine their efforts and work as a team. The objectives are reviewed and renewed every 10 years. Overall the Healthy People 2010 goals are to:

1. Increase quality and years of healthy life.
2. Eliminate health disparities.

Food safety is a focus area within Healthy People 2010 with its own set of seven goals, which are:

1. Reduce infections caused by key foodborne pathogens. For those microorganisms that have baseline data on number of infections, the goal is to reduce those rates by half, as shown in Table 4-1. For those that do not have baseline data, part of the goal is to collect that data.
2. Reduce outbreaks of infections caused by key foodborne bacteria. The goal is to reduce the number of outbreaks of *Escherichia coli* O157: H7 and *Salmonella* serotype Enteritidis by half (see Table 4-2).
3. Prevent an increase in the proportion of isolates of *Salmonella* species from humans and animals that are resistant to antimicrobial drugs.
4. Reduce deaths from anaphylaxis caused by food allergies. Currently there are no accurate statistics on the number of those who die from food allergies.
5. Increase the proportion of consumers who follow key food safety practices. The target is to increase by 10 percent from an estimated 72 percent to 79 percent those who follow food safety practices.
6. Improve food employee behaviors and food preparation practices that directly relate to foodborne illnesses in retail food establishments. No data yet exist for this goal.
7. Reduce human exposure to organophosphate pesticides from food. No data yet exist for this goal.

Healthy People 2010 also has two goals for water quality:

1. Increase the proportion of persons served by community water systems who receive a supply of drinking water that meets the regulations of the Safe Drinking Water Act. The current baseline is 73 percent; the 2010 goals aim to increase that to 95 percent.
2. Reduce waterborne disease outbreaks from drinking water among persons served by community water systems. Currently an estimated six outbreaks per year originate from community water systems. The goal is to decrease that to two outbreaks per year.

Table 4-1
Reduction in Infections Caused by Microorganisms (cases per 100,000 population)

	1997 Baseline	2010 Target
Campylobacter species	24.6	12.3
Escherichia coli O157:H7	2.1	1.0
Listeria monocytogenes	0.5	0.25
Salmonella species	13.7	6.8
Cyclospora cayetanenis	n/a	n/a
Postdiarrheal hemolytic uremic syndrome	n/a	n/a
Congenital *Toxoplasma gondii*	n/a	n/a

Table 4-2
Reduction in Infections Caused by *E. coli* 0157:H7 and *Salmonella enteritidis* (number of outbreaks per year)

	1997 Baseline	2010 Target
Escherichia coli O157:H7	22	11
Salmonella serotype Enteritidis	44	22

Dietary Guidelines for Americans

The Dietary Guidelines for Americans, sponsored by the U.S. Department of Health and Human Services and the U.S. Department of Agriculture, serve as the central dietary guidance for Americans. The federal government has issued nutrition and diet recommendations in one form or another to the American public since 1916. However, the year 2000 Dietary Guidelines for Americans are the first federal guidelines to include any recommendation about food safety. In it consumers are advised to:

- Clean. Wash hands and food surfaces often.
- Separate. Separate raw, cooked, and ready-to-eat foods while shopping, preparing, or storing.
- Cook. Cook foods to a safe temperature.
- Chill. Refrigerate perishable foods promptly.
- Follow the label.
- Serve safely.
- If in doubt, throw it out.

SOURCES

Anonymous. *Deadly Adulteration and Slow Poisoning Unmasked; or, Disease and Death in the Pot and the Bottle; in Which the Blood-empoisoning and Life-destroying Adulterations of Wines, Spirits, Beer, Bread, Flour, Tea, Sugar, Spices, Cheese-mongery, Pastry, Confectionary Medicines, &c. &c. &c. Are Laid Open to the Public with Tests or Methods for the Ascertaining and Detecting the Fraudulent and Deleterious Adulterations and the Good and Bad Qualities of Those Articles: With an Expose of Medical Empiricism and Imposture, Quacks and Quackery, Regular and Irregular, Legitimate and Illegitimate: and the Frauds and Mal-practices of the Pawn-brokers and Madhouse Keepers.* 1939. New ed. London: Sherwood, Gilbert and Piper.

deForest Lamb, Ruth. 1936. *American Chamber of Horrors.* New York: Farrar and Rinehart.

Environmental Protection Agency Office of Water. http://www.epa.gov/watrhome/.

Federal Food and Drugs Act of 1906 (The "Wiley Act"). Public Law 59–384 34 Stat. 768. 1906. http://www.fda.gov/opacom/laws/wileyact.htm.

Food and Agriculture Organization of the United Nations. 1999. *Understanding the Codex Alimentarius.* Rome: FAO/WHO. http://www.fao.org/docrep/w9114e/w9114e00.htm.

Halsall, Paul. 1988. *Internet Medieval Source Book.* http://www.fordham.edu/halsall/source/judgepillory.html.

Hutt, Peter Barton, and Peter Barton Hutt II. 1984. A History of Government Regulation of Adulteration and Misbranding of Food. *Food Drug Cosmetic Law Journal* 39: 2–73.

National Research Council (NRC). 1998. *Ensuring Safe Food: From Production to Consumption.* Washington: National Academy Press.

International Food Information Council (IFIC). Date unknown. *Food Safety and Foodborne Illness.* Washington: International Food Information Council. http://ificinfo.health.org/backgrnd/bkgr10.htm.

Janssen, Wallace F. December 1981–January 1982. The Squad that Ate Poison. *FDA Consumer* 15(10): 6–11.

Janssen, W. F. 1982. The Food and Drug Administration and the Consumer. In *Consumer Activists: They Made a Difference: A History of Consumer Action Related by Leaders in the Consumer Movement.* Mount Vernon, NY: Consumers Union Foundation.

Marmion, Daniel M. 1991. *Handbook of U.S. Colorants: Foods, Drugs, Cosmetics, and Medical Devices.* 3rd ed. New York: Wiley.

Pape, S. M. 1982. Legislative Issues in Food Safety Regulation. In *Social Regulation: Strategies for Reform.* Edited by Eugene Bardach and Robert A. Kagan. San Francisco: Institute for Contemporary Studies.

Rawson, Jean M., and Donna U. Vogt. 1998. *Food Safety Agencies and Authorities: A Primer.* Congressional Research Service report for Congress; 98–91 ENR. Washington: Congressional Research Service. http://www.cnie.org/nle/ag-40.html.

Schultz, H. W. 1981. *Food Law Handbook.* Westport, CT: AVI.

Shumsky, Michael. September 12, 1997. *Government Regulatory Policy and the Struggle for Meat Inspection, 1879–1906.* http://www.fas.harvard.edu/~shumsky/inspection.html.

Thonney, P. F., and C. A. Bisogni. 1992. Government Regulation of Food Safety: Interaction of Scientific and Societal Forces. *Food Technology* 46(1): 73–80.

U.S. Department of Health and Human Services. 2000. Healthy People 2010. http://www.health.gov/healthypeople/.

U.S. Food and Drug Administration (FDA). December 14, 1998. *Food Safety Initiative Education Component.* http://www.foodsafety.gov/~dms/fs-ltr03.html.

U.S. Food and Drug Administration (FDA). September 24, 1998. *Food Safety: A Team Approach.* http://vm.cfsan.fda.gov/~lrd/foodteam.html.

U.S. Food and Drug Administration (FDA). 1981. The Story of the Laws behind the Labels. Part I: 1906 Food and Drugs Act. *FDA Consumer* June 1981. http://vm.cfsan.fda.gov/~lrd/history1.html.

U.S. General Accounting Office (GAO). March 1996. *Food Safety: New Initiatives Would Fundamentally Alter the Existing System.* GAO/RED-96-81. Washington: U.S. General Accounting Office.

U.S. General Accounting Office (GAO). 1990. *Food Safety and Quality: Who Does What in the Federal Government.* GAO/RED-91-19A(B). Washington: U.S. General Accounting Office.

U.S. General Accounting Office (GAO). 1996. *Other Agencies that Play a Role in the Food Supply.* Washington: U.S. General Accounting Office.

Vetter, James L. 1996. *Food Laws and Regulations.* Manhattan, KS: American Institute of Baking.

Wodicka, V. O. 1996. Regulation of Food: Where Have We Been? *Food Technology* 50(3): 106–109.

CHAPTER 5

FOOD SAFETY STATISTICS

One of the hardest questions to answer about water—or foodborne illness—is, "How many people become ill?" This chapter examines why this question is difficult to answer, and then looks at some of the surveillance programs in place to gather information. Data from the following sources are summarized:

1. Foodborne Diseases Active Surveillance Network (FoodNet), a surveillance program to estimate the total number of people who become ill from foodborne illnesses.
2. CDC Surveillance For Foodborne-disease Outbreaks 1993–1997, which counts reported foodborne outbreaks and cases.
3. Waterborne Disease Outbreaks 1997–1998, which counts reported waterborne outbreaks and cases.

The latest data on medical costs of foodborne illness are presented. Food safety educators are interested in knowing what food safety behaviors people practice or don't practice. To this end, data from the Behavorial Risk Factor Surveillance Systems and Home Food Safety Survey are examined.

How many Americans become ill and/or die from foodborne or waterborne illness? Where are they getting sick and what behaviors cause them to become ill? How much does this cost society? While these sound like simple questions, finding the answers is fraught with difficulties. Any answers are at best an estimate based on a number of assumptions. However, it is important to have accurate statistics on water—and foodborne illness and pathogens to guide efforts at prevention and to assess the effectiveness of food safety regulations.

Several factors complicate the gathering of these statistics. The vast majority of foodborne and waterborne illness episodes are not reported. For an episode to be reported, and thus counted, several things must happen. First, the ill person must seek medical care. This does not happen unless the illness is severe. Most people pass off a case of diarrhea or vomiting as the "24-hour flu" or, even if they do attribute it to something they ate, still do not seek medical attention. It is estimated that for *Salmonella*, a bacterium that typically causes non-bloody diarrhea, for every case that is reported, 38 cases are not reported. For *E. coli* O157:H7, which causes a more severe bloody diarrhea, the estimation is 20 unreported cases for each case reported (Mead 1999). Second, if the person does seek medical care, the health care provider must obtain a specimen for laboratory testing. Third, the laboratory must perform the correct diagnostic test. And, finally, the health care provider must report the illness and/or laboratory results to public health officials. This chain of events is often broken somewhere along the line.

Many foodborne pathogens are also spread though water or from person to person, so it is difficult to assess whether the illness is foodborne. Some pathogens such as *Bacillus cereus* and *Clostridium perfringens* are spread exclusively through food, while the parasites *Cryptosporidium parvum* and *Giardia lamblia* are only transmitted by a food source 10 percent of the time. Finally, some foodborne illness is caused by pathogens or agents that have not yet been identified, and thus cannot be diagnosed. Major pathogens such as *Campylobacter jejuni, Escherichia coli* O157:H7, *Listeria monocytogenes*, and *Cyclospora cayetanensis* were either unknown or not even associated with foodborne illness 20 years ago.

Table 5-1 lists numbers of estimated illnesses and deaths for cases in which the pathogen is known. For many reported foodborne illness cases the pathogen is not determined. Adding together known pathogens and unknown agents, current estimates of foodborne illness in the United States are 76 million cases, 325,000 hospitalizations, and 5,194 deaths from foodborne pathogens per year. In cases when the pathogen is identified, bacteria cause 30 percent of foodborne illnesses, parasites 3 percent, and viruses 67 percent. But as far as deaths are concerned, bacteria cause 72 percent of the deaths attributable to foodborne illness, parasites 21 percent, and viruses 7 percent. While viruses cause a lot of illness, the case fatality rate, or number of sick people who die, is very low. Fatality rates for two bacteria are particularly high; for *Listeria* 20 percent of the people may die, and for *Vibrio vulnificus* 39 percent. Just six pathogens account for over 90 percent of the deaths associated with foodborne illness: *Salmonella* (31 percent), *Listeria* (28 percent), *Toxoplasma* (21 percent), Norwalk-like viruses (7 percent), *Campylobacter* (5 percent), and *E. coli* (3 percent). According to FoodNet data from the year 1996–97, each person in the United States suffers 1.4 episodes of diarrhea per year. With a U.S. population of 267.7 million persons, that adds up to 375 million episodes per year, many of them related to eating unsafe food.

FOODBORNE DISEASES ACTIVE SURVEILLANCE NETWORK (FOODNET)

FoodNet is a surveillance program for foodborne diseases that aims to determine the frequency and severity of foodborne illness; to determine how much foodborne illness results from eating specific foods such as meat, poultry, and eggs; and to describe the epidemiology of new and emerging bacterial, parasitic, and viral foodborne pathogens. Established in 1995, it is managed collaboratively by the Centers for Disease Control and Prevention (CDC), the U.S. Department of Agriculture (USDA), the U.S. Food and Drug Administration (FDA), and eight state sites. The participating states are Minnesota, Oregon, Georgia, and selected counties in California, Connecticut, Maryland, New York, and Tennessee. In all, FoodNet covers 29 million persons, or 11 percent of the American population. Comparison of data from year to year will give scientists a clearer picture of foodborne diseases and will lead to new prevention strategies for addressing the public health problem of foodborne illness. Scientists and regulators also use the data to

Table 5-1
Estimated Illnesses and Deaths Caused by Known Foodborne Pathogens, U.S.

	Illnesses			Deaths		
Disease or agent	Total	Food-borne	% of total foodborne	Total	Food-borne	% of total foodborne
Bacterial						
Bacillus cereus	27,360	27,360	0.2	0	0	0.0
Botulism. foodborne	58	58	0.0	4	4	0.2
Brucella spp.	1,554	777	0.0	11	6	0.3
Camplyobacter spp.	2,453,926	1,963,141	14.2	124	99	5.5
Clostridium perfringens	248,520	248,520	1.8	7	7	0.4
Escherichia coli O157:H7	73,480	62,458	0.5	61	52	2.9
E. coli. non-O157 STEC	36,740	31,229	0.2	30	26	1.4
E. coli. enterotoxigenic	79,420	55,594	0.4	0	0	0.0
E. coli. other diarrheogenic	79,420	23,826	0.2	0	0	0.0
Listeria monocytogenes	2,518	2,493	0.0	504	499	27.6
Salmonella typhi	824	659	0.0	3	3	0.1
Salmonella nontyphoidal	1,412,498	1,341,873	9.7	582	553	30.6
Shigella spp.	448,240	89,648	0.6	70	14	0.8
Staphylococcus food poisoning	185,060	185,060	1.3	2	2	0.1
Strephtococcus foodborne	50,920	50,920	0.4	0	0	0.0
Vibrio cholerae toxigenic	54	49	0.0	0	0	0.0
V. vulnificus	94	47	0.0	37	18	1.0
Vibrio, other	7,880	5,122	0.0	20	13	0.7
Yersinia enterocolitica	96,368	86,731	0.6	3	2	0.1
Subtotal	5,204,934	4,175,565	30.2	1,458	1,297	71.7
Parasitic						
Cryptosporidium parvum	300,000	30,000	0.2	66	7	0.4
Cyclospora cayetanenis	16,264	14,638	0.1	0	0	0.0
Giardia lamblia	2,000,000	200,000	1.4	10	1	0.1
Toxoplasma gondii	225,000	112,500	0.8	750	375	20.7
Trichinella spiralis	52	52	0.0	0	0	0.0
Subtotal	2,541,316	357,190	2.6	827	383	21.2
Viral						
Norwalk-like viruses	23,000,000	9,200,000	66.6	310	124	6.9
Rotavirus	3,900,000	39,000	0.3	30	0	0.0
Astrovirus	3,900,000	39,000	0.3	10	0	0.0
Hepatitis A	83,391	4,170	0.0	83	4	0.2
Subtotal	30,833,391	9,282,170	67.2	433	129	7.1
Grand Total	38,629,641	13,814,924	100.0	2,718	1,809	100

Source: Paul S. Mead, Laurence Slutsker, Vance Dietz, Linda F. McCaig, Joseph S. Bresee, Craig Shapiro, Patricia M. Griffin, and Robert V. Tauxe. 1999. Food-Related Illness and Death in the United States. *Emerging Infectious Diseases.* Vol. 5(5). http://www.cdc.gov/ncidod/eid/vol5no5/mead.htm

assess the effectiveness of food safety regulations in decreasing the number of cases of foodborne diseases in the United States each year.

Most systems for reporting foodborne illness statistics are passive systems, that is, they rely on clinical labs to report cases of foodborne illness to state health departments, which then report to CDC. Only a fraction of cases are actually reported through these passive surveillance systems. FoodNet is an active surveillance system, meaning that its investigators regularly contact clinical laboratories to find new cases of foodborne diseases. This ongoing active surveillance allows public health officials to better understand the epidemiology of foodborne diseases—who gets ill, how ill they get, what foods are most likely to cause illness, what times of the year foodborne illnesses are more common, and which pathogens cause illness.

Even cases reported through active surveillance represent only a fraction of the cases that occur in the community. To better estimate the total number of foodborne illness cases, FoodNet consists of five components as shown in the foodborne diseases pyramid in Figure 5-1:

Figure 5-1
FoodNet Pyramid

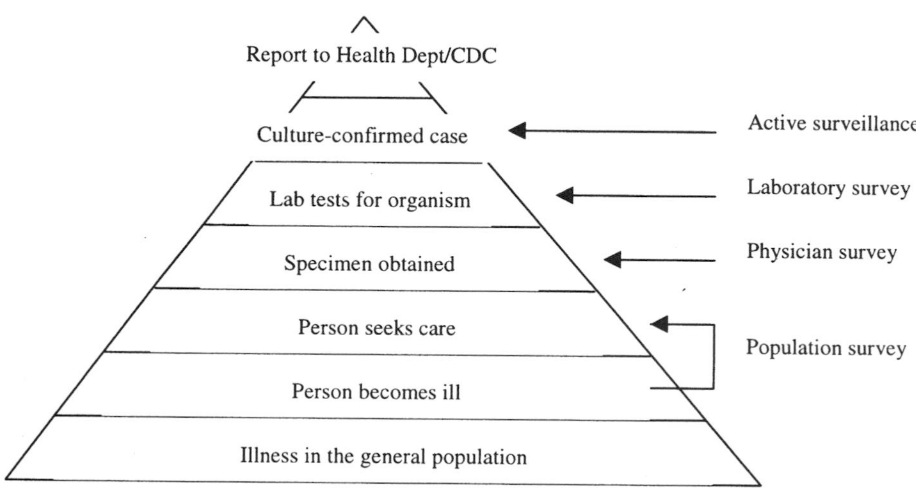

Source: Centers for Disease Control and Prevention. March 14, 2000. What Is FoodNet? http://www.cdc.gov/foodnet/what_is.htm.

1. Active surveillance. Investigators contact clinical laboratories that test stool samples in the participating sites to find cases of laboratory-confirmed cases of foodborne illness. Pathogens monitored are *Campylobacter*, *E. coli* O157:H7, *Listeria*, *Salmonella*, *Shigella*, *Vibrio*, *Yersinia*, *Cyclospora*, and *Cryptosporidium*. Rates of *Campylobacter* were higher than expected, especially in California.
2. Laboratory survey. Investigators collect information on the methods laboratories use to collect and examine specimens. Practices in clinical laboratories vary, and this can have an effect on whether the laboratory finds disease-causing bacteria. Results from this survey will assist in developing standard guidelines for laboratories to use in testing samples.
3. Physician survey. Because laboratories test stool specimens from a patient only upon the request of a physician or other health care provider, it is important to measure how often and under what circumstances health care providers order these tests. Results from this survey will allow investigators to estimate the proportion of health care providers who order a bacterial stool sample when a patient comes in with diarrheal illness.

4. Population survey. Investigators randomly contact residents in each site by telephone every month to ask if the person had recent diarrheal illness, whether he or she sought medical attention for the illness, and whether he or she consumed certain foods that have been associated with foodborne illness. This helps to determine what percentage of people who become ill with diarrhea seek medical care. Since most do not, this estimate is crucial to estimating foodborne disease in the general population.
5. Case-control studies. The case-control studies below provide new and more precise information about which foods cause disease.

   E. coli O157:H7 case-control studies. A case-control study of *E. coli* O157:H7 infections conducted at FoodNet sites in 1997 found that undercooked ground beef was the principal food source of these infections. A follow-up case-control study in 1999, which also included subtyping of isolates by pulsed-field gel electrophoresis (PFGE), again evaluated the role of undercooked ground beef and examined risk and prevention factors for *E. coli* O157:H7 infections.

   Salmonella case-control studies. Eating chicken and undercooked eggs was associated with sporadic *Salmonella enteritidis* and *Salmonella heidelberg* infections. Antimicrobial use in the month before illness was associated with multi-resistant *Salmonella typhimurium* DT104 infections. Breast-feeding was found to be protective against infant salmonellosis. Reptile contact was associated with salmonellosis.

   Campylobacter case-control study. In 1998, a FoodNet case-control study to determine risk and prevention factors for *Campylobacter* infection enrolled more than 1,200 cases and 1,200 controls. Analysis is ongoing. A pilot study in four FoodNet sites showed that domestically acquired fluoroquinolone-resistant *Campylobacter* has emerged in the United States.

   Listeria case-control study. To determine sources and risk factors for listeriosis, a FoodNet case-control study began in 1999. Data are not yet available.

   Cryptosporidium case-control study. A FoodNet case-control study is being conducted to determine sources and risk factors for *Cryptosporidium* infection.

Comparison of data from year to year can highlight successes and failures in efforts to prevent foodborne illness. As can be seen from table 5-2, the overall incidence rates for the pathogens monitored decreased from 51.2 in 1996 to 40.7 in 1999. The biggest decreases were seen in *Campylobacter* and *Shigella* infections. Infections from *Salmonella* decreased significantly from 1996 to 1998, but then rose again in 1999. Having data of this sort will allow epidemiologists to investigate why disease rates fluctuate. While the differences between the numbers in table 5-2 seem small, they are calculated in terms of 100,000 people, so of the total population of the United States even a small change in incidence rate represents many cases of foodborne illness.

FoodNet data also highlights differences in infection rates by pathogens in different parts of the country. The most notable differences are the high rates of *Campylobacter* and *Shigella* infections in California, the low rate of *Campylobacter* infections in Maryland, and the high rate of *Salmonella* infections in Georgia. Reasons for these differences are not yet clear, but now that epidemiologists recognize that there are different infection rates, they can begin to address why this is so.

There exists a seasonal variation in cases of foodborne illness, with the summer months of June, July, and August having the highest incidence of *Campylobacter*, *Salmonella*, *Shigella*, and *E. coli* (See Figure 5-2). This may be due to the hotter temperatures, which allow bacteria to multiply more rapidly, and to people participating in more outdoor eating activities such as picnics, fairs, and camping.

Table 5-2
Cases per 100,000 of Specific Bacterial Foodborne Pathogens for the Five Original Sites, FoodNet, 1996–1999

Pathogen	1996	1997	1998	1999*
Campylobacter	23.5	25.2	21.4	17.3
E. coli O157:H7	2.7	2.3	2.8	2.1
Listeria	0.5	0.5	0.6	.5
Salmonella	14.5	13.6	12.3	14.8
Shigella	8.9	7.5	8.5	5.0
Vibrio	0.2	0.3	0.3	0.2

Figure 5-2
Rate* of Laboratory-confirmed Infections Detected by the Foodborne Diseases Active Surveillance Network (Foodnet),[1] by site—United States, 1999

*Preliminary data using 1998 population estimates.
Source: Centers for Disease Control and Prevention. March 17, 2000. Preliminary FoodNet Data on the Incidence of Foodborne Illnesses—Selected Sites, United States, 1999. *Morbidity and Mortality Weekly Report*. Vol. 49(10): 201–5. http://www.cdc.gov/mmwr/preview/mmwrhtml/

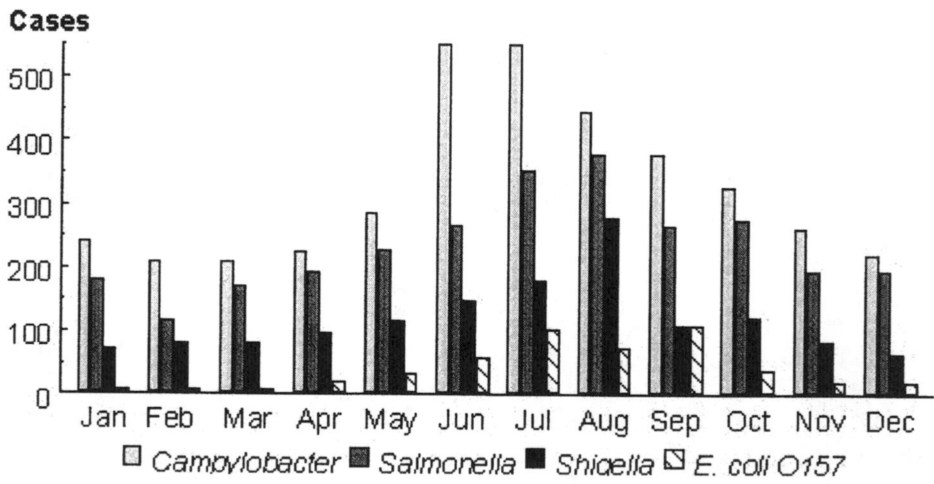

*Per 100,000 population.
[1]Reporting was statewide in Connecticut, Georgia, Minnesota, and Oregon and from selected counties in California, Maryland, and New York.
Source: Centers for Disease Control and Prevention. March 12, 1999. Incidence of Foodborne Illnesses: Preliminary Data from the Foodborne Diseases Active Surveillance Network (FoodNet)—United States, 1998. *Morbidity and Mortality Weekly Report*. Vol. 48(9): 189–94. http://www.cdc.gov/epo/mmwr/preview/mmwrhtml/00056654.htm.

CDC SURVEILLANCE FOR FOODBORNE-DISEASE OUTBREAKS, 1993–1997

Unlike the FoodNet program, the CDC Surveillance for Foodborne-Disease Outbreaks is a passive recording system, with data gathered from standardized forms sent to the CDC mainly from state and territorial health departments. As such, it represents only the tip of the iceberg of actual outbreaks and cases of foodborne disease. It counts only reported outbreaks and makes no attempt to estimate the total number of persons that become ill from foodborne illness. The 1993—1997 data reported a total of 2,751 foodborne disease outbreaks, which caused 86,058 persons to become ill. While some of these were small and only consisted of several individual cases, others affected hundreds of people. The definition of a foodborne disease outbreak is the occurrence of two or more cases of a similar illness resulting from eating a common food.

It is also interesting to know where foodborne disease outbreaks occur (Table 5-3), and what mistakes in food handling lead to them (Table 5-4). Data in Table 5-3 must be interpreted with caution, since outbreaks associated with restaurants are much more likely to be reported than those that occur in homes or other locations.

Table 5-3
Reported Foodborne Disease Outbreaks by Place Where Food Was Eaten, 1993–1997

Location	1993	1994	1995	1996	1997	Total
Home	87	130	17	108	113	585
Restaurant*	224	259	288	198	216	1185
School	14	29	8	23	17	91
Picnic	10	7	3	8	6	34
Church	14	14	16	9	10	63
Camp	5	8	10	3	4	30
Other	126	185	129	109	115	664

*Includes delicatessens and cafeterias.

Source: Sonja J. Olsen, Linda C. MacKinon, Joy S. Goulding, Nancy H. Bean, and Laurence Slutsker. March 17, 2000. Surveillance for Foodborne-Disease Outbreaks—United States, 1993–1997. *Morbidity and Mortality Weekly Report*. 49(SS-1): 1–62. http://www.cdc.gov/epo/mmwr/preview/mmwrhtml/ss490lal.htm.

Table 5-4
Factors Contributing to Foodborne Disease Outbreaks, 1993–1997

Contributing Factors	1993	1994	1995	1996	1997	Total
Improper holding temperatures	208	217	210	149	154	938
Inadequate cooking	59	60	63	44	48	274
Contaminated equipment	80	99	75	60	86	400
Food from unsafe source	33	42	35	24	19	153
Poor personal hygiene	82	124	94	90	100	490
Other	67	65	62	45	43	282

Source: Sonja J. Olsen, Linda C. MacKinon, Joy S. Goulding, Nancy H. Bean, and Laurence Slutsker. March 17, 2000. Surveillance for Foodborne-Disease Outbreaks—United States, 1993–1997. *Morbidity and Mortality Weekly Report*. 49(SS-1): 1–62. http://www.cdc.gov/epo/mmwr/preview/mmwrhtml/ss490lal.htm.

Improper holding temperature is a failure to keep hot foods hot and cold foods cold. Inadequate cooking means that food did not reach temperatures hot enough to kill pathogens. Contaminated equipment could be dirty cutting boards or utensils. Food from an unsafe source includes food purchased from unknown vendors or other questionable sources. Poor personal hygiene includes not washing hands, sneezing or coughing on food, touching face or hair, etc.

WATERBORNE DISEASE OUTBREAKS, 1997–1998

In addition to food, water may also cause people to become ill. CDC, EPA, and the Council of State and Territorial Epidemiologists collaborate to maintain a surveillance system that collects data on waterborne disease outbreaks (WBDOs) from drinking and recreational water. As with the food surveillance systems, this program seeks to determine what pathogens in the water supply cause illness and how many people become ill. Characterizing the epidemiology of WBDOs allows public health officials to identify how and why outbreaks occur, to train public health personnel in detecting and investigating WBDOs, and to design initiatives to prevent waterborne diseases. Like other data submitted on a voluntary basis, the data underestimate the true incidence of WBDOs. Reporting is dependent on public awareness, the likelihood that ill persons consult the same health care provider, that health care provider's awareness about WBDOs, availability of laboratory testing facilities, local requirements for reporting cases of particular diseases, and the capabilities of state and local agencies to investigate potential outbreaks. A total of 2,038 people became ill from drinking water, and 2,128 from recreational water in 1997–98. As with foodborne outbreaks, more WBDOs occur in summer months and the cause is often unidentified.

During 1997–1998 there were 17 outbreaks in drinking water. As seen in figure 5–3, 6 (35.3 percent) were caused by parasites (4 by *Giardia*, 2 by *Cryptosporidium*); 4 (23.5 percent) by bacteria (3 by *E. coli* O157:H7 and 1 by *Shigella sonnei*); 5 (29.4 percent) by unidentified origin; and 2 (11.8 percent) by chemical poisoning. Both chemical poisonings were from copper poisonings. Eight (47.1 percent) of the 17 WBDOs were associated with community water systems. Of these eight, three were caused by problems at water treatment plants, three were the result of problems in the water distribution systems and plumbing of individual facilities, and two were associated with contaminated, untreated groundwater. Five (29.4 percent) of the 17 WBDOs were associated with non-community water systems; all five were from groundwater (i.e., a well or spring) systems. The four outbreaks (23.5 percent) associated with individual water systems also were from groundwater.

Eighteen outbreaks associated with recreational water resulted in gastroenteritis. As seen in Figure 5-4, 9 (50 percent) were caused by the parasite *Cryptosporidium*. The other outbreaks were due to *E. coli* O157:H7 (3 outbreaks or 16.7 percent), *Shigella sonnei* (1 outbreak or 5.6 percent), Norwalk-like viruses (2 outbreaks or 11.1 percent), and unknown cause (3 three outbreaks or 16.7 percent). Slightly over half (55.6 percent) occurred in treated water-pools, hottubs, or fountains; the others occurred in fresh water—lakes, rivers, or hot springs.

WBDO reports peaked during 1979–1983 and have been declining ever since (see Figure 5-5). This decrease could be due to improved implementation of water treatment regulations, increased efforts by many water utilities to produce drinking water substantially better than EPA standards require, and efforts by public health officials to improve drinking water quality. Of the waterborne disease outbreaks re-

Figure 5-3
Waterborne-disease Outbreaks Associated with Drinking Water, by Etiologic Agent and Water System—United States, 1997–1998 (n=17)

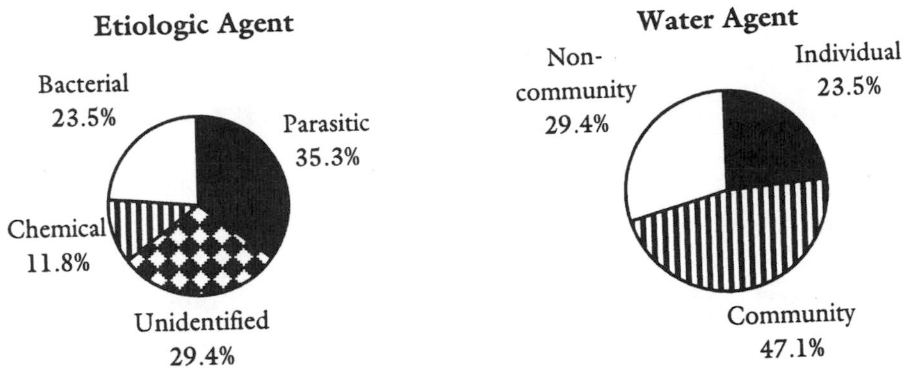

Community water system: A public water system that serves year-round residents of a community, subdivision, or mobile-home park that has greater than or equal to 15 service connections or an average of greater than or equal to 25 residents.

Noncommunity water system: A public water system that (a) serves an institution, industry, camp, park, hotel, or business that is used by the public for greater than or equal to 60 days per year; (b) has greater than or equal to 15 service connections or serves an average of greater than or equal to 25 persons; and (c) is not a community water system.

Individual water system: A small water system, not owned or operated by a water utility, that serves less than 15 residences or farms that do not have access to a public water system.

Source: Rachel S. Barwick, Deborah A. Levy, Gunther F. Craun, Michael J. Beach, and Rebecca L. Calderon. 2000. *Surveillance for Waterborne-Disease Outbreaks*—United States, 1997–1998. *May 26, 2000 / 49(SS04): 1*–35. http://www.cdc.gov/epo/mmwr/preview/mmwrhtml/ss4904al.htm.

Figure 5-4
Waterborne-disease Outbreaks Associated with Drinking Water, by Etiologic Agent and Water System—United States, 1997–1998 (n=18)

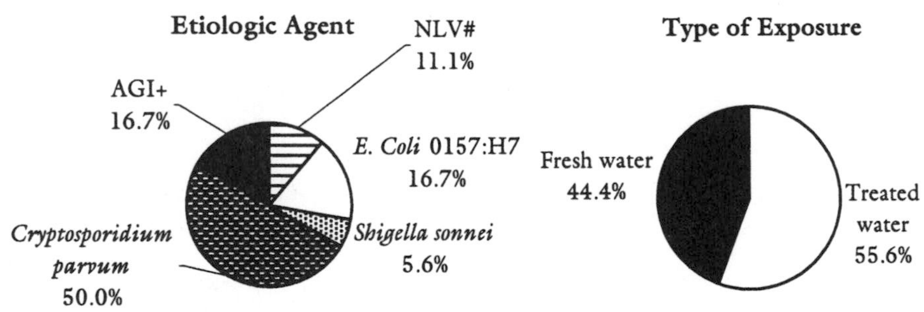

\# Norwalk-like virus
\+ Acute gastrointestinal illness of unknown etiology

Source: Barwick, Rachel S., Deborah A. Levy, Gunther F. Craun, Michael J. Beach, and Rebecca L. Calderon. 2000. *Surveillance for Waterborne-Disease Outbreaks—United States, 1997–1998.* May 26, 2000 / 49(SS04): 1–35. http://www.cdc.gov/epo/mmwr/preview/mmwrhtml/ss4904al.htm.

Figure 5-5
Number of Waterborne-disease Outbreaks Associated with Drinking Water, by Year and Etiologic Agent—United States, 1971–1998 (n=691)

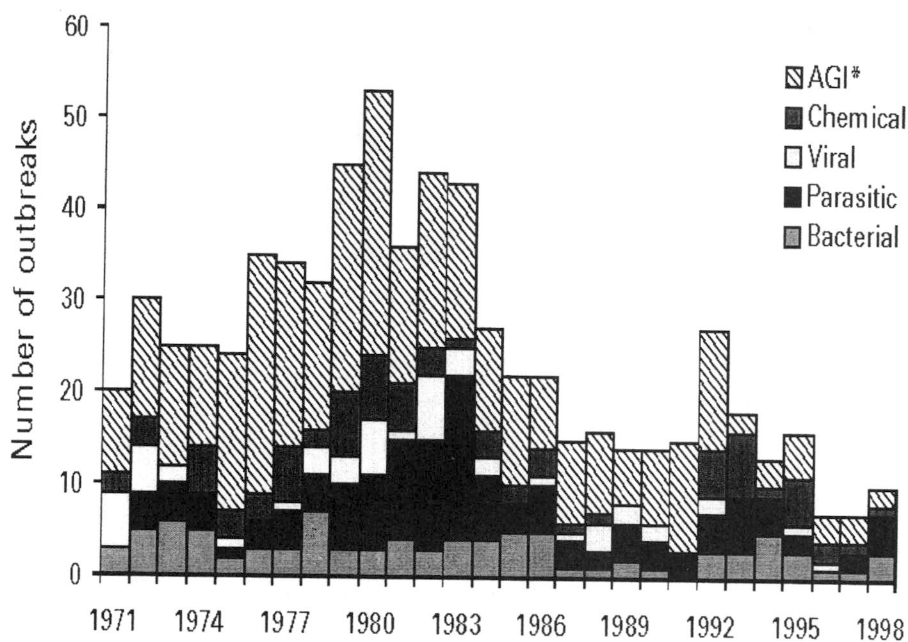

Source: Barwick, Rachel S., Deborah A. Levy, Gunther F. Craun, Michael J. Beach, and Rebecca L. Calderon. 2000. *Surveillance for Waterborne-Disease Outbreaks—United States, 1997–1998.* May 26, 2000 / 49(SS04): 1–35.

Table 5-5
Significant Waterborne Disease Outbreaks, 1985–1993

Year	State/ Territory	Cause of Disease	Number of People Affected
1985	Maine	*Giardia lamblia* (protozoan)	703 illnesses
1987	Georgia	*Cryptosporidium parvum* (protozoan)	13,000 illnesses
1987	Puerto Rico	*Shigella sonnei* (bacterium)	1,800 illnesses
1989	Montana	*E. coli* O157:H7 (bacterium)	243 illnesses, 4 deaths
1991	Puerto Rico	Unknown	9,847 illnesses
1993	Montana	*Salmonella typhimurium* (bacterium)	650 illnesses, 7 deaths
1993	Wisconsin	*Cryptosporidium parvum* (protozoan)	400,000+illnesses, 50+ deaths

Source: Environmental Protection Agency (EPA). December 1999. *25 Years of the Safe Drinking Water Act: History and Trends.* Washington: Environmental Protection Agency. http://www.epa.gov/safewater/sdwa25 /sdwa.html.

ported to CDC from 1974 to 1996, 12 percent were caused by bacterial agents, 33 percent by parasites, 5 percent by viruses, 18 percent by chemical contaminants, and 31 percent by unidentified agents. Table 5-5 highlights the larger outbreaks that occurred from 1985 to 1993. (EPA 1999)

MEDICAL COSTS OF FOODBORNE ILLNESS

What price do we pay for foodborne illness in the United States? As with other estimates of foodborne illness, available data are only an estimate. In 1996 the USDA Economic Research Service estimated the costs due to six bacterial pathogens out of the 40 that cause foodborne illness (Table 5-6). They concluded that the annual costs of illness for the six bacterial foodborne illnesses are between $2.9 billion and $6.7 billion (in 1993 dollars). This includes direct medical costs for treatment and productivity losses due to illness or early death. These figures are an underestimate of the true costs to society because only six pathogens were included in the analysis, and there are many lasting consequences to foodborne illness that are difficult to put a price on. Also missing from these estimates are the costs undertaken by industry, government, and consumers to prevent foodborne illness. Resources used to track and investigate foodborne outbreaks are not included either. Costs associated with *Salmonella* were the highest, followed by *Staphylococcus.*

Table 5-6
Cost Summary for selected bacterial pathogen in the U.S., 1993[1]

Pathogen	Foodborne Cases	Foodborne Deaths	Foodborne Costs
	Number		$ in billions
Campylobacter	1,375,000–1,750,000	110–511	0.6–1.0
Clostridium perfringens	10,000	100	-.1
E. coli O157:H7[2]	8,000–16,000	160–400	0.2–0.6
Listeria monocytogenes[3]	1,526–1,767	378–485	0.2–0.3
Salmonella (non-typhoid)	696,000–3,840,000	696–3,840	0.6–3.5
Staphylococcus aureus	1,513,000	1,210	1.2
Total	**3,603,526–7,130,767**	**2,654–6,546**	**2.9–6.7**

[1]Totals are subject to rounding.
[2]Deaths are for acute illness only and do not include chronic illness deaths.
[3]Cases that do not require hospitalization are not included due to data limitations.
Source: Jean C. Buzby, Tanya Roberts, C.-T. Jordan Lin, and James M. MacDonald. 1996. Bacterial Foodborne Disease: Medical Costs and Productivity Losses. *Agricultural Economic Report No. 741.* Washington: USDA Economic Research Service.

BEHAVIORAL RISK FACTOR SURVEILLANCE SYSTEMS (BRFSS)

It is also useful to know how people get sick from food. Behavioral surveys look at what people are doing that could cause foodborne illness. CDC, FDA, and several state health departments ask consumers a set of food safety handling, preparation, and consumption questions as part of the Behavorial Risk Factor Surveillance Systems (BRFSS). Investigators telephone adults and ask them about their health behaviors and practices for the previous 12 months. Results from the food safety section of the survey for the years 1995 and 1996 are combined in Table 5-7.

Among those practicing risky eating behaviors, eating hamburgers and especially pink hamburgers, was the most oft-reported behavior. Eating undercooked eggs and home-canned vegetables were also reported by a high number of respondents. Almost 20 percent of respondents did not appropriately wash their hands or cutting boards. Less than half remember even seeing the safe food-handling labels on meat products, but three-quarters who did remember seeing it also read it.

Table 5-7
Responses to Food Safety Survey Questions—Behavioral Risk Factor Surveillance System (BRFSS), 1995 and 1996* (n=19,356)

Consumption of high-risk foods during the previous 12 months	**%**	**(95% CI†)**
Home-canned vegetables	23.8	(±0.8)
Hamburgers	86.3	(±0.7)
Pink hamburgers	19.7	(±0.8)
Undercooked eggs	50.2	(±1.0)
Raw oysters	8.0	(±0.5)
Raw milk	1.4	(±0.2)
High-risk food-handling and preparation practices		
Not washing hands with soap after handling raw meat or chicken	18.6	(±0.8)
Not washing cutting surface with soap/bleach after using it for cutting raw meat or chicken	19.5	(±0.9)
Awareness of safe food-handling labels and the effect of those labels on meat preparation		
Remembered seeing label information on uncooked meat or poultry	45.4	(±1.2)
Of persons who remembered seeing label, remembered reading label	77.2	(±1.2)

*Twelve standard food-safety questions were added to the 1955 BRFSS in Colorado, Florida, Missouri, New York, and Tennessee and to the 1996 BRFSS in Indiana and New Jersey. Two food-consumption questions were added to the 1996 BRFSS in South Dakota.

Source: Samantha Yang, Marilyn G. Leff, Doris McTague, Kathryn A. Horvath, Jeanette Jackson-Thompson, Theophile Murayi, Georgette K. Boeselager, Thomas A. Melnik, Mark C. Gildemaster, David L. Ridings, Sean F. Altekruse, and Frederick J. Angulo. 1998. Multistate Surveillance for Food-Handling, Preparation, and Consumption Behaviors Associated with Foodborne Diseases: 1995 and 1996 BRFSS Food-Safety Questions. *Morbidity and Mortality Weekly Report.* September 11, 1998 / 47(SS-4): 33–54. http://www.cdc.gov/ epo/mmwr/preview/mmwrhtml/00054714.htm.

HOME FOOD SAFETY SURVEY

While the BRFSS collected data from a telephone interview, Audits International conducted its Home Food Safety Survey by going into consumer's homes and evaluating their food safety practices while they prepared food. The survey measured critical violations, those which in and of themselves may cause foodborne illness; and major violations, those which on their own are unlikely to cause foodborne illness but are frequently contributing factors. A home was classified as acceptable if it had no critical violations and no more than four major violations. Even though participants knew they were being evaluated, and thus were more likely to pay attention to food safety, in 1999 only 26 percent of the households achieved an acceptable rating. This was an increase over 1997 when only 4 percent of the households achieved an acceptable rating (Table 5-8). Households with young children were three times as likely to have an acceptable rating than those without.

Both the critical violations (Figure 5-6) and the major violations (Figure 5-7) are the same types of factors contributing to foodborne disease outbreaks reported to CDC (as seen in Table 5-4)—improper heating and cooling temperatures, poor personal hygiene, and contaminated equipment.

Table 5-8
Comparison of 1997 and 1998 Home Food Safety Survey Results

Result	1997	1999
Households with acceptable ratings (%)	4	26
Critical violations per household	2.3	1.7

Figure 5-6
Percent of Critical Violations Observed in Households (households observed = 121)

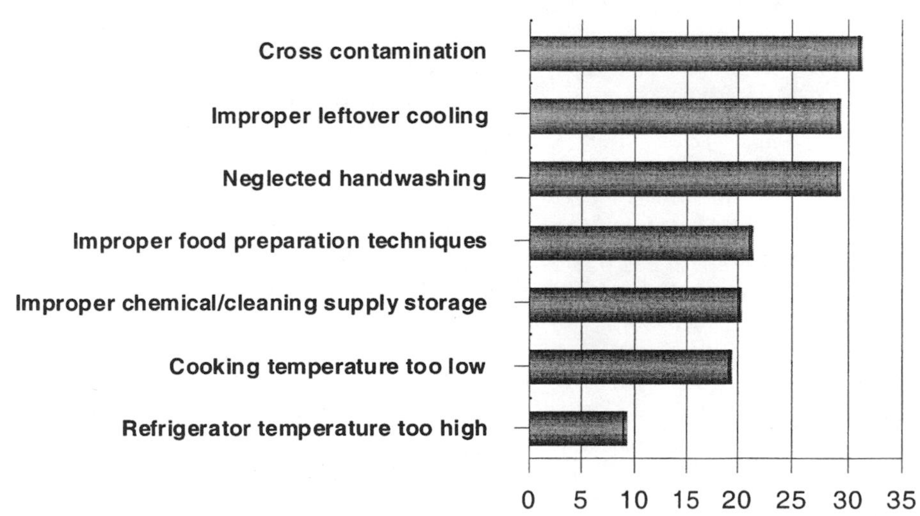

Source: Audits International's Home Food Safety Survey. Conducted Second Quarter of 1999. Audits International. http://www.audits.com/Report.html.

Figure 5-7
Percent of Major Violations Observed in Households (households observed = 121)

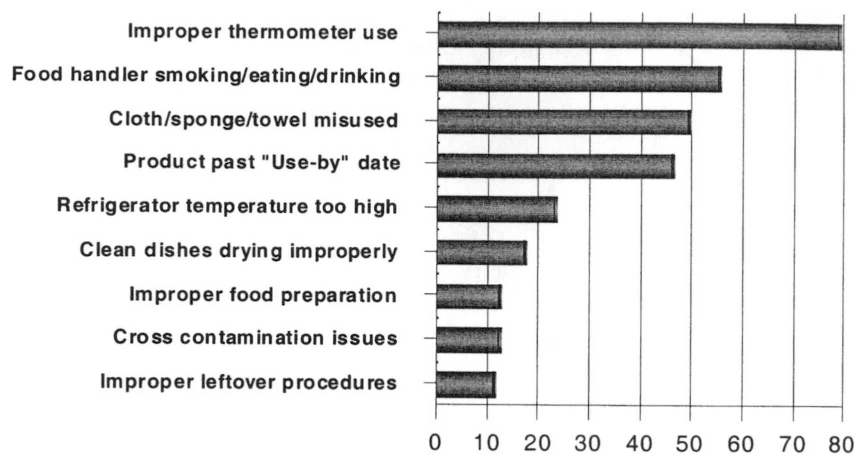

Source: Audits International's Home Food Safety Survey. Conducted Second Quarter of 1999. Audits International. http://www.audits.com/Report.html.

To effectively design research and educational programs to reduce foodborne illness, it is important to know the numbers of people who become ill, what pathogens are causing illness, and which practices are responsible. To evaluate whether implemented programs are successful, it is necessary to compare the situation before and after. The surveillance systems described in this chapter are a means of providing such data.

SOURCES

Audits International's Home Food Safety Survey. Conducted Second Quarter of 1999. Audits International. http://www.audits.com/Report.html.

Barwick, Rachel S., Deborah A. Levy, Gunther F. Craun, Michael J. Beach, and Rebecca L. Calderon. 2000. Surveillance for Waterborne-Disease Outbreaks—United States, 1997–1998. May 26, 2000 / 49(SS04): 1–35. http://www.cdc.gov/epo/mmwr/preview/mmwrhtml/ss4904a1.htm.

Buzby, Jean C., Tanya Roberts, C.-T. Jordan Lin, and James M. MacDonald. 1996. Bacterial Foodborne Disease: Medical Costs and Productivity Losses. *Agricultural Economic Report No. 741*. Washington: USDA Economic Research Service.

Centers for Disease Control and Prevention (CDC). March 17, 2000. Preliminary FoodNet Data on the Incidence of Foodborne Illnesses—Selected Sites, United States, 1999. *Morbidity and Mortality Weekly Report*. Vol. 49(10): 201–205. http://www.cdc.gov/epo/mmwr/preview/mmwrhtml/mm4910a1.htm.

Centers for Disease Control and Prevention (CDC). March 14, 2000. What Is FoodNet? http://www.cdc.gov/ncidod/dbmd/foodnet/what_is.htm.

Centers for Disease Control and Prevention (CDC). March 12, 1999. Incidence of Foodborne Illnesses: Preliminary Data from the Foodborne Diseases Active Surveillance Network (FoodNet)—United States, 1998. *Morbidity and Mortality Weekly Report*. Vol. 48(9): 189–194. http://www.cdc.gov/epo/mmwr/preview/mmwrhtml/00056654.htm.

Environmental Protection Agency (EPA). December 1999. *25 Years of the Safe Drinking Water Act: History and Trends.* Washington: Environmental Protection Agency. http://www.epa.gov/safewater/sdwa25/sdwa.html.

Mead, Paul S., Laurence Slutsker, Vance Dietz, Linda F. McCaig, Joseph S. Bresee, Craig Shapiro, Patricia M. Griffin, and Robert V. Tauxe. 1999. Food-Related Illness and Death in the United States. *Emerging Infectious Diseases.* Vol. 5(5). http://www.cdc.gov/ncidod/eid/vol5no5/mead.htm.

Olsen, Sonja J., Linda C. MacKinon, Joy S. Goulding, Nancy H. Bean, and Laurence Slutsker. March 17, 2000. Surveillance for Foodborne-Disease Outbreaks—United States, 1993–1997. *Morbidity and Mortality Weekly Report.* 49(SS-1): 1–62. http://www.cdc.gov/epo/mmwr/preview/mmwrhtml/ss4901a1.htm.

Yang, Samantha, Marilyn G. Leff, Doris McTague, Kathryn A. Horvath, Jeanette Jackson-Thompson, Theophile Murayi, Georgette K. Boeselager, Thomas A. Melnik, Mark C. Gildemaster, David L. Ridings, Sean F. Altekruse, and Frederick J. Angulo. 1998. Multistate Surveillance for Food-Handling, Preparation, and Consumption Behaviors Associated with Foodborne Diseases: 1995 and 1996 BRFSS Food-Safety Questions. *Morbidity and Mortality Weekly Report.* September 11, 1998 / 47(SS-4): 33–54. http://www.cdc.gov/epo/mmwr/preview/mmwrhtml/00054714.htm.

CHAPTER 6

CAREERS IN FOOD SAFETY

There is no one path to a career in food safety, mainly because food safety is a part of so many jobs. Being a researcher requires a high level of education with extensive knowledge of science, while managing a restaurant requires much less education and not necessarily a background in science. This chapter outlines some of the job possibilities and makes general recommendations on how the reader should prepare for them. While no schools currently offer a degree in food safety, a number of credentials do exist. All food safety credentials for food professionals existing at the time of publication are outlined:

Certified Food Safety Professional (CFSP)
Registered Environmental Health Specialist/Registered Sanitarian (REHS/RS)
Certified Food Protection Professional (CFPP)
National Certified Professional Food Manager (NCPFM)
Food Safety Manager Certificate (FSMC)
National Restaurant Association ServSafe

Recommendations for finding continuing education (CE) courses and distance learning courses in food safety are given. The chapter closes with ideas on where to find scholarships, internships, and fellowship opportunities.

Food safety is a broad field, with widely varying jobs requiring various levels of education. Researchers from academia, industry, and government work to develop and assess new technologies, unravel disease mechanisms of foodborne pathogens, and control microorganisms causing foodborne illness from the farm to the table, all to ensure that the food we eat is safe and wholesome. Food processing is the largest manufacturing industry in the United States. Many food protection specialists are needed to ensure that food is produced safely. Finally, while most consumers do not see much of the research and manufacturing aspects of food, we all have experience with the retail food service industry—restaurants, grocery stores, convenience stores, and institutions. Food safety specialists also work in the retail food arena to make sure food in these establishments is produced and served safely.

Food scientists study the physical, microbiological, and chemical nature of foods; the causes of their deterioration; methods to analyze foods and microorganisms; and the principles underlying food processing. Microbiologists, chemists, food engineers, and veterinarians are also a part of the food safety research team. Some of these researchers carry out basic research at universities. Others work for the government to develop policies, guidance, and regulations that serve to protect the food supply. Industry is the largest employer of food safety researchers. Every processed food purchased in food stores or served in retail food service establishments is the result of research into how to produce and serve it without causing foodborne illness. At the pre-processing level, veterinarians work with food animals to ensure that they are healthy and wholesome. They also deal with problems of microbial resistance to antibiotics and animal drug residues and are experts in pathology, parasitology, and epidemiology.

Food technologists apply information from researchers to the selection, preservation, processing, packaging, and distribution of food. Food technologists need a thorough understanding of food science, chemistry, microbiology, quality assurance, and statistics. Most food manufacturers hire quality assurance (QA) personnel to ensure that products meet legal, industry, and company standards; to perform microbiological testing on raw materials during processing and on finished products; and to maintain quality assurance records. Most QA personnel have a food science or other science degree from a four-year college, but technicians may have a two-year degree from a technical program with an emphasis on the sciences. Food engineers design equipment for the production of new food products; that equipment has to produce food safely, not harbor microorganisms, and be easy to clean.

Food service workers also play a large role in food safety. Since they are the ones who handle food, they too need to have food safety knowledge. Many states, counties, and cities now require food service establishments to have a certified food manager present. A college degree may not be necessary to obtain food manager certification or other food safety credentials. The food service industry employs almost 12 million people. Such a large number of employees represents a great need for educational trainers to teach principles of food safety.

The government is a large employer of food safety specialists, both at the federal and local levels. Health inspectors enforce sanitation regulations dealing with food, water, and sewage to protect the food supply and the public. Inspectors employed by states, counties, and cities are responsible for inspecting restaurants, grocery stores, convenience stores, institutions, fairs, festivals, and special events. They also investigate foodborne illness outbreaks and teach food safety principles to owners and managers of food establishments. At the national level, the Food and Drug Administration (FDA) and U.S. Department of Agriculture (USDA) employ food technologists, food inspectors, and scientists in the fields of chemistry, microbiology, and epidemiology. USDA also has more than 1,300 veterinary medical officers. USDA inspectors work in meat and poultry slaughter and processing plants, while FDA inspectors work in food processing and manufacturing facilities to ensure that they adhere to approved food safety standards.

Other professions are also involved in food safety. There are lawyers specializing in food law, product package designers to develop new packaging technologies, risk assessment specialists, and food toxicologists.

EDUCATION

Currently there are no universities offering an undergraduate degree in food safety. The wide variety of different career choices in food safety necessitates that educational preparation for those careers vary. In general, food safety involves the study of microbes, the interaction between properties of food and microorganisms, and the interaction between microorganisms and man or other animals, and as such is a science. Those wishing to pursue a career in food safety would be well served to have a good general science background. A college curriculum in food science, microbiology, chemistry, dietetics, general biology, zoology, veterinary science, environmental health, epidemiology, and health sciences serves as good preparation. Still others have entered the field of food safety with educational backgrounds in cooking, education, and policy making.

George Washington University in Washington, D.C., offers a professional advancement program in food studies for those pursuing a career in food and food-related businesses, including government regulators, trade association executives, food service professionals, and owners and managers of food-related businesses. Courses include food regulation and policy, food safety, food writing, food trends, and consumer advocacy in food safety.

The Institute of Food Technologists maintains a list on its Web site at www.ift.org of universities in the United States and Canada offering graduate degrees in food science. For a list of veterinary colleges and schools see the Association of American Veterinary Medical Colleges Web page at aavmc.org.

Credentials

Although it is not possible to obtain a degree in food safety, several credentials are available to the food safety professional.

Certified Food Safety Professional (CFSP)

The National Environmental Health Association (NEHA) and Experior Assessments offer this advanced credential for health inspectors, quality assurance inspectors, food managers and trainers, commercial food processors, food protection supervisors, chefs, and dietitians. The exam can be taken at the annual NEHA meeting each July, at Experior Testing Centers, and at Sylvan Testing Centers. To be eligible for the Certified Food Safety Professional credential a candidate must meet the criteria for either A or B as follows:

A. Degree Track: Bachelor's degree in Food Science or Environmental Health from an accredited degree program, or bachelor's degree with at least two years of experience in food protection, or bachelor's degree and possession of the REHS/RS credential.

B. Experience Track: Candidate must meet the criteria for 1 or 2 as follows:

1. High school diploma or GED and
    - a. Five years progressive experience in food-related work
    - b. Successful passage of the Certified Professional Food Manager exam, or ServSafe exam, or membership in a food-related professional organization and accumulation of 24 hours of continuing education experience. (Presenting a paper or having a paper published can be substituted for four hours of continuing education experience up to a maximum of two papers.)

2. Associates degree and

    a. Four years of progressive experience in food related work.

    b. Successful passage of the Certified Professional Food Manager exam, or ServSafe exam, or membership in a food related professional organization and accumulation of 16 hours of continuing education experience. (Presenting a paper or having a paper published can be substituted for four hours of continuing education experience up to a maximum of two papers.)

The CFSP exam is based on the following content areas. Next to each subject heading is the approximate percentage of questions in that content area on the exam.

Causes and Prevention of Foodborne Illness (51 percent). Knowledge of HACCP; microbiology and epidemiology; and food protection including: cooling and holding, heating and holding, cooking, equipment sanitation, approved vs. unapproved sources, and personal hygiene.

Inspection of Food Establishments (8 percent). Knowledge of inspection requirements and procedures.

Enforcement (8 percent). Knowledge of statutes and regulations (federal, state, and local), constitutional protections, and plan review.

Equipment and Utensils (8 percent). Knowledge of proper installation, use, and maintenance of equipment and utensils.

Management and Personnel (6 percent). Rights and obligations of food establishment management and personnel. Liability relative to foodborne illness.

Sampling Procedures and Interpretation of Results (4 percent). Knowledge of product sampling practices and techniques for both routine investigation and foodborne illness, interpretation of laboratory results, and corrective actions.

Physical Facilities, Water, Plumbing, and Waste (4 percent). Knowledge of design, use, and maintenance.

Cleaning and Sanitizing (4 percent). Knowledge of proper use of approved chemicals and the impact of cleaning and sanitizing agents on microorganisms.

Vector and Pest Control (4 percent). Knowledge of pests, their life cycles, and control measures—biological, physical and chemical.

Purchasing, Shipping, Receiving, and Storing (3 percent). Knowledge of proper procedures and regulatory requirements for food products.

Registered Environmental Health Specialist/Registered Sanitarian (REHS/RS)

The National Environmental Health Association and Experior Assessments also offer the REHS/RS credential. While a Registered Sanitarian covers other areas of public health in addition to food safety, many food safety inspectors are also Registered Sanitarians. To be eligible for the Registered Environmental Health Specialist/Registered Sanitarian credential, a candidate must meet one of the following conditions:

A. Candidate holds an Environmental Health Degree: Bachelor's, master's, or Ph.D. in environmental health from an accredited college or university.

B. Candidate holds a bachelors degree, which includes:

1. An algebra course or higher level math.

2. Thirty semester/45 quarter hours in the basic sciences, i.e., courses in biology, chemistry, physics, or other physical sciences, as well as sanitary engineering or environmental engineering.

3. Two or more years of experience in environmental health.

The REHS/RS exam is based on the following content areas. Next to each subject heading is the approximate percentage of questions in that content area on the exam.

General Environmental Health (12 percent). Knowledge of health inspection procedures, disease-causing agents, epidemiology, sampling techniques, field tests and methodology, land use planning, construction plans, permit/license process, and public education.

Statutes and Regulations (5 percent). Knowledge of legal authority, law concerning inspections, agency administrative actions (embargo, seizure, nuisance abatement, etc.), federal environmental health acts, laws, agencies, and regulations.

Food Protection (13 percent). Knowledge of inspection/investigation procedures of food establishments. Knowledge of food safety principles, protection, quality, and storage. Knowledge of temporary food service events. Knowledge of proper food transport.

Potable Water (8 percent). Knowledge of sanitary survey principles regarding potential or existing water systems and watersheds. Understand testing/sampling methods, water supply systems, water treatment processes, and diseases associated with contaminated water.

Wastewater (9 percent). Knowledge of inspection/investigation procedures of wastewater systems. Knowledge of soil characteristics and analysis methods, land use issues, wastewater treatment systems and processes, and disease-causing organisms associated with wastewater.

Solid and Hazardous Waste (9 percent). Knowledge of waste management systems, waste classifications, landfill methods, hazardous waste disposal methods, and health risks associated with poor waste management.

Hazardous Materials (4 percent). Knowledge of inspection/investigation of hazardous materials, self-protection procedures, and types of hazardous materials.

Vectors, Pests, and Weeds (7 percent). Knowledge of control methods for vectors, pests, and weeds; life cycle; different types of vectors, pests, and weeds; diseases and organisms associated with vectors, pests, and weeds; and public education methods.

Radiation Protection (3 percent). Knowledge of inspection/investigation of radiation hazards, types of radiation, common sources of exposure, protection methods, health risks of radiation exposure, and testing equipment/sampling methods used to detect radiation.

Occupational Safety and Health (3 percent), Knowledge of inspection/investigation procedures of occupational settings, common health and safety hazards at work sites, and general OSHA principles.

Air Quality and Noise (4 percent). Knowledge of inspection/investigation procedures to assess ambient air quality and environmental noise, air pollution sources, air/noise sampling methods and equipment, air/noise pollution control equipment and techniques, and health risks associated with poor air quality and excessive noise.

Housing (5 percent). Knowledge of inspection/investigation procedures of public/private housing and mobile home/recreational vehicle parks; health/safety risks of substandard housing; housing codes; heating, ventilation, and cooling systems; child safety hazards such as lead; and utility connections.

Institutions and Licensed Establishments (9 percent). Knowledge of the health hazards and sanitation problems commonly associated with correctional facilities; medical facilities; licensed establishments (tanning salons, massage clinics, tattoo parlors, and cosmetology salons); child care facilities and schools; common disease-causing organisms and transmission modes; epidemiology; heating, ventilation, and cooling systems.

Swimming Pools and Recreational Facilities (6 percent). Knowledge of inspection/investigation procedures for swimming pools/spas, recreational areas/facilities, amusement parks, temporary mass gatherings (concerts, county fairs, etc.). Knowledge of common organisms and resultant diseases associated with swimming pools/spas, water treatment systems, water chemistry, safety issues, and sampling/test methods.

Disaster Sanitation (3 percent). Knowledge of disaster preparation, site management of disaster situations, and post-disaster management. Knowledge of emergency response procedures, chain of command, supply needs, temporary shelter/facilities and services, and remediation methods.

Certified Food Protection Professional (CFPP)

The Dietary Managers Association (DMA) offers the CFPP credential. After completion of DMA's food protection course, participants are eligible to take the CFPP exam. Options for the course are a 16–hour classroom food safety training course, independent study via print materials through the DMA, or independent online study through the DMA. Geared towards the food service professional, as of 1999 the CFPP is accepted in 20 states, and is under consideration in 9 more. Check DMA's Web site at http://www.dmaonline.org/legis/legislate5.html for current status.

National Certified Professional Food Manager (NCPFM)

The National Certified Professional Food Manager (NCPFM) exam, offered by Experior Assessments, tests knowledge, skills, and abilities related to food protection. It also tests a manager's ability to organize and supervise employees within the work environment. A major focus is on application of the principles and procedures of the Hazard Analysis and Critical Control Points (HACCP) system. The NCPFM exam is appropriate for those who work as site supervisors, managers, or first-line supervisors in establishments that prepare and serve food, including the following:

Restaurants
Fast-food establishments
Retail grocery delicatessens
Convenience stores
Institutional settings
Nursing homes
Hospitals
Day care centers
Correctional facilities

The NCPFM exam is based on the following content areas. Next to each subject heading is the approximate percentage of questions in that content area on the exam.

HACCP (35 percent). Includes foodborne illness, application of principles of safe food management, time/temperature requirements, and methods for handling and monitoring food protection procedures.

Health and Hygiene (30 percent). Includes managerial responsibility for policy, employee personal health and hygiene, illness and injury procedures.

Cleaning and Sanitizing Equipment and Utensils (20 percent).

Facilities and Pest Control (5 percent).

Accident Prevention (5 percent).

Crisis Management (5 percent).

Food Safety Manager Certificate (FSMC)

This certification, administered by the National Registry of Food Safety Professionals, Inc., serves the food service industry, regulatory agencies, and academia. The Food Safety Manager Certification Examination is designed to be used with any food safety training program available on the market. The following is the test content list and the number of questions for each area. There are 80 multiple-choice questions on the test.

Ensure Food Protection	12
Purchase and Receive Food	11
Store Foods and Supplies	11
Prepare Foods	9
Serve and Display Foods	9
Use and Maintain Tools and Equipment	2
Clean and Sanitize Equipment, Utensils, and Food Contact Services	4
Select, Monitor, and Maintain Water Sources	1
Monitor and Maintain Plumbing Fixtures	1
Monitor and Maintain Ventilation Systems	1
Select, Monitor, and Maintain Waste Disposal Facilities and Equipment	1
Clean and Maintain Toilet and Hand-washing Equipment and Facilities	1
Perform General Maintenance and Housekeeping Duties	2
Monitor the Location of Equipment and Facilities	1
Assure Proper Ventilation Equipment	1
Monitor Personal Hygiene of Personnel	3
Assure Personnel are Appropriately Trained	2
Monitor Personnel Behaviors Related to Food Safety	7
Ensure Regulatory Compliance and Minimize Legal Violations	1
Total Items on Examination	**80**

National Restaurant Association ServSafe

The ServSafe program of the Educational Foundation of the National Restaurant Association provides food safety education and training materials for the restaurant and food service industry. More federal, state, and local jurisdictions recognize and accept the ServSafe program than any other food safety program. More than one million individuals have been certified in the last 25 years. ServSafe provides comprehensive training adhering to the most recent FDA Food Code. This training prepares students to earn the industry-recognized ServSafe credential through passing the ServSafe Food Protection Manager Certification Examination. The Conference for Food Protection recognizes the ServSafe Food Protection Manager Certification Examination. Visit the foundation's Web site for a list of instructors and course locations. Their site also maintains a list of training requirements for food service workers and managers in jurisdictions around the country.

Continuing Education Courses in Food Safety

Many organizations for a particular segment of the food industry offer food safety courses geared towards that segment. The organizations below offer food safety courses and training. Contact and Web site information can be found in chapter 11.

American Institute of Baking
Association of Food and Drug Officials
Chartered Institute of Environmental Health
Food Processors Institute
Institute of Food Technologists
International Inflight Food Service Association
NSF International
Office of Continuing Professional Education at Rutgers University
U.S. Department of Commerce, National Oceanic and Atmospheric Administration
U.S. Food and Drug Administration, Office of Regulatory Affairs

Many University Cooperative Extension agents from the state land-grant universities teach food safety courses for industry, retail, or consumers. Some state health and/or agriculture departments also offer food safety training, or have lists of local trainers. To find companies that offer HACCP training, search the USDA/FDA Foodborne Illness Education Information Center's HACCP Training Programs and Resources Database at http://www.nal.usda.gov/foodborne/. Consultants who offer HACCP training for the food service and retail industry can be found on the foodservice.com Web site.

Distance Learning Courses

This promises to be a growing area with trade associations, universities, government agencies, and others involved in food safety developing new courses.

American Institute of Baking
Food Sanitation, Food Safety, HACCP
Description: Courses are designed to provide technical instruction for bakers at all levels of the industry.
Web site: http://www.aibonline.org

Dietary Managers Association
Food Protection Training Program
Description: To earn this credential, individuals must demonstrate competency in a variety of areas such as planning and implementing an HACCP system; receiving and storing food; preparing food safely; holding, serving, and reheating food; applying knowledge to create procedures and policies; and conducting employee training. It is based on the FDA Food Code, and can be taken online, or through a 16-hour course. After completing the course, individuals are qualified to take the Certified Food Protection Professional (CFPP) exam.
Web site: http://dmaonline.org

Food Safety Project at Iowa State University Extension
Safe Food: It's Your Job Too!
Description: The Food Safety Project at Iowa State University Extension developed these food safety lessons to provide consumers and future consumers with the tools they need to help minimize their risk from harmful pathogens in the food supply. They will help participants understand how knowledge about pathogen reduction, time and temperature abuse, and cleanliness will help decrease their incidence of foodborne illness. It will help consumers to understand their role in keeping food safe.

Web site: http://www.extenion.iastate.edu/foodsafety/Lesson/

Institute of Food Technologists
Introduction to the Food Industry
Description: Introduction to the Food Industry is a self-study learning tool designed to assist high school students in their exploration into the food industry and its career opportunities. It consists of eight lessons. While designed to be self-taught and self-paced, the course may be enhanced by including previewing and post-viewing tests to be administered by an instructor as part of a more formal learning experience. Lesson topics are Food Safety and Quality Assurance; Processing Food; Nutrition, Labeling and Packaging; Integrated Resource Management; From the Plant to the Store; From the Store to the Shopper; The Customer Service Chain; and Food Preparation at Home.
Web site: http://www.ift.org/careers/

Kansas State University
Various courses available
Description: K-State degree programs and credit courses offered through distance education are taught by the same faculty members who teach K-State on-campus courses. Course offerings include Introduction to Food Science, Principles of Animal Science, Fundamentals of Food Processing, Food Chemistry, Food Microbiology, and Quality Assurance of Food Products.
Web site: http://www.dce.ksu.edu/dce/distance/

Michigan State University
Emerging Food Safety Issues in the International Retail Market
Description: This advanced-level course is especially designed for middle to upper level managers with responsibility for local, national, or international food operations and M.S./Ph.D. candidates in food science, food service, or related areas. This course focuses on emerging food safety issues identified by the multi-university team of food professionals and includes the latest information in food microbiological epidemiology, national and international food law, irradiation, and retail and institutional food concerns in relation to issues of safe and healthy food supply.
Web site: http://www.vu.msu.edu/preview/fsc891/

Michigan State University
International Food Laws and Regulations
Description: This course covers domestic and international food laws including EU, Asia, Canada, and Latin America. Region-specific instruction may be provided as requested. It will meet the needs of attorneys, producers, processors, and researchers by providing knowledge of international regulatory requirements essential to the food industry professional.
Web site: http://www.vu.msu.edu

National Universities Degree Consortium (NUDC)
Various courses available
Description: NUDC is composed of nine accredited member institutions. Course offerings include Food Production Management, Food Science, Fundamentals of Food Processing, Food Microbiology, and Quality Assurance of Food Products.
Web site: http://www.nudc.org/

University of Florida and the Florida Restaurant Association
On-line Food Safety Training Manual
Description: Contains all the basic food safety information needed to teach employees or students the basics. Available full-text online, including posters that can be downloaded in pdf format. Also available as a book.
Web site: http://www.foodsafety.ufl.edu

University of Illinois, College of Veterinary Medicine
Food Safety Computer Assisted Instruction
Description: The "Food Safety CAI" Web site is intended to provide distance learning exercises in "farm to table" food safety for those whose current or future employment includes direct or indirect involvement in foods of animal origin. This would include the following audiences:

Veterinary students as part of their professional curriculum.

Food animal veterinarians as part of a continuing education program.

FSIS inspectors and trainees as part of their normal training and CE programs.

Individuals working in local and state public health departments whose professional responsibilities include food safety.

Others (students and academics, military, industry) in related food safety/public health programs.

Users may choose from four pre-harvest lessons, five processing (meat inspection) lessons, and four foodborne disease outbreak investigation lessons. The lessons are also intended to demonstrate how the Web can be used to provide continuing education credit. The program can be downloaded.
Web site: http://sable.cvm.uiuc.edu/

Professor Ronald LaPorte, Graduate School of Public Health, University of Pittsburgh and National Library of Medicine, National Institutes of Health
Investigation and Control of Outbreaks of Foodborne Illness
Description: This course is designed to provide an overview on epidemiology and the Internet for students in medical- and health-related fields around the world. It uses foodborne outbreaks as examples and presents two hypothetical outbreaks describing how data from epidemiologic and laboratory studies are linked in outbreak investigations. Included is a list of steps taken in a generalized outbreak investigation.
Web site: http://www.pighealth.com/Scourse/lecture/lec0161/index.htm

USDA Food Safety and Inspection Service
Food Safety Virtual University (FSVU)
Description: The FSVU is an effort to utilize a rapidly advancing technology to deliver training and education in the area of food safety to a widely dispersed and very diverse audience. The FSVU will make it possible for almost anyone to access training and educational materials. Courses include: Animal Production Food Safety, Animal and Meat Science courses, Microbial Ecology of Foods, Food Laws and Regulations, HACCP training, and Sanitation Standard Operating Procedures.
Web site: http://www.fsis.usda.gov/OFO/HRDS/fsvu.html

SCHOLARSHIPS, INTERNSHIPS, AND FELLOWSHIPS

Many trade associations and professional societies offer scholarships, internships, or fellowship opportunities. The organizations below offer scholarships and/or fellowships and internships. Contact and Web site information can be found in chapter 11. Those seeking scholarships, internships, or fellowships are encouraged to check the local chapters of organizations in addition to the national offices.

American Culinary Federation, Inc.

American Dietetic Association

American Institute of Baking

American School Food Service Association

American Society for Healthcare Food Service Administrators

Centers for Disease Control and Prevention

Institute of Food Technologists

International Association of Culinary Professionals

International Food Service Executives Association

Joint Institute for Food Safety and Applied Nutrition

National Association of College and University Food Services

National Environmental Health AssociationNational Grocers Association

National Meat Association

National Restaurant Association Educational Foundation

Part 2

Resources

CHAPTER 7

REPORTS AND BROCHURES

This chapter lists more than 100 reports and almost 50 brochures. The reports tend to be detailed investigations from a variety of organizations on specific topics relating to food safety. Most organizations make their reports available on the World Wide Web. An exception to this is the Congressional Research Service (CRS), which prepares reports for members of Congress, congressional committees, or congressional staff. These reports are prepared to further the legislative process, not for the general public. While the National Council for Science and the Environment does make some of these reports available on their Web site, these are not authorized for posting by CRS. Those who want CRS reports should contact their congressperson or senator. As the investigative arm of Congress, the Government Accounting Office (GAO) helps Congress oversee federal programs and operations to assure accountability to the American people. As part of their mission they investigate a wide variety of food safety topics. Their reports are published and archived on the GAO Web site. Reports from FDA, USDA, EPA, and CDC that deal with food safety can also be found on www.foodsafety.gov, the government gateway to food safety information. The organizations below are the major publishers of food safety reports. Readers wanting the most current reports should search their Web sites.

Center for Science in the Public Interest (CSPI) http://www.cspinet.org

Council for Agricultural Science and Technology (CAST) http://www.cast-science.org

Environmental Working Group (EWG) http://www.ewg.org

Food and Agriculture Organization http://www.fao.org

Institute of Food Science & Technology http://www.ifst.org

National Research Council http://www.nationalacademies.org/nrc/

U.S. Environmental Protection Agency http://www.epa.gov

U.S. Food and Drug Administration http://vm.cfsan.fda.gov

U.S. General Accounting Office http://www.gao.gov

USDA, Economic Research Service http://www.ers.usda.gov

World Health Organization http://www.who.int

Brochures tend to be short-lived items, printed and available until copies are gone. As they are consumer-level publications that provide basic information in an easy-to-read format, their content is self-evident from the title, making a description of their content unnecessary. Due to the very basic nature of the information, it does not become out of date as quickly as does more technical information, therefore dates are not listed. Most organizations will supply single copies of their brochures for free. Many of the brochures are also available on the Web, and some agencies have made reproducible masters available for organizations that would like to use them with their own logo.

REPORTS

American Academy of Microbiology. February 2000. *Food Safety: Current Status and Future Needs.* Washington, DC: American Academy of Microbiology.
Web site: Available full-text at http://www.asmusa.org/acasrc/pdfs/Foodsafetyreport.pdf

This report from the American Academy of Microbiology's Critical Issues Colloquia program discusses factors that influence the incidence of foodborne disease, sampling and surveillance, risk assessment, and the food safety community.

Center for Public Integrity. June 2, 1998. *Unreasonable Risk: The Politics of Pesticides.* Washington, DC: The Center for Public Integrity. Web site: Available full-text at http://www.publicintegrity.org/unreasonable_risk.html

A comprehensive study that examines how Congress and the EPA regulate the pesticide industry and its products.

Center for Science in the Public Interest (CSPI). August 1999. *Outbreak Alert! Closing the Gaps in Our Federal Food-Safety Net.* Washington, DC: Center for Science in the Public Interest.
Web site: Available full-text at http://www.cspinet.org/reports/outbreak_alert/index.htm

Available full-text online, this report criticizes the federal government for failing to adequately maintain and analyze a comprehensive list of food safety outbreaks. To help fill that gap, CSPI compiled and analyzed an inventory of foodborne illness outbreaks from 1990 to 1999. That list and the findings are the subject of this report.

Center for Science in the Public Interest (CSPI). January 2000. *Unexpected Consequences: Miscarriage and Birth Defects from Tainted Food.* Washington, DC: Center for Science in the Public Interest.
Web site: Available full-text at http://www.cspinet.org/foodsafety/conseqco.pdf

In this report, CSPI covers *Listeria monocytogenes* and *Toxoplasma gondii* as they relate to foodborne illness and pregnant women. The report concludes with recommendations for government agencies, the food industry, consumers, and medical professionals to minimize these two pathogens.

Centers for Disease Control and Prevention. 1999. *Prevention of Hepatitis A through Active or Passive Immunization: Recommendations of the Advisory Committee on Immunization Practices (ACIP).* MMWR 48(RR12);1–37. October 1, 1999. Washington, DC: Centers for Disease Control and Prevention.
Web site: Available at http://www.cdc.gov/epo/mmwr/preview/mmwrhtml/rr4812a1.htm

This update of the 1996 recommendations on the prevention of hepatitis A through immunization includes new data about the epidemiology of hepatitis A, recent findings about the effectiveness of community-based hepatitis A vaccination programs, and recommendations for the routine vaccination of children.

Congressional Research Service. Continually updated. *Food Safety Issues in the 107th Congress.* IB98009. Washington, DC: Congressional Research Service.
Web site: Available full-text at http://www.cnie.org/nle/ag-38.html

This report looks at food safety issues faced by the 106th Congress and how Congress responded to the issues. This report is periodically updated.

Congressional Research Service. Updated periodically. *Food Biotechnology in the United States: Science, Regulation, and Issues.* Report no.

RL30198. Washington, DC: Congressional Research Service.
Web site: Available full-text at http://www.cnie.org/nle/st-41.pdf

This report provides basic information on the science of food biotechnology, regulatory policies, and issues of concern about the use of biotechnology.

Congressional Research Service. 2001. *Antimicrobial Resistance: An Emerging Public Health Issue*. RL30814. Washington: Congressional Research Service.

This report is an in-depth analysis on antimicrobial resistance and its relation to human health.

Congressional Research Service. 2000. *Labeling of Genetically Engineered Foods*. Washington, DC: Congressional Research Service.
Web site: Available full-text at http://www.cnie.org/nle/ag-98.html

This report covers the issues relating to labeling of genetically enginereed (GE) foods.

Congressional Research Service. Updated December 9, 1999. *The European Union's Ban on Hormone-Treated Meat*. RS20142. Washington, DC: Congressional Research Service.
Web site: Available full-text at http://www.cnie.org/nle/ag-63.html

This report examines the World Trade Organization (WTO) dispute settlement panel that ruled that the European Union's (EU) ban on imports of meat derived from animals treated with growth hormones is inconsistent with the Uruguay Round Agreement on health and safety measures used to restrict imports, the so-called Sanitary and Phytosanitary (SPS) agreement. The issues behind the ruling are examined.

Congressional Research Service. August 30, 2000. *Fruits and Vegetables: Ongoing Issues for Congress*. IB10031. Washington, DC: Congressional Research Service.
Web site: Available full-text at http://www.cnie.org/nle/ag-70.html

This report looks at the current food safety issues with produce, including irradiation, pesticides, organic produce, and international trade issues.

Congressional Research Service. June 8, 2000. *Meat and Poultry Inspection Issues*. IB10037. Washington, DC: Congressional Research Service.
Web site: Available full-text at http://www.cnie.org/nle/ag-30.html

This report prepared for Congress examines USDA HACCP inspection, irradiation of meat, labeling of organically produced meats, inspection authority and requirement, the zero tolerance policy, testing procedures, and more.

Congressional Research Service. Updated October 21, 1999. *Country-of-Origin Labeling for Foods: Current Law and Proposed Changes*. Washington, DC: Congressional Research Service. 97–508.
Web site: Available full-text at http://www.cnie.org/nle/inter-5.html

This report looks at the country-of-origin labeling requirements for meat products, fruits, and vegetables at the retail level. Trade issues and food safety issues are examined.

Congressional Research Service. Updated August 27, 1999. *Science Behind the Regulation of Food Safety: Risk Assessment and the Precautionary Principle*. RS20310. Washington, DC: Congressional Research Service.
Web site: Available full-text at http://www.cnie.org/nle/rsk-29.html

This report looks at the use of science as a basis for food safety regulatory activities and the controversies about how science can best be used for this purpose.

Congressional Research Service. Updated August 24, 1999. *Food Safety: A Chronology of Selected Recent Events, 1992–1999*. Report no. 98–119 C. Washington, DC: Congressional Research Service.
Web site: Available full-text at http://www.cnie.org/nle/crsag.html

This is a chronology of selected federal actions and proposals related to food safety and specific outbreaks or instances of foodborne illness. Also included are links to food safety information on the Internet and addresses and telephone numbers of the major federal food safety agencies. This report will be updated periodically as significant events occur.

Congressional Research Service. August 3, 1999. *Pesticide Residue Regulation: Analysis of Food Quality Protection Act Implementation*. Report no. RS20043. Washington, DC: Congressional Research Service.
Web site: Available full-text at http://www.cnie.org/nle/crspest.html

This report examines the progress made on implementing the Food Quality Protection Act of 1996. It reviews the mandates of the act, implementation issues, and stakeholder involvement.

Congressional Research Service. Updated February 8, 1999. *Safe Drinking Water Act Amendments of 1996: Overview of P.L. 104–182.* 96–722 ENR. Washington, DC: Congressional Research Service.
Web site: Available full-text at http://www.cnie.org/nle/h2o-17.html

The 104th Congress made extensive changes to the Safe Drinking Water Act (SDWA) with the Safe Drinking Water Act Amendments of 1996 (P.L. 104–182), bringing to a close a multiyear effort to amend a statute that was widely criticized as having too little flexibility, too many unfunded mandates, and an arduous but unfocused regulatory schedule. Among the many changes to the SDWA, the 1996 amendments added provisions to provide funding to communities for drinking water mandates, focus regulatory efforts on contaminants posing health risks, and add some flexibility to the regulatory process. Congress also added programs to improve the capacity of public water systems to comply with drinking water regulations, prevent contamination of source waters, strengthen the science underlying drinking water regulations, and increase information provided to the public water system customers. This report reviews selected provisions of these amendments.

Congressional Research Service. October 21, 1998. *U.S.-European Agricultural Trade: Food Safety and Biotechnology Issues.* 98–861 ENR. Washington, DC: Congressional Research Service.
Web site: Available full-text at http://www.cnie.org/nle/ag-51.html

This report looks at the issues of meat hormones and bioengineered products from U.S. and European Union perspectives as they related to food safety and international trade.

Congressional Research Service. February 5, 1998. *Food Safety Agencies and Authorities: A Primer.* Report no. 98–91 ENR. Washington, DC: Congressional Research Service.
Web site: Available full-text at http://www.cnie.org/nle/crsag.html

In the wake of an outbreak of foodborne illness and the largest recall of suspected contaminated meat in U.S. history in August 1997, several policy makers have reopened the debate on creating a single, independent, federal food safety agency. As background for further discussion on this and related food safety issues, this report describes the roles of the primary federal and cooperating state agencies responsible for food safety, and enumerates the major legislative authorities currently governing them.

Congressional Research Service. Updated July 9, 1997. *"Mad Cow Disease" or Bovine Spongiform Encephalopathy: Scientific and Regulatory Issues.* Report no. 96–641 SPR. Washington, DC: Congressional Research Service.
Web site: Available full-text at http://www.cnie.org/nle/crsag.html

This report provides background information on BSE, or "mad cow disease," and Creutzfeldt-Jakob disease (CJD) and their relation to each other. It reviews the BSE situation in the United Kingdom and the rest of Europe, U.S. federal government actions, and the policy issues involved.

Congressional Research Service. 1993. *Selected Recommendations for Changes in the Federal Organization of Food Safety Responsibilities, 1949–1993.* Report no. 93–955 SPR. Washington, DC: Congressional Research Service.

This report summarizes 18 recommendations made throughout the last five decades for changing the federal organization of food safety responsibilities. Most recommendations fit into one of three categories: 1) a single independent food safety institution should be given responsibility for all food safety; 2) responsibility for all food products should be returned to USDA; or 3) responsibility for all food products should be given to FDA. The history and pros and cons of each of these are examined.

Consultative Group on International Agricultural Research (CGIAR). 1999. *Agricultural Biotechnology and the Poor: Conference Proceedings.* Washington, DC: Consultative Group on International Agricultural Research (CGIAR).
Web site: Available full-text at http://www.cgiar.org/biotech/rep0100/contents.htm

This report is from an international conference held in October 1999 that focused on agricultural biotechnology and its potential impact in developing countries. the conference was held to convene an open, inclusive, and participatory debate on potential benefits and risks of agricultural biotechnology grounded in scientific evidence and concerned with the common good.

Consumers Union. February 1999. *Do You Know What You're Eating?* New York: Consumers Union.
Web site: Available full-text at http://www.ecologic-ipm.com/findings.html

This technical report is an analysis of the U.S. Department of Agriculture's Pesticide Data Program to compare the relative amounts and toxicity of pesticide residues in different foods. Readers can learn with foods have the highest and which have the lowest toxicity index.

Consumers Union. September 1998. *WORST FIRST: High-risk Insecticide Uses, Children's Foods and Safer Alternatives.* New York: Consumers Union.
Web site: Available full-text at http://www.ecologic-ipm.com/findings

This report identifies 40 specific insecticide uses on nine fruit and vegetable crops that account for a large portion of children's overall dietary insecticide exposure and risk.

Council for Agricultural Science and Technology (CAST). September 2000. *Transmissible Spongiform Encephalopathies in the United States.* Ames: Council for Agricultural Science and Technology (CAST).
Web site: Available full-text at http://www.cast-science.org

This report from CAST characterizes the overall U.S. risk for the occurrence of bovine spongiform encephalopathy (BSE), commonly called "mad cow" disease, as extremely low. The report summarizes the latest information and disease statistics in its new report on transmissible spongiform encephalopathies (TSEs), a unique group of fatal diseases that can affect the nervous systems of animals and humans worldwide.

Council for Agricultural Science and Technology (CAST). February 6, 2000. *Liability and Labeling of Genetically Modified Organisms.* Ames: Council for Agricultural Science and Technology.
Web site: Available full-text at http://www.cast-science.org/0002abab.htm

This is a report from the May 26, 1999, roundtable, entitled "Liability and Labeling of Genetically Modified Organisms." The roundtable brought together representatives of the scientific and legal communities, corporate and trade associations, consumer groups, and others to share their perspectives on the issue of liability and labeling of genetically modified organisms.

Council for Agricultural Science and Technology (CAST). December 1999. *Applications of Biotechnology to Crops: Benefits and Risks.* Issue Paper 12. Ames: Council for Agricultural Science and Technology.
Web site: Available full-text at http://www.cast-science.org/biotc_ip.htm

The purpose of this paper is to summarize the recent scientific developments that underpin modern biotechnology and to discuss the potential risks and benefits when these are applied to agricultural crops. This introductory paper is intended for those who are not specialists in the area but who are interested in participating in the current debate about the future of genetically modified crops.

Council for Agricultural Science and Technology (CAST). March 1999. *Agricultural Impact of the Sudden Elimination of Key Pesticides under the Food Quality Protection Act.* Issue Paper no. 11. Ames: Council for Agricultural Science and Technology.
Web site: Available full-text at http://www.cast-science.org/fqp1_ip.htm

In analyzing the potential impact on agricultural producers from sudden elimination of key pesticides under implementation of the Food Quality Protection Act (FQPA), this report examines what the impact would be on integrated pest management programs, resistance management, food production, and competitiveness of U.S. food products.

Council for Agricultural Science and Technology (CAST). October 1998. *Foodborne Pathogens: Review of Recommendations.* Special Publication no.22. Ames: Council for Agricultural Science and Technology.
Web site: Available full-text at http://www.cast-science.org/pat2/pat2.htm

Reviewing the recommendations contained in the CAST report, Foodborne Pathogens: Risks and Consequences, published in 1994, this report updates and adds to the earlier recommendations.

Council for Agricultural Science and Technology (CAST). June 23, 1998. *Food Safety, Sufficiency, and Security.* Ames: Council for Agricultural Science and Technology.

Web site: Available full-text at http://www.cast-science.org/fsss/fsss.htm

A November 1997 conference sponsored by CAST explored complex relationships among food safety, sufficiency, and security on a national and global basis. This report of that conference highlights new and changing circumstances that require examination of policy options by governments, agribusinesses, food producers and processors, and consumers.

Council for Agricultural Science and Technology (CAST). April 1998. *Naturally Occurring Antimicrobials in Food.* Task force report no. 132. Ames: Council for Agricultural Science and Technology.
Web site: http://www.cast-science.org/anti_is.htm

This report examines naturally occurring antimicrobials in food products and their role in food preservation, production, and safety.

Council for Agricultural Science and Technology (CAST). April 1996. *Radiation Pasteurization of Food.* Issue Paper no. 7. Ames: Council for Agricultural Science and Technology.
Web site: Available full-text at http://www.cast-science.org/past_ip.htm

This report examines irradiation as it applies to fruits and vegetables; wheat and flour; beef, lamb, pork, and poultry; fish and shellfish; and commercially sterile foods. It outlines consumer acceptance of irradiation, technology, and endorsements of the process.

Council for Agricultural Science and Technology (CAST). January 1995. *Public Perceptions of Agrichemicals.* Task force report no. 123. Ames: Council for Agricultural Science and Technology.
Web site: Summary available at http://www.cast-science.org/pper_is.txt

This report reviews relevant research findings and develops recommendations for policy and for future research. It looks at the public's perceptions of risks from residues of agrichemicals in food, including pesticides and animal drugs.

Council for Agricultural Science and Technology (CAST). September 1994. *Foodborne Pathogens: Risks and Consequences.* Task force report no. 122. Ames: Council for Agricultural Science and Technology.
Web site: Summary available at http://www.cast-science.org/path_is.htm

Written by a collaboration of scientists, this report outlines the risks associated with foodborne pathogens and gives recommendations for reducing foodborne illness.

Environmental Working Group (EWG). January 1998. *Overexposed: Organophosphate Insecticides in Children's Food.* Washington, DC: Environmental Working Group.
Web site: Available full-text at http://www.ewg.org/pub/home/reports/ops/oppress.html

This EWG report is a comprehensive analysis of exposure to organophosphate pesticides in the U.S. food supply. It is based on more than 80,000 samples of food tested by the U.S. Department of Agriculture and the Food and Drug Administration, and dietary records for more than 4,000 children collected by the USDA.

Environmental Working Group (EWG). May 1996. *Just Add Water.* Washington, DC: Environmental Working Group.
Web site: Available full-text at http://www.ewg.org/pub/home/reports/JustAddWater/JustAdd.html

To produce *Just Add Water*, EWG analyzed more than 16 million records submitted by public water supplies to state water agencies and the EPA and stored in the computerized system known as the Safe Drinking Water Information System (SDWIS). *Just Add Water* analyzed only health standard violations, showing that Americans are exposed to chemical, radiation, or biological contamination at levels that federal health authorities consider unsafe.

Environmental Working Group (EWG). November 1995. *A Shopper's Guide to Pesticides in Produce.* Washington, DC: Environmental Working Group.
Web site: Available full-text at http://www.ewg.org/pub/home/reports/Shoppers/Shoppers.html

To help consumers minimize their exposure to pesticides in produce, and maximize the nutritional benefits of the fruits and vegetables they eat, EWG analyzed the results of 15,000 samples of food tested for pesticides by the Food and Drug Administration during 1992 and 1993. The guide provides easy-to-understand ranking of fruits and vegetables from those with the highest and most toxic contamination to those with the fewest and least toxic levels of contamination.

Environmental Working Group (EWG). August 17, 1995. *Weed Killers by The Glass*. Washington, DC: Environmental Working Group.
Web site: Available full-text at http:// www.ewg.org/pub/home/reports/Weed_Killer/Weed_Home.html

This report examines the magnitude of tap water contamination with weed killers, including the severity and duration of peak levels of exposure that routinely exceed federal health standards during the three- to four-month peak runoff period. The results of these tests reveal widespread contamination of tap water with many different pesticides at levels that present serious health risks.

Environmental Working Group (EWG). July 26, 1995. *Pesticides in Baby Food*. Washington, DC: Environmental Working Group.
Web site: Available full-text at http://www.ewg.org/pub/home/reports/Baby_food/Baby_home.html

This report examines the extent of pesticide contamination of baby food. After a review of infant risks from pesticides, data is presented on EWG's analysis of eight foods (applesauce, garden vegetables or pea-and-carrot blend, green beans, peaches, pears, plums, squash, and sweet potatoes) made by the three major baby food producers that account for 96 percent of all baby food sales.

Environmental Working Group (EWG). February 1995. *Forbidden Fruit: Illegal Pesticides in the U.S. Food Supply*. Washington, DC: Environmental Working Group.
Web site: Available full-text at http:// www.ewg.org/pub/home/reports/Fruit/Contents.html

Forbidden Fruit analyzes 14,923 computerized records from the Food and Drug Administration's (FDA) routine pesticide monitoring program for the fiscal years 1992 and 1993. Violations of pesticide laws are reported in excess of what U.S. government agencies claim.

Environmental Working Group (EWG). October 18, 1994. *Tap Water Blues*. Washington, DC: Environmental Working Group, Physicians for Social Responsibility.

This report is an analysis of pesticide contamination of drinking water supplies in the Midwest. It identifies more than 10 million individuals exposed to five herbicides (atrazine, cyanazine, simazine, alachlor, and metolachlor) at levels that exceed EPA's negligible cancer risk standard of one additional cancer case per million individuals.

Joint FAO/WHO Expert Committee on Food Additives (JECFA). February 2000. *Veterinary drugs residues*. Rome: Food and Agriculture Organization.
Web site: Available full-text at http://www.fao.org/waicent/faoinfo/ECONOMIC/esn/jecfa/jecfa54.pdf

The result of an FAO Expert Committee on Food Additives held in Geneva February 15–24, 2000, this report elaborates on principles for evaluating the safety of veterinary drug residues in food and for establishing acceptable daily intakes and maximum residue limits.

FAO/NACA/WHO Study Group. 1999. *Food Safety Issues Associated with Products from Aquaculture*. Technical Report Series, No. 883. Rome: Food and Agriculture Organization.
Web site: Available full-text at http://www.who.int/fsf/trs883.pdf

This report is the result of an expert assessment of risks to human health that may arise from the consumption of farmed finfish and crustaceans. The core of the report provides a complete assessment of all potential biological and chemical hazards. Included are strategies for controlling biological and chemical hazards and recommendations and conclusions reached during the assessment.

FAO/WHO Expert Consultation. March 1999. *Risk Assessment of Microbiological Hazards in Foods*. Rome: Food and Agriculture Organization.
Web site: Available full-text at http:// www.fao.org/waicent/faoinfo/ECONOMIC/esn/hazard/hazard.htm

The result of a Joint FAO/WHO Expert Consultation on the Risk Assessment of Microbiological Hazards in Foods held in Geneva March 15–19, 1999, the objectives of the consultation were to examine current scientific knowledge concerning microbiological risk assessment for food and related issues, recommend an overall strategy and framework for risk assessment, recommend methodologies for risk assessment suitable for use at an international level to estimate the risk that microbiological hazards pose to human health, and suggest priority issues in risk assessment.

FAO/WHO Expert Consultation. February 1998. *Application of Risk Communication to Food Standards and Safety Matters*. Report no. 70. Rome: Food and Agriculture Organization.

Web site: Available full-text at http:// www.fao.org/waicent/faoinfo/ECONOMIC/esn/riskcomm/HTTOC.htm

This report is the result of a Joint FAO/WHO Expert Consultation on the Application of Risk Communication to Food Standards and Safety Matters held in Rome February 2–6, 1998. The goals of the consultation were to identify the elements of, and recommend guiding principles for, effective risk communication; to examine the barriers to effective risk communication and to recommend means by which they can be overcome; to identify strategies for effective risk communication within the risk analysis framework; and to provide practical recommendations to FAO, WHO, Member Governments, Codex Alimentarius Commission (CAC), other international and national organizations, industry, and consumers to improve their communication on matters related to the risk assessment and management of food safety hazards.

FAO Expert Consultation. March 1997. *Animal Feeding and Food Safety*. Report no. 69. Rome: Food and Agriculture Organization.
Web site: Available full-text at http://www.fao.org/waicent/faoinfo/ECONOMIC/esn/animal/animapdf/contents.htm

The result of an FAO Expert Consultation on Animal Feeding and Food Safety held in Rome March 10–14, 1997, this report includes a draft code of practice for good animal feeding; an overview of the control of health factors in the production of animal feed; an overview of infections and intoxications of farm livestock associated with feed and forage; and standards, guidelines, and other recommendations related to the quality and safety of feed and foods from the Codex Alimentarius Commission.

FAO/WHO Expert Consultation. January 1997. *Risk Management and Food Safety*. Report no. 65. Rome: Food and Agriculture Organization.
Web site: Available at http://www.fao.org/waicent/faoinfo/ECONOMIC/esn/risk/riskcont.htm

This report is the result of a Joint FAO/WHO Expert Consultation on the Application of Risk Management to Food Safety Matters held in Rome January 27–31, 1997. The main goal of this consultation was to arrive at a series of recommendations on the application of risk management to food safety, dealing with the management of risk from both chemical and biological hazards in food and covering the full range of acute and chronic adverse health effects.

FAO/WHO Expert Consultation. October 1996. *Biotechnology and Food Safety*. Report no. 61. Rome: Food and Agriculture Organization.
Web site: Available full-text at http://www.fao.org/waicent/faoinfo/ECONOMIC/esn/biotech/tabconts.htm

This Expert Consultation addressed the evaluation of the safety, for purposes of consumption, of all food and food components produced using techniques involving biotechnology, whether plant, animal, or microbial in origin.

Food & Water. 1998. *Meat Monopolies: Dirty Meat and the False Promises of Irradiation*. Walden, VT: Food & Water.

This special report takes a critical look at food irradiation.

FAO Panel of Experts on Pesticide Residues in Food and the Environment. Ongoing. *Pesticide Residues in Food and the Environment*. Report no. 148. Rome: Food and Agriculture Organization.
Web site: Available full-text at http:// www.fao.org/waicent/faoinfo/AGRICULT/agp/agpp/Pesticid/jmpr/pm_jmpr.htm

The Joint FAO/WHO Meeting on Pesticide Residues has met annually since 1963 to conduct scientific evaluations of pesticide residues in food. It provides advice on the acceptable levels of pesticide residues in food moving in international trade.

Food Marketing Institute and Grocery Manufacturers Association. 1998. *Consumer's Views on Food Irradiation*. Washington, DC: Food Marketing Institute and Grocery Manufacturers Association.

A one-stop shop for information about irradiation, this report provides background information as well as insight into consumers' attitudes about irradiation. It contains many charts and graphs to explain the data and is easy to read.

Food Marketing Policy Center. 1998. *Mandatory vs. Voluntary Approaches to Food Safety*. Research Report No. 36. Storrs, CT: University of Connecticut.
Web site: Available full-text at http:// vm.uconn.edu/~cotteril/rr36.pdf

This report examines whether a voluntary approach to food safety is likely to lead to adequate consumer protection.

Food Marketing Policy Center. June 1995. *Regulatory Targets and Regimes for Food Safety: A Comparison of North American and European Approaches.* Storrs, CT: University of Connecticut.
Web site: Available full-text at http://agecon.lib.umn.edu/ne165/ne165c01.pdf

This report, from the proceedings of the NE-165 conference on the Economics of Reducing Health Risks from Food, examines the effect of international trade agreements on the supply and safety of food products.

Institute of Food Science & Technology. September 1999. *Bovine Somatotropin (BST).* London: Institute of Food Science & Technology.
Web site: Available full-text at http://www.ifst.org/hottop8a.htm

This position statement on BST examines issues related to human health, antibiotic residues in milk, socioeconomic concerns, legal considerations, animal health and welfare, and labeling.

Institute of Food Science & Technology. September 1999. *Genetic Modification and Food.* London: Institute of Food Science & Technology.
Web site: Available full-text at http:// www.ifst.org/hottop10.htm

Topics included in this position statement on genetic modification (GM) of food are GM across the species barrier, techniques of GM, benefits of GM, examples of GM foods and food ingredients, safety and regulation of GM foods, antibiotic resistance concerns, environmental issues, labeling, and public perception of GM foods.

Institute of Food Science & Technology. June 1999. *Bovine Spongiform Encephalopathy (BSE).* London: Institute of Food Science & Technology.
Web site: Available full-text at http://www.ifst.org/hottop5.htm

This position statement begins with background and a summary on BSE and then examines origin and transmission in cattle, the infective agent, measures to prevent transmission to humans, transmission to other species, the risk of BSE transmission to humans, and whether vCJD is linked to BSE.

Institute of Food Science & Technology. June 1999. *Food Allergens.* London: Institute of Food Science & Technology.
Web site: Available full-text at http://www.ifst.org/hottop19.htm

Topics covered in this position statement include background information about food allergies; the responsibilities of individuals, food manufacturers, caterers, and retailers; labeling of foods; novel foods, including genetically modified foods; and research in food allergens.

Institute of Food Science & Technology. December 1998. *The Use of Irradiation for Food Quality and Safety.* London: Institute of Food Science & Technology.
Web site: Available full-text at http://www.ifst.org/hottop11.htm

After a brief introduction to the food irradiation process, this position statement on irradiation covers food irradiation applications, international perspectives on food irradiation, nutritional quality of irradiated foods, detection of irradiated foods, and high-dose food irradiation.

Institute of Food Technologists. August 2000. *IFT Expert Panel on Biotechnology and Foods.* Chicago: Institute of Food Technologists.
Web site: Available full-text at http://www.ift.org/resource/policy/biotechreport.shtml

Following an introduction to food biotechnology, this report examines the issues of safety, labeling, and benefits and concerns. Its purpose is to provide science-based information about food biotechnology to the general public, journalists, and members of IFT.

International Agricultural Trade Research Consortium (IATRC). May 1998. *Implementation of the WTO Agreement on the Application of Sanitary and Phytosanitary Measures: The First Two.* Working Paper 98-4. International Agricultural Trade Research Consortium (IATRC).
Web site: Available full-text at http://agecon.lib.umn.edu/iatrc/wp9804.pdf

This paper examines the implementation of the 1995 Sanitary and Phytosanitary Agreement, providing an overview of the agreement, looking at the international dispute over hormones and how it was handled, and offering a view of the future of the agreement.

Life Sciences Research Office, Federation of American Societies for Experimental Biology. 1995. *Analysis of Adverse Reactions to Monosodium Glutamate (MSG).* Bethesda, MD: American Institute of Nutrition.

This report, prepared for the FDA, seeks to ascertain whether MSG, as used in the American food supply, contributes to Chinese Restaurant Syndrome or any other adverse symptoms.

National Performance Review. 1996. *Reinventing Food Regulations.* Washington, DC: National Performance Review.

This report provides an overview of food safety regulations in the United States and discusses in detail FSIS and FDA initiatives with regard to HACCP and regulatory reform.

National Research Council, Committee on Genetically Modified Pest-Protected Plants. April 2000. *Genetically Modified Pest Protected Plants.* Washington, DC: National Academy of Sciences-National Research Council.
Web site: Available full-text at http://www.nap.edu/catalog/9795.html

This technical report investigates the benefits and risks of genetically modified pest-protected plants, providing an overview on improving pest resistance, health-related concerns, environmental concerns, and the regulatory framework.

National Research Council, Committee on Drug Use in Food Animals. 1999. *The Use of Drugs in Food Animals: Benefits and Risks.* Washington, DC: National Academy of Sciences-National Research Council.
Web site: Available full-text at http://books.nap.edu/html/foodanim/

This report provides an overview of why and how drugs are used in the major food-producing animal industries. It discusses the prevalence of human pathogens in foods of animal origin, the transfer of resistance in animal microbes to human pathogens, and the resulting risk of human disease.

National Research Council, Committee to Ensure Safe Food from Production to Consumption. 1998. *Ensuring Safe Food: From Production to Consumption.* Washington, DC: National Academy of Sciences-National Research Council.
Web site: Available full-text at http://books.nap.edu/catalog/6163.html

The Committee to Ensure Safe Food from Production to Consumption was formed by the Institute of Medicine (IOM) and National Research Council (NRC). The committee reviewed mechanisms now in place at the federal level to ensure safe food, assessed the extent to which they are effective in addressing food safety issues from production to consumption, and developed recommendations about changes needed to move towards a more effective food safety system. This volume reports the deliberations, conclusions, and recommendations of the committee.

National Research Council, Committee on Pesticides in the Diet of Infants and Children. 1993. *Pesticides in the Diets of Infants and Children.* Washington, DC: National Academy Press.
Web site: Available full-text at http://books.nap.edu/catalog/2126.html

This oft-quoted report examines what is known about exposures to pesticide residues in the diets of infants and children, the adequacy of risk assessment methods and policies, dietary intakes of infants and children, pesticide residues in the food supply, and toxicologic issues of concern. In addition, the committee looked at research priorities and scientific and policy issues faced by government agencies.

Natural Resources Defense Council (NRDC). February 1999. *Bottled Water: Pure Drink or Pure Hype?* New York: Natural Resources Defense Council.
Web site: Available full-text at http://www.nrdc.org/nrdcpro/fppubl.html

NRDC did a four-year study of the bottled water industry, including its bacterial and chemical contamination problems. They report on available information on bottled water and its sources, an in-depth assessment of government programs that regulate bottled water safety, and an analysis of government and academic bottled water testing results. In addition, NRDC commissioned independent lab testing of more than 1,000 bottles of 103 types of bottled water from many parts of the country.

North Carolina Biotechnology Center and USDA Office of Agricultural Biotechnology. 1993. *Conference Proceedings: Symbol, Substance, Science: The Societal Issues of Food Biotechnology.* Research Triangle Park, NC: North Carolina Biotechnology Center.

These proceedings are from a two-day conference held in June 1993 in which participants from a variety of backgrounds discussed issues related to food biotechnology. Sessions included benefits and likely reality, ethical considerations, scientific and philosophical considerations, allergenicity, safety, novel foods, and regulatory policy.

Public Voice for Food & Health Policy. February 18–19, 1998. *Identifying, Addressing and Overcoming Consumer Concerns: A Roundtable on Food Irradiation.* Washington, DC: Public Voice

for Food & Health Policy.
Web site: Available full-text at http://www.publicvoicedc.com/download/foodirradiation.doc

Public Voice, together with the National Food Processors Association and the International Food Information Council, convened a roundtable discussion to address consumer concerns about food irradiation. Participants included many of the top government and academic experts on irradiation, representatives of consumer organizations with an interest in food irradiation, and representatives of the food and irradiation industries. The group included both critics and advocates of irradiation, and participants were encouraged to ask tough questions of those on opposing sides. The agenda for the roundtable included the capabilities of irradiation; current uses in this country and worldwide; different irradiation technologies and their application to various foods; safety, nutritional, and organoleptic issues; and labeling, consumer acceptance, and education.

Regional Research Project NE-165. June 1996. *Strategy and Policy in the Food System: Emerging Issues.* Storrs, CT: Food Marketing Policy Center.
Web site: Available full-text at http://www.ncfap.org/foodsafe.htm

These conference proceedings from the Strategy and Policy in the Food System: Emerging Issues conference include papers on Modeling the Costs of Food Safety Regulation, Improving Cost/Benefit Analysis for HACCP and Microbial Food Safety: An Economist's Overview, A Policy Perspective on Improving Benefit/Cost Analysis: The Case of HACCP and Microbial Food Safety, and Improving Benefit-Cost Analysis for Policy Makers.

South Centre. July 1999. *WTO Agreement on Sanitary and Phytosanitary Measures: Issues for Developing Countries.* Geneva, Switzerland: South Centre.
Web site: Available full-text at http://www.southcentre.org/publications/s&p/toc.htm

U.S. Environmental Protection Agency (EPA). July 12, 2000. *Available EPA Information on Assessing Exposure to Pesticides in Food—A User's Guide.* Washington, DC: Environmental Protection Agency.
Web site: Available full-text at http://www.epa.gov

This document provides the reader with a comprehensive listing and discussion of federal guidance, policy documents, and databases that provide detailed, specific "how-to" information or data on assessing exposure to pesticides from foods that we eat.

U.S. Environmental Protection Agency (EPA), Office of Water. December 1999. *25 Years of the Safe Drinking Water Act: History and Trends.* Report no. EPA 816-R-99-007. Washington, DC: U.S. Environmental Protection Agency.
Web site: Available full-text at http://www.epa.gov/safewater/sdwa25/sdwa.html

This report examines the changes that have taken place in the Safe Drinking Water Act over the last 25 years.

U.S. Environmental Protection Agency (EPA). February 1997. *Drinking Water Infrastructure Needs Survey.* Washington, DC: U.S. Environmental Protection Agency.
Web site: Available full-text at http://www.epa.gov/ogwdw/needs.html

The 1996 Safe Drinking Water Act amendments directed EPA to conduct a survey to find out how much money public drinking water systems nationwide will have to invest in order to comply with existing and proposed regulations, and to replace aging infrastructure. The first survey was released in 1997, with updates to be released every four years. Results from the survey are used to develop a formula to allot funds for Drinking Water State Revolving Fund grants to states.

U.S. Food and Drug Administration (FDA). Ongoing. *FDA Pesticide Program Residue Monitoring.* Washington, DC: U.S. Food and Drug Administration.
Web site: Available full-text at http://vm.cfsan.fda.gov/~dms/pesrpts.html

Since 1987 annual reports have been prepared to summarize results of the FDA's pesticide residue monitoring program. Annual reports since 1993 are available full-text on the FDA's Web site.

U.S. Food and Drug Administration (FDA). August 10, 2000. *Report of the FDA Retail Food Program Database of Foodborne Illness Risk Factors.* Washington, DC: U.S. Food and Drug Administration.

Web site: Available full-text at http://vm.cfsan.fda.gov/~dms/retrsk.html

This project is designed to establish a national baseline on the occurrence of foodborne disease risk factors within the retail segment of the food industry. This report presents the methodology used to establish a baseline and reports the results of the data collected. It is provided to regulators and industry with the expectation that it will be used to focus greater attention and increased resources on the control of foodborne illness risk factors.

U.S. Food and Drug Administration, Center for Food Safety and Applied Nutrition. September 1999. *Evaluation of Risks Related to Microbiological Contamination of Ready-to-eat Food by Food Preparation Workers and the Effectiveness of Interventions to Minimize Those Risks.* Washington, DC: U.S. Food and Drug Administration, Center for Food Safety and Applied Nutrition.
Web site: Available full-text at http://vm.cfsan.fda.gov/~ear/rterisk.html

This white paper begins with an exhaustive literature review of outbreaks caused by food workers from 1975 to 1998. The second section covers bare-hand contact with ready-to-eat foods and examines handwashing procedures and products.

U.S. Food and Drug Administration, Center for Food Safety and Applied Nutrition, Imports Branch. March 25, 1999; Modified May 20, 1999. *FDA Survey of Imported Fresh Produce.* Washington, DC: U. S. Food and Drug Administration.
Web site: Available full-text at http://vm.cfsan.fda.gov/~dms/prodsurv.html

The objective of this survey was to determine the incidence of microbial contamination on imported fresh produce to reduce foodborne illnesses from contaminated fresh product.

U.S. Food and Drug Administration (FDA), U.S. Department of Agriculture (USDA), U.S. Environmental Protection Agency (EPA), and Centers for Disease Control and Prevention (CDC). May 1997. *Food Safety from Farm to Table: A National Food Safety Initiative: A Report to the President.* HE 20.4002:SA 1/3. Washington, DC: U.S. Food and Drug Administration (FDA), U.S. Department of Agriculture (USDA), U.S. Environmental Protection Agency (EPA), and Centers for Disease Control and Prevention (CDC).
Web site: Available full-text at http://www.foodsafety.gov/~dms/fsreport.html

The President directed three Cabinet members-the Secretary of Agriculture, the Secretary of Health and Human Services, and the Administrator of the Environmental Protection Agency—to identify specific steps to improve the safety of the food supply. He directed them to consult with consumers, producers, industry, states, universities, and the public, and to report back to him. In this response to the President's request the agencies outline a comprehensive new initiative to improve the safety of the nation's food supply.

U.S. General Accounting Office (GAO). August 24, 2000. *Food Irradiation: Available Research Indicates That Benefits Outweigh Risks.* Report no. GAO/RCED-00-217. Washington, DC: U.S. General Accounting Office.
Web site: Available full-text at http://www.gao.gov

This report analyzes the extent and the purpose for which food irradiation is being used in the United States and the scientifically supported benefits and risks of food irradiation.

U.S. General Accounting Office (GAO). February 25, 2000. *Food Safety: FDA's Use of Faster Tests to Assess the Safety of Imported Foods.* Report no. GAO/RCED-00-65. Washington, DC: U.S. General Accounting Office.
Web site: Available full-text at http:// www.gao.gov

This report examines the Food and Drug Administration's (FDA) use of faster technologies, known as rapid tests, to screen and identify potentially unsafe imported foods, particularly at ports of entry, before they make it to grocery store shelves. This report describes: (1) the rapid tests used to screen foods for pathogens, such as bacteria, parasites, and viruses; (2) FDA's use of these tests, particularly at ports of entry; and (3) the factors that may limit FDA's greater use of rapid tests for foodborne pathogens.

U.S. General Accounting Office (GAO). February 22, 2000. *School Meal Programs: Few Outbreaks of Foodborne Illness.* Report no. GAO/RCED-00-53. Washington, DC: U.S. General Accounting Office.
Web site: Search for full-text of report at http://www.gao.gov

This report looked at the extent of foodborne illness related to meals served in schools; how often USDA-donated foods in schools were removed, replaced, or disposed of because of the potential to cause foodborne illness; and USDA procurement policies and procedures for ensuring the safety of foods it donates to the programs.

U.S. General Accounting Office (GAO). December 8, 1999. *Meat and Poultry: Improved Oversight and Training Will Strengthen New Food Safety System.* Report no. GAO/RCED-00-16. Washington, DC: U.S. General Accounting Office.
Web site: Available full-text at http://www.gao.gov

GAO reviewed the Department of Agriculture's (USDA) efforts to improve the safety of meat and poultry products, focusing on whether the system adopted by USDA in its regulations is consistent with the seven Hazard Analysis and Critical Control Points (HACCP) principles endorsed by the National Advisory Committee on Microbiological Criteria for Foods, whether the HACCP training program for USDA inspectors is adequate and science-based, and whether there is an adequate dispute resolution (appeals) process between plants and USDA under the new HACCP inspection system.

U.S. General Accounting Office (GAO). October 27, 1999. *Food Safety: Agencies Should Further Test Plans for Responding to Deliberate Contamination.* Report no. GAO/RCED-00-3. Washington, DC: U.S. General Accounting Office.
Web site: Available full-text at http://www.gao.gov

GAO reviewed the preparedness of the federal food safety regulatory agencies to respond to acts or threats of deliberate food contamination, including those by terrorists, focusing on the extent to which food has been deliberately contaminated with a biological agent (bacteria, virus, or toxin) or threatened to be contaminated with such an agent; and plans and procedures that federal food safety regulatory agencies have for responding to threats and acts of deliberate food contamination.

U.S. General Accounting Office (GAO). August 4, 1999. *Food Safety: U.S. Needs a Single Agency to Administer a Unified, Risk-Based Inspection System.* Report no. T-RCED-99-256. Washington, DC: U.S. General Accounting Office.
Web site: Available full-text at http://www.gao.gov

In this report GAO looks at the need to revamp the current U.S. food safety system into a single food agency. The existing system suffers from inconsistent and inflexible oversight and enforcement, inefficient use of resources, and ineffective coordination. In GAO's view, a single food safety inspection agency responsible for administering a uniform set of laws is the most effective way to resolve these long-standing problems, deal with emerging food safety issues, and help ensure a safe food supply. GAO recognizes, however, that there are short-term costs and other considerations associated with establishing a new government agency. A second, though less desirable, option would be to consolidate food safety activities in an existing department.

U.S. General Accounting Office (GAO). July 1, 1999. *Food Safety: U.S. Lacks a Consistent Farm-to-Table Approach to Egg Safety.* Report no. GAO/ RCED-99-232. Washington, DC: U.S. General Accounting Office.
Web site: Available full-text at http://www.gao.gov

Concerned about the risks of eating eggs contaminated with *Salmonella enteritidis*, GAO looks at the adequacy of the current system for ensuring the safety of eggs. Specifically, GAO examined whether a prevention-based approach to food safety has been applied to egg production and processing, a new federal policy on egg refrigeration will effectively reduce the risks associated with contaminated eggs, federal and state policies on serving eggs to vulnerable populations and dating egg cartons are consistent, and federal egg safety resources are used efficiently and policies are coordinated effectively.

U.S. General Accounting Office (GAO). April 28, 1999. *Food Safety: The Agricultural Use of Antibiotics and Its Implications for Human Health.* Report no. GAO/RCED-99-74. Washington, DC: U.S. General Accounting Office.
Web site: Search for at http://www.gao.gov

Pursuant to a congressional request, GAO provided information on antibiotic resistance issues that may stem from the use of antibiotics in agriculture, focusing on the use of antibiotics in agriculture and the implications of that use for human health, federal roles and responsibilities for overseeing the use of antibiotics in agriculture, and issues surrounding the debate over whether to further regulate or restrict the use of antibiotics in agriculture.

U.S. General Accounting Office (GAO). April 20, 1999. *Food Safety: Experiences of Four Countries in Consolidating their Food Safety Systems.* Report no. GAO/RCED-99-80. Washington, DC: U.S. General Accounting Office.
Web site: Search for at http://www.gao.gov

Pursuant to a congressional request, GAO reviewed the experiences of foreign countries that are consolidating their food safety responsibilities, focusing on reasons for and approaches taken to consolidation; the costs and savings, if any, associated with consolidation; efforts to assess the effectiveness of the revised food safety systems; and lessons that the United States might learn from these countries' experiences in consolidating their food safety functions.

U.S. General Accounting Office (GAO). September 9, 1998. *Food Safety: Weak and Inconsistently Applied Controls Allow Unsafe Imported Food to Enter U.S. Commerce.* Report no. GAO/RCED-98-271. Washington, DC: U.S. General Accounting Office.
Web site: Available full-text at http://www.gao.gov

In this report GAO found that the Food and Drug Administration's current controls provide little assurance that shipments targeted for inspection are actually inspected or that shipments found to violate U.S. safety standards are destroyed or re-exported.

U.S. General Accounting Office (GAO). August 6, 1998. *Food Safety: Opportunities to Redirect Federal Resources and Funds Can Enhance Effectiveness.* Report no. GAO/RCED-98-224. Washington, DC: U.S. General Accounting Office.
Web site: Available full-text at http://www.gao.gov

In this report GAO analyzed the federal food safety agencies' budgets to determine whether the appropriated funds could be spent more effectively, and provided its views on whether the food safety initiatives proposed would address underlying problems.

U.S. General Accounting Office (GAO). April 1998. *Food Safety: Federal Efforts to Ensure the Safety of Imported Foods are Inconsistent and Unreliable.* Report no. GAO/RCED-98-103. Washington, DC: U.S. General Accounting Office.
Web site: Available full-text at http://www.gao.gov

GAO questions whether the Food Safety and Inspection Service and FDA are targeting their inspection resources at those imported foods posing the greatest safety risks.

U.S. General Accounting Office (GAO). April 10, 1998. *Food Safety: Agencies' Handling of a Dioxin Incident Caused Hardships for Some Producers and Processors.* Report no. GAO/RCED-98-104. Washington, DC: U.S. General Accounting Office.
Web site: Available full-text at http://www.gao.gov

In response to the discovery by federal agencies of elevated levels of dioxin in poultry samples, this report determined: (1) the basis for the federal agencies' decisions to require producers to demonstrate that their food products did not contain unacceptable levels of dioxin; (2) federal agencies' effectiveness in working together to make decisions to address the problem of dioxin-contaminated feed and in communicating their decisions to state agencies, producers, and processors; and (3) the impact of the food safety system on the handling of this dioxin incident.

U.S. General Accounting Office (GAO). October 8, 1997. *Food Safety: Fundamental Changes Needed to Improve the Nation's Food Safety System.* Report no. GAO/RCED-98-24. Washington, DC: U.S. General Accounting Office.
Web site: Available full-text at http://www.gao.gov

This testimony discusses fundamental weaknesses—namely, regulatory fragmentation and inconsistency—that, in GAO's view, need to be corrected to achieve a fully effective food safety system. GAO believes that the existing federal food safety structure needs to be replaced with a uniform, risk-based inspection system under a single food safety agency.

U.S. General Accounting Office (GAO). May 23, 1996. *Food Safety: Information on Foodborne Illnesses.* Report no. GAO/RCED-96-96. Washington, DC: U.S. General Accounting Office.
Web site: Available full-text at http://www.gao.gov

This report summarizes information on the frequency of foodborne illness, health consequences and economic impacts of foodborne illness, and the adequacy of knowledge about foodborne illness to develop effective control strategies.

U.S. General Accounting Office (GAO). May 23, 1996. *Food Safety: Reducing the Threat of Foodborne Illnesses.* Report no. GAO/RCED-96-185. Washington, DC: U.S. General Accounting Office.
Web site: Available full-text at http://www.gao.gov

This report focuses on what is and is not known about the scope, severity, and cost of foodborne illnesses in the United States at the time of publication. It also summarizes prior GAO work on the structural problems that limit the federal government's ability to ensure food safety.

U.S. General Accounting Office (GAO). March 27, 1996. *Food Safety: New Initiatives Would Fundamentally Alter the Existing System.* Report no. GAO/RCED-96-81. Washington, DC: U.S. General Accounting Office.
Web site: Available full-text at http://www.gao.gov

In response to continuing outbreaks of food poisoning, Congress and federal agencies are considering new approaches to ensuring food safety. This report discusses the federal food safety system, particularly the current responsibilities, budgets, staffing, and workloads of the federal agencies involved.

U.S. General Accounting Office (GAO). June 30, 1995. *Meat and Poultry Inspection: Impact of USDA's Food Safety Proposal on State Agencies and Small Plants.* Report no. GAO/RCED-95-228. Washington, DC: U.S. General Accounting Office.
Web site: Search for full-text at http://www.access.gpo.gov/su_docs/aces/aces160.shtml

This report describes state meat and poultry inspection programs, provides information on the expected effects of USDA's proposal on state inspection programs, and discusses the proposal's likely effects on small plants.

U.S. General Accounting Office (GAO). December 1994. *Pesticides: Reducing Exposure to Residues of Canceled Pesticides.* Report no. GAO/RCED-95-23. Washington, DC: U.S. General Accounting Office.
Web site: Search for full-text at http://www.access.gpo.gov/su_docs/aces/aces160.shtml

This report investigates whether marketed foods contain unsafe levels of residues from canceled pesticides and evaluates the EPA's procedures for revoking tolerances for canceled food-use pesticides.

U.S. General Accounting Office (GAO). September 26, 1994. *Food Safety: Changes Needed to Minimize Unsafe Chemicals in Food.* Report no. GAO/RCED-94-192. Washington, DC: U.S. General Accounting Office.
Web site: Search for full-text at http://www.access.gpo.gov/su_docs/aces/aces160.shtml

In this report GAO identified five basic weaknesses in the overall federal structure and systems for monitoring chemicals in food.

U.S. General Accounting Office (GAO). May 25, 1994. *Food Safety: A Unified, Risk-based Food Safety System Needed.* Report no. GAO/T-RCED-94-223. Washington, DC: U.S. General Accounting Office.
Web site: Search for full-text at http://www.access.gpo.gov/su_docs/aces/aces160.shtml

This report examines the federal food safety system and whether this system should be revamped. It details the need for a uniform, scientific, risk-based system and concludes that the current food safety system hampers efforts to address public health concerns and is slow to respond to changing health risks.

U.S. General Accounting Office (GAO). May 19, 1994. *Food Safety: Risk-based Inspections and Microbial Monitoring Needed for Meat and Poultry.* Report no. GAO/RCED-94-110. Washington, DC: U.S. General Accounting Office.
Web site: Search for full-text at http://www.access.gpo.gov/su_docs/aces/aces160.shtml

Concerned about the effectiveness of FSIS' meat and poultry inspection system, GAO evaluated whether the system makes the most effective use of its resources to ensure food safety, whether meat and poultry plants have programs to test for microorganisms, and whether the Hazard Analysis and Critical Control Points system is an effective approach for ensuring food safety.

U.S. General Accounting Office (GAO). December 1990. *Food Safety and Quality: Who Does What in the Federal Government.* Report no. GAO/RCED-91-19A(B). Washington, DC: U.S. General Accounting Office.

A companion volume to the GAO's report on the subject of food safety and quality, this book contains a more detailed description of the food safety and quality activities of the 12 federal agencies discussed in the first volume.

U.S. House of Representatives, Committee on Science. April 2000. *Seeds of Opportunity.* Washington, DC: U.S. House of Representatives.
Web site: Available full-text at http://www.house.gov/science/smithreport_041300.pdf

A culmination of a series of hearings held on agricultural biotechnology issues, this report contains 13 specific findings and makes six recommendations. It presents the science behind the U.S. government's decision to proceed with the applications of this biotechnology to the benefit of food, agriculture, and the environment, while also giving clear and fair attention to the safety concerns expressed by the critics of agricultural biotechnology.

USDA, Animal and Plant Health Inspection Service, Centers for Epidemiology and Animal Health. 1999. *Antimicrobial Resistance Issues in Animal Agriculture.* Fort Collins, CO: USDA, Animal and Plant Health Inspection Service.
Web site: Available full-text at: http://www.aphis.usda.gov

This report provides a knowledge base related to antimicrobial resistance that will assist decision makers in assigning research priorities and resources. The report describes the origins and mechanisms of antimicrobial resistance, antimicrobial use in food animals in the United States, the epidemiology of antimicrobial resistance, implications of antimicrobial resistance for human and animal health, and current activities and future needs related to antimicrobial resistance.

USDA, Economic Research Service (ERS). July 1997. *Estimated Annual Costs of* Campylobacter*-Associated Guillian-Barré Syndrome.* Agricultural Economic Report No. 756. Washington, DC: USDA, Economic Research Service.
Web site: Available full-text at http://www.ers.usda.gov/epubs/pdf/aer756/

Of an estimated 2,628 to 9,575 new U.S. cases of Guillian-Barré Syndrome annually, between 526 and 3,830 are triggered by infection with *Campylobacter*, the most frequently isolated cause of foodborne diarrhea. This report estimates the annual cost-of-illness of GBS caused by all *Campylobacter* infections and by foodborne *Campylobacter* infections in the United States.

USDA, Economic Research Service (ERS). July 1997. *An Economic Assessment of Food Safety Regulations: The New Approach to Meat and Poultry Inspection.* Agricultural Economic Report No. 755. Washington, DC: USDA, Economic Research Service.
Web site: Available full-text at http://www.ers.usda.gov/epubs/pdf/aer755/

USDA is now requiring all federally inspected meat and poultry processing and slaughter plants to implement the Hazard Analysis and Critical Control Points system to reduce potentially harmful microbial pathogens in the food supply. This report finds that the benefits of the regulation, which are the medical costs and productivity losses that are prevented when foodborne illnesses are averted, will likely exceed the costs, which include spending by firms on sanitation, temperature control, planning and training, and testing.

USDA, Economic Research Service (ERS). June 1997. *The Benefits of Safer Drinking Water: The Value of Nitrate Reduction.* Agricultural Economic Report No. 752. Washington, DC: USDA, Economic Research Service.
Web site: Available full-text at http://www.ers.usda.gov/epubs/pdf/aer752/

This report evaluates the potential benefits of reducing human exposure to nitrates in the drinking water supply. In a survey, respondents were asked a series of questions about their willingness to pay for a hypothetical water filter that would reduce their risk of nitrate exposure.

USDA, Economic Research Service (ERS). August 1996. *Bacterial Foodborne Disease: Medical Costs and Productivity Losses.* Agricultural Economic Report No. 741. Washington, DC: USDA, Economic Research Service.
Web site: Available full-text at http://www.ers.usda.gov/epubs/pdf/aer741/

This report documents ERS analyses for six bacteria—*Salmonella, Campylobacter jejuni, Escherichia coli* O157:H7, *Listeria monocytogenes, Staphylococcus aureus,* and *Clostridium perfringens*—providing a comprehensive, detailed accounting of how the cost-of-illness estimates were calculated.

USDA, Economic Research Service (ERS). January 1996. *Pesticide Residues: Reducing Dietary Risks.* Agricultural Economic Report No. 728. Washington, DC: USDA, Economic Research Service.

Consumers' dietary intake of pesticide residues comes from three identifiable sources: on-farm pesticide use, pesticides used on imported foods, and canceled pesticides that persist in the environment. This report shows how each of these sources contributes to dietary risk from pesticide residues and ranks pesticides according to their contribution to dietary risk.

USDA, Economic Research Service (ERS). February 1995. *Economic Issues Associated with Food Safety.* Staff Paper AGE-9506. Washington, DC: USDA, Economic Research Service.

This document outlines, in graphs and figures, ERS research findings about the incidences and costs of foodborne illness in meat and poultry and exposure to pesticide residues on fresh fruit and vegetables.

Water Infrastructure Network (WIN). April 12, 2000. *Clean and Safe Water for the 21st Century.* Washington, DC: Water Infrastructure Network (WIN).
Web site: Available full-text at http://www.amwa-water.org/

Chapters in this report are: The Value of Clean and Safe Water, A Historic and Future Perspective on Investment in Water and Wastewater, Water and Wastewater Investment Needs of the Next Century, The Federal Role in Water and Wastewater Infrastructure, and The Path Forward—A National Dialogue on Water and Wastewater Infrastructure Investment.

World Health Organization (WHO). June 1999. *Strategies for Implementing HACCP in Small and/or Less Developed Businesses.* WHO/SDE/PHE/FOS/99.7. Geneva: World Health Organization.
Web site: Available full-text at http://www.who.int/fsf

This report offers guidance for applying HACCP principles to food businesses with less-developed food safety management systems. Sections include benefits and barriers to implementing HACCP, overcoming barriers, advice on development of sector-specific industry guides, and guidelines for the applications of the HACCP system.

World Health Organization (WHO). 1999. *Basic Food Safety for Health Workers.* WHO/SDE/PHE/FOS/99.1. Geneva: World Health Organization.
Web site: Available full-text at http://www.who.int/fsf

This publication was prepared with a view to strengthening the education and training of health professionals in food safety. As the primary health care system is one of the most important vehicles for health education in food safety, health workers need to know the epidemiology of foodborne diseases, the sociocultural conditions that encourage them, and how to investigate foodborne disease outbreaks.

World Health Organization (WHO). 1994. *Safety and Nutritional Adequacy of Irradiated Food.* Geneva: World Health Organization.
This report reviews scientific studies that have been carried out on the safety and nutritional quality of irradiated food. After describing the chemistry and potential applications of food irradiation, it reviews toxicological studies, studies on the effects of irradiation on microorganisms, and studies on the nutritional quality of irradiated food.

BROCHURES

American Academy of Allergy, Asthma and Immunology
Tips to Remember—Food Allergies
Cost: Single copies free.
Also available in Spanish.

American Council on Science and Health
Feeding Baby Safely: Facts, Fads and Fallacies
Cost: $5
Available full-text at http://www.acsh.org/publications/booklets/feedingbaby.html

American Council on Science and Health
Traces of Environmental Chemicals in the Human Body: Are They a Risk to Health?
Cost: $5
Available full-text at http://www.acsh.org/publications/booklets/traceChem.html

Centers for Disease Control and Prevention (CDC)
An Ounce of Prevention: Keeps the Germs Away
Cost: Single copy free, order at 800–995–9765. For multiple copies: ncid@cdc.gov or NCID Office of Health Communication, CDC, 1600 Clifton Rd., C14, Atlanta GA 30333.

Centers for Disease Control and Prevention (CDC)
Safe Food and Water: A Guide for People with HIV Infection

Cost: Single copy free from the CDC National AIDS Clearinghouse, 800–458–5231.
Available full-text at http://www.cdc.gov/hiv/pubs/brochure

Centers for Disease Control and Prevention (CDC)
You Can Prevent Cryptosporidiosis: A Guide for People with HIV Infection
Cost: Single copy free the CDC National AIDS Clearinghouse, 800–458–5231.
Available full-text at http://www.cdc.gov/nchstp/hiv_aids/pubs/brochure/oi_cryp.htm

Cornell University Cooperative Extension
Drinking Water Alternatives: Bottled Water
Cost: $2. Call 607–255–2080 to order or visit Web site at http://www.cce.cornell.edu

Environmental Protection Agency
Children and Drinking Water Standards
Cost: Single copy free from the EPA's Safe Drinking Water Hotline at 800–426–4791.
Available full-text at http://www.epa.gov/safewater/kids/child.pdf

Environmental Protection Agency
Drinking Water and Health: What You Need to Know
Cost: Single copy free from the EPA's Safe Drinking Water Hotline at 800–426–4791.
Available full-text at http://www.epa.gov/ogwdw000/dwhealth.html

Environmental Protection Agency
It's Your Drinking Water: Get to Know It and Protect It
Cost: Single copy free from the EPA's Safe Drinking Water Hotline at 800–426–4791.
Available full-text at http://www.epa.gov/ogwdw000/consumer/itsyours.html

Environmental Protection Agency
Lead In Your Drinking Water
Cost: Single copy free from the EPA's Safe Drinking Water Hotline at 800–426–4791.
Available full-text at http://www.epa.gov/safewater/Pubs/lead1.html

Environmental Protection Agency
Tap Into It
Cost: Single copy free from the EPA's Safe Drinking Water Hotline at 800–426–4791.

Environmental Protection Agency
Water on Tap: A Consumer's Guide to the Nation's Drinking Water
Cost: Single copy free from the EPA's Safe Drinking Water Hotline at 800–426–4791.
Available full-text at http://www.epa.gov/OGWDW/wot/introtap.html

EPA/FDA/USDA
Pesticides and Food: What You and Your Family Need to Know
Cost: $0.50 from the Consumer Information Center
Available full-text at http://www.pueblo.gsa.gov/food.htm and at Evironmental Protection Agency Web site.

Food and Drug Administration
Can Your Kitchen Pass the Food Safety Test?
Cost: Single copy free from the Consumer Information Center.
Available full-text at http://www.pueblo.gsa.gov/food.htm

Food and Drug Administration
Critical Steps Toward Safer Seafood
Cost: Single copy free from the Consumer Information Center.
Available full-text at http://www.pueblo.gsa.gov

Food and Drug Administration
Fresh Look At Food Preservatives
Cost: Single copy free from the Consumer Information Center.
Available full-text at http://www.pueblo.gsa.gov/food.htm

Food and Drug Administration
Irradiation: A Safe Measure for Safer Food
Cost: Single copy free from the Consumer Information Center.
Available full-text at http://www.pueblo.gsa.gov/food.htm

Food and Drug Administration
Keep Your Food Safe
Cost: Single copy free from the Consumer Information Center.
Also available in Spanish. Available full-text at http://www.pueblo.gsa.gov/food.htm

Food and Drug Administration
Preventing Food-Borne Illness

Cost: Single copy free from the Consumer Information Center.
Available full-text at http://www.pueblo.gsa.gov/food.htm

Food and Drug Administration
Playing It Safe with Eggs: What Consumers Need to Know
Cost: Single copy free by calling 1-800-332-4010.
Available full-text at http://www.cfsan.fda.gov

Food and Drug Administration
To Your Health! Food Safety for Seniors
Cost: Single copy free from Consumer Information Center.
Available full-text at http://www.pueblo.gsa.gov/food.htm

Food and Drug Administration and the U.S. Department of Agriculture
American Meat Institute and in cooperation with the National Live Stock and Meat Board, the *Food Service Guide to Safe Handling and Preparation Of Ground Meat and Ground Poultry*
Cost: $5

Food Marketing Institute
Bioengineered Food and You
Cost: Free to download camera-ready copy.
Available full-text at http://www.fmi.org

Food Marketing Institute
A Consumer Guide to Food Quality and Safe Handling: Dairy Products and Eggs
Cost: $5

Food Marketing Institute
A Consumer Guide to Food Quality and Safe Handling: Deli and Fresh Prepared Foods
Cost: $0.50

Food Marketing Institute
A Consumer Guide to Food Quality and Safe Handling: Fresh Fruits and Vegetables
Cost: $0.50

Food Marketing Institute
A Consumer Guide to Safe Handling and Preparation: Ground Meat and Ground Poultry
Cost: $0.50
Also available in Spanish.

Food Marketing Institute
A Consumer Guide to Food Quality and Safe Handling: Meat and Poultry
Cost: $0.50

Food Marketing Institute
A Consumer Guide to Food Quality and Safe Handling: Seafood
Cost: $0.50

Food Marketing Institute
Facts About Food and Floods: A Consumer Guide to Food Quality and Safe Handling After a Flood or Power Outage
Cost: $0.50

Food Marketing Institute in cooperation with Cornell University in cooperation with USDA and Cooperative Extension Service
The Food Keeper
Cost: $0.75

Food Marketing Institute with Food and Drug Administration, American Meat Institute, Grocery Manufacturers of America, National Cattlemen's Beef Association, National Food Processors Association, and The American Dietetic Association
Food Irradiation-A Safe Measure
Cost: $0.50
Available full-text at http://www.fmi.org

The Groundwater Foundation
Is My Water Safe to Drink?
Cost: Single copy free

International Food Information Council Foundation
A Consumer's Guide to Pesticides and Food Safety
Cost: Single copy free
Available full-text at http://ificinfo.health.org/brochure/cgfs&p.htm

International Food Information Council Foundation
Everything You Need to Know About Glutamate and Monosodium Glutamate
Cost: Single copy free
Available full-text at http://ificinfo.health.org/brochure/msg.htm

International Food Information Council Foundation
Food Additives

Cost: Single copy free
Available full-text at http://ificinfo.health.org/brochure/food-add.htm

International Food Information Council Foundation
Food Biotechnology: Enhancing Our Food Supply
Cost: Single copy free.
Available full-text at http://ificinfo.health.org/brochure/bioenhancing.htm

International Food Information Council Foundation
Food Biotechnology: Health and Harvest For Our Times
Cost: Single copy free
Available full-text at http://ificinfo.health.org/brochure/biobroch.htm

International Food Information Council Foundation
Understanding Food Allergy
Cost: Single copy free
Available full-text at http://ificinfo.health.org/brochure/allergy.htm

March of Dimes Birth Defects Foundation
Food-borne Risks in Pregnancy
Cost: Order from Web site, $5 for a package of 50.
Available full-text at http://www.modimes.org/HealthLibrary2/FactSheets/Food_Born_Risks.htm

Mothers & Others
The Mothers' Milk List and rBGH Factsheet
Cost: $2

National Cattlemen's Beef Association
Plating It Safe
Cost: Single copy free
Available full-text at http://www.beef.org/library/safety/plating.htm

National Consumers League
Irradiation . . . What You Need to Know
Order for $1 from NCL at 202-835-3323.
Available full-text at http://www.natlconsumersleague.org/brochures.html

National Consumers League
Keep It Clean, Keep it Healthy
Cost: $1
Order from NCL at 202–835–3323

National Pork Producers Council
Serving Up Safely
Cost: Single copy free. Order from http://www.nppc.org/catalog/

National Restaurant Association
Food Allergy Brochure for Restaurant Employees
Cost: Sold in packets of 25 for $24

North Carolina Biotechnology Center
Food Biotechnology
Cost: Single copy free from North Carolina Biotechnology Center, 919–541–9366
Available full-text at http:/ www.ncbiotech.org/news/foodbt.cfm

Partnership for Food Safety Education, USDA/FDA/CDC
Fight BAC!: Four Simple Steps to Food Safety
Cost: Single copy free from the Consumer Information Center
Available full-text at http://www.pueblo.gsa.gov/food.htm

USDA Food Safety and Inspection Service
Listeriosis and Food Safety Tips
Cost: Single copy free from the Consumer Information Center
Also available in Spanish. Available full-text at http://www.fsis.usda.gov

USDA Food Safety and Inspection Service
Safe Handling of Complete Meals to Go
Cost: Single copy free
Available full-text at http://www.fsis.usda.gov

USDA Food Safety and Inspection Service
Take the Guesswork Out of Roasting a Turkey
Cost: Single copy free
Available full-text at http://www.fsis.usda.gov

USDA Food Safety and Inspection Service
Use a Food Thermometer
Cost: Single copy free from the Consumer Information Center.
Available full-text at http://www.pueblo.gsa.gov/cic_text/food/therm/thermy.htm

CHAPTER 8

BOOKS AND NEWSLETTERS

This chapter consists of books and newsletters covering all aspects of food safety. There is a mix of general food safety works, and many that deal only with a specific food safety topic. There are books for consumers without a background in science, more technical works that are better understood with some science knowledge, and books for children. The books are arranged in the following order:

A. Reference books

B. General food safety books
   1. Children's general food safety books

C. Books on specific food safety topics
   1. Additives
   2. Animal health
   3. Bovine spongiform encephalopathy (BSE)
   4. Food allergy
   5. Food allergy books for children
   6. Food biotechnology
   7. Food irradiation
   8. Food preservation
   9. Food safety regulations
   10. Naturally occurring, environmental, and chemical toxins
   11. Pesticides
   12. Water

D. Texts

The newsletters are smaller, harder-to-find, and not usually indexed in major databases. While there are some newsletters written for the consumer, the bulk of the newsletters are geared towards educators, food sanitarians, and food professionals. With the trend towards electronic publishing, some newsletters are now available only online, while some are available both in hard copy and online. Those that are only available in hard copy will probably move toward electronic distribution. The newsletters are organized as follows:

Food biotechnology

Food regulations

General food safety for consumers

General food safety for educators and food professionals

Pesticides

BOOKS

Reference Books

Francis, Jack J., ed. 1999. *Wiley Encyclopedia of Food Science and Technology*. 2nd ed. New York: John Wiley.

This edition of the comprehensive four-volume encyclopedia reflects major advances in the field, with an emphasis on emerging areas in food and nutrition delivery systems, including chemical and microbiological food safety, risk management in food safety, functional foods and neutraceuticals in food formulation, food substitutes, and advances in food biotechnology.

Igoe, Robert S. 1999. *Dictionary of Food Ingredients*. 3rd rev. ed. New York: Chapman and Hall.

Concise, easy-to-use dictionary provides definitions of more than 1,000 commonly used food additives, including natural ingredients, FDA approved artificial ingredients, and compounds used in food processing. This is a good tool to make label reading easier for those with food allergies.

Meister, Richard T., ed. 1999. *Farm Chemicals Handbook '99*. Willoughby, OH: Meister.

This handbook lists fertilizers, pesticides, chemical manufacturers, federal and state regulations, chemical application procedures, and storage and disposal options. The pesticide dictionary includes action, use, formulations, combinations, environmental guidelines, safety guidelines, toxicity class, hazards, solubility, emergency guidelines, and first aid treatments. Quick reference tables are included. Also comes in software version: Electronic Pesticide Dictionary 99.

Robinson, Richard, Carl A. Batt, and Pradip Patel, eds. 1999. *Encyclopedia of Food Microbiology*. Lake Oswego, OR: Academic Press.

This technical reference work has as its purpose to offer the largest comprehensive reference source of current knowledge available in the field of food microbiology. It addresses a wide audience of academic and professional/industrial microbiologists, e.g., analysts in industry seeking an authoritative source of information on a branch of microbiology peripheral to their own; and it is also a useful source of course material for undergraduate students and postgraduate students as well as teachers and lecturers. Consisting of nearly 400 articles written by the world's leading scientists, the encyclopedia presents a highly structured distillation of the whole field, its alphabetical sequence ranging from acetobacter to zymomonas. An online version with extensive hypertext linking and advanced search tools is also available.

Maizell, Robert E. 1998. *How to Find Chemical Information: A Guide for Practicing Chemists, Educators, and Students*. 3rd ed. New York: John Wiley.

This book is a practical and easy-to-use guide on how to quickly find sources of chemical information through the use of CD-ROMs, electronic databases, the Internet, and numerous new print publications.

National Academy of Sciences, Committee on Food Chemicals Codex. 1996. *Food Chemical Codex*. 4th ed. Washington, DC: National Academy Press.

Food Chemical Codex is the accepted standard for defining the quality and purity of food chemicals. It is frequently referenced by the U.S. Food and Drug Administration and other international food regulatory authorities. Entries include a description of substances and their use in foods; tolerable levels of contaminants; appropriate tests to determine compliance, packaging, and storage guidelines; and more. The Codex will be of interest to producers and users of food chemicals, including processed-food manufacturers, food technologists, quality control chemists, research investigators, teachers, students, and others involved in the technical aspects of food safety. Frequent supplements are printed to update material. Also available in a CD-ROM version.

U.S. Environmental Protection Agency. 1994. *Drinking Water Glossary—A Dictionary of Technical and Legal Terms Related to Drinking Water.* Washington: U.S. Environmental Protection Agency.

This book serves as a reference document for drinking water treatment operators, technical assistance providers, state and local drinking water officials, and the general public on commonly used drinking water terms to enhance their understanding of program issues. Order from: National Technical Information Service, Telephone: 703-605-6000 or Web site: www.ntis.gov, NTIS Order Number: PB94-203486INZ.

Cress, D., K. P. Penner, and F. Aramouni. 1993. *Food Safety: Common Terms, Acronyms, Abbreviations, Agencies and Laws.* Manhattan, KS: North Central Regional Extension.

This 16-page publication defines many of the terms and acronyms related to food safety. It explains the functions and responsibilities of the various agencies that regulate agricultural and food products. It is intended to serve as a reference for professionals as well as for interested consumers.

Frank, Hanns K. 1992. *Dictionary of Food Microbiology.* 1st English ed. Lancaster, PA: Technomic.

Although somewhat dated, this book listing common and technical terms used in the fields of food science and safety is still a valuable reference tool.

General Food Safety Books

Egendorf, Laura K., ed. 2000. *Food Safety (At Issue).* San Diego: Greenhaven Press.

The potential threats to the world's food supply, and ways to reduce those threats, are considered in this volume. Topics include how bacteria, pesticides, and unclean processing plants can make some foods dangerous, or even deadly, to eat.

Matthews, Dawn. 2000. *Food Safety Sourcebook: Basic Consumer Health Information about the Safe Handling of Meat (Health Reference Series).* Detroit: Omnigraphics.

This book contains basic consumer health information about the safe handling of meat, poultry, seafood, eggs, fruit juices, and other food items; facts about pesticides and drinking water; food safety overseas; and the onset, duration, and symptoms of foodborne illnesses. It clarifies the role of the consumer, the food handler, and the government in food safety. A glossary is included.

Redman, Nina E. 2000. *Food Safety: A Reference Handbook.* Santa Barbara: ABC-Clio.

This consumer-level book contains information about current and historical issues in food safety, along with biographies, a directory of organizations, and resources.

Cliver, Dean O. 1999. *Eating Safely: Avoiding Foodborne Illness.* 2nd ed. New York: American Council on Science and Health.

This consumer-level book attempts to combat media hype on food safety and redirect the nation's attention away from additives, pesticides, and chemicals to the real dangers in food—naturally occurring pathogens, disease-producing pathogens, and their products. It is a basic primer on the definition of foodborne illness; sources and prevention of foodborne illness; and the role of industry, government, and consumers. Available full-text at: http://www.acsh.org/publications/booklets/eatsaf.html.

Fox, Nicols. 1999. *It Was Probably Something You Ate: A Practical Guide to Avoiding and Surviving Food-Borne Illness.* New York: Viking Penguin.

This short but dense treatment of foodborne illness contains a wealth of information, but is not presented in a manner interesting enough to capture the attention of the average consumer. After an explanation of why food is not as safe as it used to be, the author discusses foodborne pathogens and offers advice on how to avoid foodborne disease.

Satin, Morton. 1999. *Food Alert! The Ultimate Sourcebook for Food Safety.* New York: Facts on File.

A text-laden book, *Food Alert!* includes descriptions of the key food groups and the contaminants that affect each one; tips on handling, preparing, and storing food; checklists of the 20 most common causes of contamination in the kitchen; instructions on how to recognize the symptoms of foodborne illness; and more. It contains a special reference section detailing the different foodborne pathogens and how they thrive, how they cause harm, and how to stop them.

Van der Heijden, Kees, ed. 1999. *International Food Safety Handbook: Science, International Regulation, and Control.* New York: Marcel Dekker.

Although geared more towards the food professional than the average consumer, this collection of papers by international food safety experts from industry, government, academia, consumer groups, and the media contains a wealth of information on just about every topic of food and water safety.

Acheson, David, W. K. MD, and Robin K. Levinson. 1998. *Safe Eating.* New York: Dell.

This easy-to-read book for consumers covers the range of what consumers need to know to protect themselves and their family from foodborne illness. Topics covered include an overview of foodborne illness; how pathogens cause foodborne illness; diagnosis and treatment; and how to reduce the risk of becoming ill at home, when dining out, and when traveling.

International Food Information Council Foundation (IFIC). 1998. *Food Insight Media Guide on Food Safety and Nutrition.* Washington: IFIC Foundation.

Primarily designed for media, this resource guide is useful for health communicators and educators as well. In addition to providing background papers on topics throughout the field of food safety, it identifies nearly 200 independent scientific experts who are willing to be media sources and provide perspective on new scientific studies in their areas of expertise.

Lieberman, Adam J., and Simona C. Kwon. 1998, rev. *Facts Versus Fears. A Review of the Greatest Unfounded Health Scares of Recent Times.* 3rd ed. New York: American Council on Science and Health.

The authors examine some of the most noteworthy unfounded health scares of the past half-century. Included are the scares about cranberries, red dye, cyclamates, saccharin, and alar. In each case the charges made against a product or substance are reviewed, as well as the basis for the charges, the reactions of the public and the media, and the actual facts as to what risk (if any) ever existed. Available full-text at: http://www.acsh.org/publications/reports/facts3.pdf.

Scott, Elizabeth, and Paul Sockett. 1998. *How to Prevent Food Poisoning: A Practical Guide to Safe Cooking, Eating, and Food Handling.* New York: John Wiley.

This easy-to-read book offers basic information about the causes of food poisoning, its symptoms and complications, and how to prevent it. A detailed index makes it easy to find specific information. A case study food safety quiz at the end tests readers' knowledge.

Tollefson, Linda, ed. 1998. *Microbial Food Borne Pathogens.* Philadelphia: Saunders.

This book gives an overview of foodborne pathogens from a public health standpoint. Chapters cover individual pathogens, factors in the emergence of foodborne pathogens, transmissible spongiform encephalopathies in food animals, and overviews of the National Animal Health Monitoring System and the National Antimicrobial Monitoring System. Although the material presented is of a technical nature, readers with a general background in science will understand the concepts.

Eisnitz, Gail A. 1997. *Slaughterhouse: The Shocking Story of Greed, Neglect, and Inhumane Treatment inside the U.S. Meat Industry.* Amherst, NY: Prometheus.

Eisnitz' book is investigative shock reporting of what goes on in U.S. slaughterhouses. Written by an animal rights activist.

Fox, Nicols. 1997. *Spoiled: The Dangerous Truth about a Food Chain Gone Haywire.* New York: Basic Books.

This journalistic treatment of foodborne illness documents how changes in the way food is produced, processed, and distributed, along with changes in our lifestyle and culture, have created new niches for foodborne pathogens. Well-researched and drawn from interviews with physicians, farmers, food safety experts from various government agencies, and victims of foodborne illness, it traces the background epidemiology and rise of some of the latest food safety problems. The author maintains that we need to look at the complex synergies and connections of the natural world and alter how we interact with nature.

Lehmann, Robert H. 1997. *Cooking for Life: A Guide to Nutrition and Food Safety for the HIV-Positive Community.* New York: Dell.

Written for people with HIV or AIDS, their friends, families, and healthcare professionals, this book offers nutrition and food safety information that can help to lengthen and improve the quality of many lives. Written by a professional chef in consultation with a team of AIDS-knowledgeable medical advisors.

Powell, Douglas, and William Leiss. 1997. *Mad Cows and Mother's Milk: The Perils of Poor Risk Communication.* Montreal: McGill Queens University Press.

Using a series of case studies, including mad cow disease, *E. coli* outbreaks, agricultural biotechnology, and rBST (bovine somatotropin), the authors outline the crucial role of risk management in dealing with such public controversies. They argue that the failure to inform the public about the scientific basis of risks makes it difficult and costly for governments, industry, and society to manage risk controversies sensibly.

Cody, Mildred M. 1996. *Safe Food for You and Your Family.* Minneapolis: Chronimed.

This easy-to-read pocket-size book for consumers contains basic food safety information such as how foods become contaminated, which foods are potentially unsafe, how to prevent spreading bacteria in your kitchen, how to store and serve leftovers, and how to pack lunches safely.

Heersink, Mary. 1996. *E.coli O157: The True Story of a Mother's Battle with a Killer Microbe.* Far Hills, NJ: New Horizon Press.

Mary Heersink has written an emotionally charged, true-life medical drama about her 11-year-old son, Damion, who is struck down by *E.coli.* It details her struggle to save her son's life from a disease that at the time was little understood.

Nielson, Sheri. 1996. *Everybody's FOODSAFE Kitchen. Your Step-by-Step Guide to the Safe Preparation of Food.* British Columbia, Canada: Everybody's Kitchen Ventures, Ltd.

Written for the consumer audience, this book deals with basic food safety circumstances that one is likely to encounter in one's home kitchen. It includes food safety for special circumstances such as camping, barbecues, parties, and picnics.

Bellenir, Karen, and Peter D. Dresser, eds. 1995. *Food and Animal Borne Diseases Sourcebook: Basic Information about Diseases That Can Be Spread to Humans through the Ingestion of Contaminated Food or Water or by Contact with Infected Animals and Insects.* Detroit: Omnigraphics.

This is a collection of non-technical papers about diseases that are transmitted to humans by pathogens found in food and water, or carried by animals and insects. Chapters include why immune system problems raise the risk of foodborne illness; information on how to prevent foodborne illness; food handling information; and food advice for emergencies, traveler's diarrhea, and food irradiation.

Light, Louise. 1994. *The Risk of Getting Sick from Bacteria in Meat and Poultry.* Kensington, MD: Institute for Science in Society.

Written in easy-to-understand language, this work covers which disease-causing bacteria are in meat and poultry, how pathogens in meat and poultry are transmitted to people, who gets sick, and how widespread the problem is. It pulls together information from numerous experts, reports, and the scientific literature, and presents it in a clear, concise manner.

Arnold, Andrea. 1990, Reissued 1998. *Fear of Food: Environmentalist Scams, Media Mendacity, and the Law of Disparagement.* Bellevue, WA: Merril Press.

This book examines the gullibility and manipulation of the American public by the media and environmental groups on issues such as pesticide use, with a focus on the Alar controversy. The author seeks to develop in the public a sense of balance and perspective that can be used to judge campaigns by overly enthusiastic advocacy groups.

Children's General Food Safety Books

Latta, Sara L. 1999. *Food Poisoning and Foodborne Diseases.* Berkeley Heights, NJ: Enslow Publishers.

In this large-type book for ages 12 and up, author Sara Latta covers food poisoning and foodborne pathogens from a historical analysis to directions for the future, including along the way chapters on microbes, diagnosis and treatment, prevention, and the cost to society. She covers safe food handling practices and explains how different bacteria can cause illness. Included are real-life, current stories of people affected by foodborne diseases.

Kalbacken, Joan. 1998. *Food Safety.* New York: Children's Press.

This children's book discusses food sickness and how to avoid it. It is written in large print with multiethnic color photos that also show boys and men involved in food preparation.

Colombo, Luann. 1997. *Gross But True Germs.* New York: Simon and Schuster.

For children ages six through 12, this book focuses on the scientific inquiry into viruses, fungi, and bacteria. It includes two petri dishes and directions to grow a germ garden.

Rice, Judith. 1997. *Those Mean Nasty Dirty Downright Disgusting but Invisible Germs.* Saint Paul, MN: Redleaf Press.

A little girl, who accumulates germs on her hands during her busy day, defeats them by washing her hands before meals. Teaches children ages four through eight about the importance of handwashing. Also available in Spanish.

Berger, Melvin, and Marylin Hafner. 1996. *Germs Make Me Sick!* Rev. ed. New York: HarperCollins Children's Books.

This richly illustrated children's book explains how bacteria and viruses affect the human body and how the body fights them. While not strictly about foodborne microorganisms, it uses simple language to convey a great deal of general information about microbes and how they make people sick. The audience is children from 4 to 8.

Katz, Bobbi. 1996. *Germs! Germs! Germs!* New York: Scholastic.

Germs tell their side of the story in rhyme in this book for children ages four through eight. It introduces young readers to germs and where they live, from food left out of the refrigerator to the inside of the body, and offers gentle rhyming instructions on how to keep germs away.

Patten, Barbara J. 1996. *Food Safety.* Vero Beach, FL: Rourke Corporation.

This children's book discusses how to keep food safe, covering such topics as careful food preparation, different kinds of food poisoning, and the safe packing of lunches. Includes lots of color pictures and not very much text.

International Food Information Council Foundation (IFIC). 1993. *Food Risks: Perception vs. Reality.* Rockville, MD: Food and Drug Administration.

This educational guide presents food safety information to high school students and encourages critical thinking skills. Prepared by the U.S. Food and Drug Administration and The International Food Information Council Foundation. It is also available full-text at: http://ificinfo.health.org/brochure/frtop.htm.

Books on Specific Food Safety Topics

Additives

Fallow, Christine H. 2001. *Food Additives: A Shopper's Guide to What's Safe and What's Not.* Revised ed. Escondido, CA: KISS For Health.

This book classifies commonly used food additives according to safety, whether they may cause allergic reactions, and whether they are generally recognized as safe (GRAS) by the FDA. It uses easy language to give the bottom line on how many of the common chemicals that are used in food processing affect the human body.

Lewis, Richard J. 1999. *Food Additives Handbook.* New York: John Wiley.

More than 1,350 food additives, including direct and indirect additives, packaging materials, pesticides, and selected animal drugs. Listed in alphabetical order. Each entry covers physical properties, usage information, occupational restrictions, and toxicological data. The additive's uses in food or food packaging materials is highlighted.

Renders, Eileen. 1999. *Food Additives, Nutrients, and Supplements A-to-Z: A Shopper's Guide.* Santa Fe: Clear Light.

This reference book on food additives boils down the essential information from published research, the author's ongoing work in the field, and standard dietary and chemical references to provide consumers with the knowledge to make healthy choices in eating.

Winter, Ruth. 1999. *Consumer's Dictionary of Food Additives.* 5th ed. New York: Three Rivers.

Describing more than 8,000 ingredients found in foods, the dictionary format of this easy-to-read book allows users look up an ingredient alphabetically and learn what it is, how and why it's used, and its benefits and risks.

Sergeant, Doris, and Karen Evans. 1998. *Hard to Swallow: The Truth about Food Additives.* Blaine, WA: Alive Books.

This guide contains an alphabetical listing of nearly 300 chemical additives that are found in the American food supply. The authors explain the health and environmental dangers of genetic engineering and other modern methods of production that adulterate the foods Americans eat. They offer solutions for consumers who want to halt the production trends in farming (genetic engineering, pesticides, insecticides) and food processing (irradiation) by rolling up their sleeves and demanding changes be made to food and labeling laws.

Animal Health

Animal Health Institute. 1999. *1999-2000 Source Book.* Washington: Animal Health Institute.

A comprehensive directory of organizations related to the animal health industry and food safety issues. Contains more than 1,000 updated listings of federal and state agencies, animal food safety experts, trade associations, animal science and veterinary schools, and manufacturers of animal health products.

Crawford, Lester M., and Don A. Franco, eds. 1994. *Animal Drugs and Human Health.* Lancaster, PA: Technomic.

This collection of technical articles covers animal drugs from the public health perspective, residue programs in meat and poultry inspection, methods of detection, and more.

Bovine Spongiform Encephalopathy (BSE)

Lacey, Richard. 1998. *Poison on a Plate: The Dangers in the Food We Eat, and How to Avoid Them.* London: Metro.

Dr. Lacey traces the rise of several foodborne pathogens in Britain—*Listeria monocytogenes, Salmonella enteritidis, E. coli* O157:H7—pointing out efforts by the British government and food industry to discredit him and to cover up the evidence of unsafe food. He then concentrates on bovine spongiform encephalopathy (BSE), looking at how changes in the food manufacturing industries and farming processes gave rise to the BSE problem, how the government could have realized what was going on, and how it refused to accept information or advice from external sources. He finishes by advising consumers on what they can do to protect themselves from unsafe food.

Rhodes, Richard. 1998. *Deadly Feasts: The "Prion" Controversy and the Public's Health.* New York: Simon and Shuster.

Written as a medical detective story, this book traces the path and social milieu of mad cow disease in Britain from its inception, to beef producers, to the British government, to the consumers who have died from the new variant of Creutzfeldt-Jakob disease. Also available as an audiocassette.

Socialist Equality Party Staff. 1998. *Human BSE/CJD: Anatomy of a Health Disaster.* Oak Park, MI: Mehring Books.

This is the book of testimonies by speakers at the Workers Inquiry convened in 1997 by the Socialist Equality Party of Britain to investigate the fatal illness contracted from eating infected beef. Jean Shaoul, an economic lecturer, explains how the economic setup of the various industries in the United Kingdom was likely to lead to problems. Richard Lacey lectures on how the human risk had been present for many years and how the U.K. government should have known about it. Several relatives of victims relate how they were treated. This is an opportunity to look at the reasons behind the BSE epidemic, explained with a political and economic slant.

Rhodes, Richard. 1997. *Deadly Feasts: Tracking the Secrets of a Terrifying New Plague.* New York: Simon and Schuster.

Written for the general public, this book is about the transmissible spongiform encephalopathies (of which BSE is a type) . It begins with the kuru work done in Papua New Guinea, then discusses cases of Creutzfeldt-Jakob disease (CJD), research into scrapie, and transmissible mink encephalopathy. Rhodes describes the transmission experiments of kuru and CJD to monkeys and primates that took place starting in the 1960s. He examines the BSE epidemic in the UK and Europe, and some of the recent research and theories on the nature of the infective agent. Also available on audiocassette.

Rampton, Sheldon, and John C. Stauber. 1997. *Mad Cow U.S.A.: Could the Nightmare Happen Here?* Monroe, ME: Common Courage Press.

The authors argue that both the American and British governments colluded with beef producers to suppress important facts about interspecies transmission of bovine spongiform encephalopathy (BSE), or "mad cow disease"—facts that might have prevented gruesome deaths. They ask, "Could a British-style BSE epidemic happen in America?"

Food Allergy

Emsley, John, and Peter Fell. 2000. *Was It Something You Ate? Food Intolerance, What Causes It and How to Avoid It.* Los Angeles: Getty Center for Education in the Arts.

The authors explain the difference between food intolerance and food allergy. They identify the common chemicals that cause food intolerance and list the foods containing both high and low (or nonexistent) levels of them. Throughout there are case studies of people who have been badly affected by their diet until the cause was identified.

Walsh, William E. 2000. *Food Allergies: The Complete Guide to Understanding and Relieving Your Food Allergies.* New York: John Wiley.

This consumer-level book covers the basics of food allergies and how to avoid them.

Collins, Lisa Cipriano. 1999. *Caring for Your Child with Severe Food Allergies: Emotional Support and Practical Advice from a Parent Who's Been There.* New York: John Wiley.

This book is geared towards parents, grandparents, and other caregivers of children with food allergies. The author writes from her own experiences raising a child with severe nut allergies, including practical observations, interviews with parents, and data from recent medical studies. It also helps families cope with the emotional aspects of raising a child at risk for severe food reactions.

Food Allergy Network (FAN). 1999. *College Guide for Students with Food Allergies: It's Not All Pizza and Ice Cream.* Fairfax, VA: Food Allergy Network.

This guide for high school students who have food allergies provides a time line and questions to ask when looking at colleges, hard-learned lessons from those who have been there, tips for handling an allergic reaction, and strategies for dining out.

Wedman-St. Louis, Betty. 1999. *Living with Food Allergies: A Complete Guide to a Healthy Lifestyle.* Lincolnwood, IL: Contemporary Books.

This authoritative guide will help readers determine if they have a food sensitivity and, if they do, how to avoid those foods through lifestyle changes and rotation diets. Includes more than 150 recipes.

Barnes Koerner, Celide, and Anne Munoz-Furlong. 1998. *Food Allergies: Up-to-Date Tips from the World's Foremost Nutrition Experts.* New York: John Wiley.

This consumer level primer on food allergies covers diagnosing food allergies, managing food allergies, and avoiding problem foods. Recipes, trial elimination menu plans, and a sample food diary are included.

Dumke, Nicolette M. 1998. *5 Years without Food: The Food Allergy Survival Guide: How to Overcome Your Food Allergies and Recover Good Health.* Louisville: Allergy Adapt, Inc.

This book for consumers covers diagnosis of food allergies, health problems that can be caused by food allergies, and treatment options. Many recipes are included, as is guidance on personalizing a standard rotation diet.

Vickerstaff Joneja, Janice. 1998. *Dietary Management of Food Allergies and Intolerances: A Comprehensive Guide.* 2nd ed. Burnaby, British Columbia: J A Hall.

Designed for the layperson, this book teaches readers about the immune system and the current controversies regarding diagnosis and treatment of food allergies.

Food Allergy Network. 1997. *The Food Allergy News Cookbook: A Collection of Recipes from Food Allergy News and Favorite Recipes from Members of the Food Allergy Network.* 2nd ed. Fairfax, VA: Food Allergy Network.

More than a cookbook, this collection contains tips for shopping, substituting foods, cooking, and a glossary of ingredient terms. Recipes are carefully tested and labeled for easy identification of allergens.

Gioannini, Marilyn. 1997. *The Complete Food Allergy Cookbook: The Foods You've Always Loved without the Ingredients You Can't Have.* Rocklin, CA: Prima.

In addition to many recipes, this book includes information on detecting food allergy symptoms, avoiding problems at dinner parties and restaurants, substituting foods, and altering recipes.

Metcalfe, Dean D., Hugh A. Sampson, and Ronald A. Simon, eds. 1997. *Food Allergy: Adverse Re-*

actions to Foods and Food Additives. 2nd ed. Cambridge, MA: Blackwell Science.

This clinical book covers both pediatric and adult adverse reactions to foods and food additives. It discusses food biotechnology and genetic engineering as they relate to allergic diseases and oral tolerance.

Food Allergy Books for Children

Food Allergy Network (FAN). 1999. *Alexander series.* Fairfax, VA: Food Allergy Network.

This series of food allergy books for elementary school children targets different food eating activities and includes the titles: *A Special Day At School, Alexander and His Pals Visit the Main Street School, Alexander Goes to a Birthday Party, Alexander Goes Trick-or-Treating, Alexander's Fun and Games Activity Book, Andrew and Maya Learn About Food Allergies, Alexander the Elephant Who Couldn't Eat Peanuts Coloring Books.*

Smith, Nicole. 1999. *Allie the Allergic Elephant.* Colorado Springs, CO: Jungle Communications, Inc.

This book is geared towards preschool age through first grade. It explains why an allergic child will say "no thank you" to foods offered, what an allergic reaction looks like (hives, coughing, swelled lips), and which foods "hide" peanuts. All this, and an elephant with hives too.

Weiner, Ellen. 1999. *Taking Food Allergies to School.* Valley Park, MO: JayJo Books.

Written for children, this book is also an important tool for teachers, parents, school nurses, caregivers, and classmates on the special needs of children with food allergies. Topics covered include sharing lunches, special parties and events, and appropriate snacks. It will give understanding as to the symptoms and dangers of food allergies. A quiz for kids is included along with tips for teachers.

Zevy, Aaron, and Susan Tebbutt. 1999. *No Nuts for Me!* Tampa, FL: Tumbleweed Press.

Written for children ages 3 to 8, this story is narrated by a very active little boy who doesn't let his nut allergy get in the way of having fun. Readers will meet Noah, who carries on a running conversation throughout the story and explains, in a matter-of-fact tone, what it's like to be allergic to nuts.

Habkirk, Lauri, and Les Habkirk. 1995. *Preschoolers Guide to Peanut Allergy.* Medford, MA: PeanutAllergy.Com.

The authors created this book to educate their daughter who is allergic to peanuts. It follows four-year-old Meagan Myers through the discovery of what it means to have a peanut allergy and how to manage it.

Food Biotechnology

Cummins, Ronnie and Ben Lilliston. 2000. *Genetically Engineered Food: A Self-Defense Guide for Consumers.* New York: Marlowe and Co.

The book takes a critical look at genetically engineered foods, emphasizing why consumers are right to oppose these products. Included is information on the types of foods most likely to be genetically engineered, where major supermarket chains stand on such foods, possibly altered ingredients to watch out for, how to avoid GE foods in restaurants, and more.

Jack, Alex. 2000. *Imagine a World without Monarch Butterflies: Awakening to the Hazards of Genetically Altered Foods.* Beckett: One Peaceful World Press.

Author Alex Jack details 50 reasons why genetically engineered foods don't make sense. He covers health, environmental, social, and ethical arguments against GE foods.

McHughen, Alan D. 2000. *Biotechnology and Food.* 2nd ed. New York: American Council on Science and Health.

This consumer-level book describes what food biotechnology is, examining genetic modification of foods, crop improvement, pest and weed control, animals for food production, and issues such as safety and labeling of biotech foods. The complete text is available online at: http://www. acsh.org/publications/booklets/biotechnology 2000.html.

Anderson, Luke. 1999. *Genetic Engineering, Food, and Our Environment.* White River Junction, VT: Chelsea Green.

This book highlights the negative social, environmental, and health implications arising from the use of genetically engineered crops.

Boyens, Ingeborg. 1999. *Unnatural Harvest: How Corporate Science Is Secretly Altering Our Food.* Toronto: Doubleday Canada.

Canadian journalist Ingeborg Boyens has a clear agenda-challenging the corporate line that genetically engineered foods are just an extension of centuries of breeding to make heartier wheat, leaner cows, or more flavorful fruits. She asserts that inserting genes from one type of organism into another raises entirely new questions, and that creating these new "frankenfoods" is not wise.

Kneen, Brewster. 1999. *Farmageddon: Food and the Culture of Biotechnology.* Gabriola Island, BC: New Society.

In this critical book, readers learn about genetically engineered products that are subtly introduced into our supermarkets, health food stores, and home-gardening outlets. Without presuming readers have a scientific background, Brewster provides a multidisciplinary account of what biotechnology is, how it is affecting the world's food supply, where it came from, the direction it's heading, and how to resist it.

Marshall, Elizabeth L. 1999. *High-Tech Harvest: A Look at Genetically Engineered Foods.* Danbury, CT: Franklin Watts.

This overview of food biotechnology written for grades seven through 10 covers genetic engineering techniques used to create crop plants and farm animals. The author explains recombinant DNA technology in a clear, concise manner and then examines its application to crop plants and farm animals to produce foods that are more appealing in taste and appearance, or have a longer shelf life. Also covered are government regulation, labeling, and ethical questions. Lists of books, articles, and Web sites facilitate further learning in this rather dry presentation of the subject.

Teitel, Martin, and Kimberly A. Wilson. 1999. *Genetically Engineered Food: Changing the Nature of Nature: What You Need to Know to Protect Yourself, Your Family, and Our Planet.* Rochester: Park Street.

Authors Martin Teitel and Kimberly Wilson explain what genetic engineering is and how it works, then explore the health risks involved with eating newly created life forms. They address the ecological catastrophe that could result from these modified plants crossing with wild species.

Lappe, Marc, and Britt Bailey. 1998. *Against the Grain: Biotechnology and the Corporate Takeover of Your Food.* Monroe, ME: Common Courage Press.

In this critical introduction to the topic of agricultural biotechnology, the authors reveal the science and politics behind transgenic foods to show how biotech companies increasingly engineer what you eat to be compatible with their chemicals-but not necessarily good for human health. Contains a glossary to define technical terms.

Nill, Kimball R. 1998. *Glossary of Biotechnology Terms.* 2nd ed. Lancaster, PA: Technomic.

With more than 2,000 definitions of biotechnology terms, this book serves as a handy reference for those with little or no training in the bio and chemical sciences. Written in as non-technical language as possible, it accommodates a wide range of audience needs, from high school students to scientists.

Nottingham, Stephen. 1998. *Eat Your Genes: How Genetically Modified Food Is Entering Our Diet.* New York: Zed Books.

This book examines the techniques used to genetically modify crops and livestock, why such products are produced, how they can remain unlabeled, how they are entering our diet, and who is responsible for producing and marketing them. It explores the food industry's commercial motivations and examines the potential ecological and health risks involved, the ethical issues, and the likely impact on developing countries. The author argues that the promises held out by genetic engineering of ending world hunger and making possible a more eco-friendly agriculture are far from being fulfilled.

Ticciati, Laura, and Robin Ticciati. 1998. *Genetically Engineered Foods: Are They Safe? You Decide.* New Canaan, CT: Keats.

In this consumer-level book by founders of the organization, Mothers for Natural Law, readers learn what genetic engineering is, which foods are genetically engineered, and what the side effects may be. The authors aim to warn the public about the dangers inherent in genetically modified foods.

Dawkins, Kristin. 1997. *Gene Wars: The Politics of Biotechnology.* New York: Seven Stories Press.

Gene Wars is an impassioned, activist argument against corporate control of food plant genes. The author discusses monoculture crops, pesticide use, government agricultural subsidies, NAFTA, and genetic diversity in building her case against globalization and the patenting of genes. Dawkins encourages citizens to become involved through political activity and teaming up with local growers to move away from the big, monoculture crop model and ensure the safety and security of the world's food supply.

Grace, Eric S. 1997. *Biotechnology Unzipped: Promises and Realities.* Washington: National Academy Press.

This large-type, easy-to-read book explains biotechnology in simple and clear terms, adding enough historical and scientific context for the reader to be able to see the big picture. It covers how biotechnology came about and early discoveries, genetic engineering, biotechnology on the farm, and ethical issues.

Thompson, Paul B. 1997. *Food Biotechnology in Ethical Perspective.* New York: Blackie Academic and Professional.

This scholarly treatment of the subject examines food safety, animal health and welfare, environmental impact, social consequences, and religious opposition to biotechnology in depth. It looks at the implications of manipulating genes in plants and animals in terms of food safety and environmental risk, and whether it is justifiable to attempt to control nature.

Institute of Food Science and Technology. 1996. *Guide to Food Biotechnology.* London: Institute of Food Science and Technology.

The aim of this guide for the food industry professional is to encourage a greater understanding of biotechnology and its application. Topics covered include genetic modification of traits, fermentation, enzymology, biochemical engineering, and microbiology and the application to crops, animals, and food production. The guide also discusses the issues of ethics, consumer acceptability, regulations, labeling, and communications.

Mausberg, Burkhard, and Maureen Press-Merkur. 1995. *The Citizen's Guide to Biotechnology.* Toronto: Canadian Institute of Environmental Law and Policy (CIELAP).

This comprehensive and easy-to-read book about biotechnology and genetic engineering focuses on biotechnology as it relates to crops, animals, fisheries, pest control, industrial applications, and milk. Order from CIELAP at 416-923-3529.

Food Irradiation

Greenberg, Richard A. 1996. *Irradiated Foods.* 4th ed. New York: American Council on Science and Health.

This book introduces consumers to the process of food irradiation and answers common questions about the quality and safety of irradiated foods. Available full-text at: http:// www.acsh.org/publications/booklets/irradiated.pdf.

Satin, Morton. 1996. *Food Irradiation: A Guidebook.* 2nd ed. Lancaster, PA: Technomic.

This book written for the consumer audience examines what food irradiation is and how it affects foods. It contains chapters on pasteurization, foodborne diseases and the use of irradiation to prevent their spread, the prevention of food losses after harvesting, advocacy objections to food irradiation, and consumer reaction to irradiated foods.

Wilkinson, V. M., and G. W. Gould. 1996. *Food Irradiation. A Reference Guide.* Oxford, England: Butterworth-Heinemann.

This book provides comprehensive information on all aspects of food irradiation. Written in dictionary style with extensive cross-references, it is a good reference work for those in industry, as well as for teachers and students.

Hayes, D. J., E. A. Murano, P. S. Murano, D. G. Olson, and S. G. Sapp. 1995. *Food Irradiation: A Sourcebook.* Edited by E. A. Murano. Ames, IA: Iowa State University Press.

Written at the consumer level, this book looks at irradiation processing, microbiology of irradiated foods, quality of irradiated foods, consumer acceptance of irradiated foods, and the economics of marketing irradiated foods.

Gibbs, Gary. 1993. *The Food That Would Last Forever: Understanding the Dangers of Food Irradiation.* Garden City Park, NY: Avery.

This book presents information on food irradiation, examines research documenting the dangers of eating irradiated foods, and exposes abuses of the irradiation industry. It evaluates the history of food irradiation and discusses the motives of those who promote it.

Food Preservation

Andress, Elizabeth. 1999. *So Easy to Preserve.* 4th ed. Athens, GA: University of Georgia.

The definitive text for canning, pickling, jellying, freezing, and drying foods, this book offers step-by-step instructions for more than 150 recipes. Much of the information in the book is available from the University of Georgia's Web site at: http://www.fcs.uga.edu/pubs/index.php3?foodsafepres/foodpres/

VanGarde, Shirley J., and Margy Woodburn. 1994. *Food Preservation and Safety: Principles and Practice.* Ames, IA: Iowa State University Press.

From harvest to table, the authors examine quality and microbial changes during drying, acidification, canning, refrigeration, freezing, curing, and sugaring. They answer the "how to" and "why" questions of preserving and storing food and discuss the basic criteria for keeping food palatable and safe.

Food Safety Regulations

Coppin, Clayton A., and Jack High. 1999. *The Politics of Purity: Harvey Washington Wiley and the Origins of Federal Food Regulation.* Ann Arbor: University of Michigan.

Although Harvey Washington Wiley is often lauded as a champion of public interests, the authors propose that Wiley was in fact surreptitiously allied with business. They postulate that in drafting the Pure Food and Drugs Act of 1906 Wiley was working with firms that would benefit from regulation and, moreover, would help him build his government agency, the Federal Bureau of Chemistry. Broader than just the issue of food safety, this book will interest scholars concerned with government regulation, including those in economics, political science, history, or business.

FCN Publishing. 1999. *FCN Insider's Directory of Food Safety Regulators.* Washington, DC: FCN Publishing.

This directory contains a comprehensive listing of the federal and state agencies and regulatory officials involved in food safety, along with the international organizations that are becoming increasingly influential both domestically and outside the United States. Included are the names of key members of Congress and congressional committees that oversee food regulation, in addition to more than 100 trade and professional organizations.

U.S. Food and Drug Administration. 1999. *FDA Food Code.* Washington, DC: U.S. Food and Drug Administration.

The Food and Drug Administration publishes the Food Code, a reference that guides restaurants, grocery stores, and institutions such as nursing homes on how to prevent foodborne illness. Local, state, and federal regulators use the FDA Food Code as a model to help develop or update their own food safety rules and to be consistent with national food regulatory policy. The Food Code is updated every two years and is available full-text at: http://vm.cfsan.fda.gov/~dms/ foodcode.html. A Spanish version can be ordered from Ceti Translations at 703-560-4499.

Food Institute. 1999. *Regulatory Directory.* Washington, DC: Food Institute.

This directory is a concise and up-to-date compilation of federal and state agencies, legislators and committees, and industry and consumer representatives who deal with food products. Includes organizational charts, contact names, phone numbers, faxes, and email addresses. Available in print and on a searchable CD-ROM with links to Web sites. Published yearly.

Goodwin, Lorine Swainston. 1999. *The Pure Food, Drink, and Drug Crusaders, 1879-1914.* Jefferson, NC: McFarland.

Based in large part on primary sources, this work examines the origins of the movement to pass the Pure Food and Drugs Act of 1906, the many groups involved in the law's passage, and how their work affected American society. Swainston pays particular attention to the women's groups that were involved in the struggle.

National Food Processors Association (NFPA). 1999. *Sourcebook of State Laws and Regulations for Food Processors.* 2nd ed. Washington: National Food Processors Association.

The sourcebook is a publication that helps food companies determine the food laws with which they need to comply in every state. It is a state-by-state, issue-by-issue reference guide to the complex state laws and regulations affecting food processors. Also available in electronic format.

Wilson, Andrew, and William Wilson. 1998. *Wilson's Practical Meat Inspection.* 6th ed. Malden, MA: Blackwell Science.

This textbook is the classic handbook for persons involved in meat inspection and the meat industry, describing anything a meat inspector might see on the job. This edition reflects the developing knowledge of BSE and *E.coli* O157:H7 and the changes in slaughter practices.

Schumann, Michael S., Thomas D. Schneid, and B. R. Schumann. 1997. *Food Safety Law*. New York: John Wiley.

Written for professionals involved in food processing, food preparation, food service, and students, this book covers U.S. laws, regulations, and procedures governing food safety, quality, and sanitation, with a special focus on the red meat and poultry industry. It describes and interprets the laws, highlights compliance methods, offers case histories, and includes the complete texts of major mandates.

Vetter, James L. 1996. *Food Laws and Regulations*. Manhattan, KS: American Institute of Baking.

This easy-to-read book provides an overview of federal regulations for producing, handling, and marketing food products in the United States. It is intended to be a reference source for people with a wide variety of responsibilities in the food and allied industries, and as a text for a college-level course.

Antle, John M. 1995. *Choice and Efficiency in Food Safety Policy*. Washington, DC: American Enterprise Institute for Public Policy Research.

In this look at public policy the author asks what economic principles should guide food safety regulation and what changes should be made in U.S. policies. Beyond bureaucratic considerations, the author questions the appropriate role of government in food safety. He argues that a 100 percent safe food supply is an unattainable goal, and that choices must be made between different aspects of food safety.

Codex Alimentarius Commission. Ongoing. *Codex Alimentarius*. Rome: Codex Alimentarius Commission.

The Codex serves as the international reference for food safety standards, guidelines, and practices. It is developed by the Codex Alimentarius Commission, a joint committee of the Food and Agriculture Organization of the United Nations and the World Health Organization.

Naturally Occurring, Environmental, and Chemical Toxins

Coker, Raymond. 1999. *Mycotoxins: The Silent Threat to Human and Animal Health*. London: University of Greenwich.

Although technical enough to require some science background on the part of the reader, this publication on mycotoxins is more reader-friendly than most on the topic. It explains what mycotoxins are, describes those that are of major importance to public health, and suggests how they can be controlled.

Moffat Colin F., and Kevin J. Whittle, eds. 1999. *Environmental Contaminants in Food*. Boca Raton, FL: CRC Press.

Topics covered in this technical reference guide include radioactivity, trace metal contaminants, pesticides, veterinary drugs, dioxins and risk assessment of contaminants.

Watson, David H., ed. 1998. *Natural Toxicants in Food*. Boca Raton, FL: CRC Press.

This book is a reference tool for professionals in food science and technology, ingredient supply, and quality assurance who have a basic understanding of chemistry. It examines the chemistry and toxicology of natural toxicants in foods and reports on developing issues in the field.

Benjamin, Denis R. 1995. *Mushrooms: Poisons and Panaceas. A Handbook for Naturalists, Mycologists, and Physicians*. New York: W.H. Freeman.

This comprehensive book covers the cultural attitudes and history of mushroom eating, as well as the biology, nutritional and medicinal properties, and poisons of mushrooms. With regard to mushroom poisoning it covers diagnosis, symptoms, testing, and treatment.

Millichap, J. Gordon. 1993. *Environmental Poisons in Our Food*. Chicago: PNB Publisher.

Although dated, the large type and ease in reading make this book still worthwhile reading for consumers who want to become more informed about toxins such as lead, trace metals, additives, caffeine, excess vitamins, and other environmental poisons. A detailed index makes finding information easy.

Watson, David H., ed. 1993. *Safety of Chemicals in Food: Chemical Contaminants*. New York: Ellis Horwood.

This book describes scientific work on chemical contamination of food. Groups of contaminants covered are veterinary drug residues; dioxins and other environmental organic chemicals; nitrate, nitrite, and N-nitrosamines; naturally occurring toxicants; chemicals from food packaging; metals; and pesticides. Also featured is a detailed description of how food chemical surveillance is carried out and of the fundamentals of estimating consumer intake of contaminants. Written for food scientists, biochemists, chemists, nutritionists, dietitians, and medical and other health professionals.

Pesticides

Kegley, Susan E., and Laura J. Wise. 1998. *Pesticides in Fruits and Vegetables.* Sausalito, CA: University Science Books.

This three-to-four-week laboratory module introduces university students to risk assessment in the context of pesticides in food. Concepts covered include structure and solubility of organic compounds, gas chromatography, biodegradation, bioaccumulation, and organic extraction techniques. As a final assignment, two groups of students (one playing the role of an agribusiness group and the other the role of environmentalists) debate the use of pesticides.

Knight, Chris. 1998. *Pesticide Controls in the Food Chain.* Chipping Campden, UK: Campden and Chorleywood Food Research Association.

This guide is designed to help farmers and food processors with the control of pesticides in the food chain. Even though written for a British audience, it contains valuable information for others too.

Elderkin, Susan, Richard Wiles, and Christopher Campbell. 1995. *Forbidden Fruit: Illegal Pesticides in the U.S. Food Supply.* Washington: Environmental Working Group.

Forbidden Fruit analyzes 14,923 computerized records from the Food and Drug Administration's routine pesticide-monitoring program for the years 1992 and 1993. Results are displayed in easy-to-read graphs. Recommendations for the future are included.

Garland, Anne Witte, with Mothers & Others for a Livable Planet. 1993. *The Way We Grow: Good-Sense Solutions for Protecting Our Families from Pesticides in Food.* New York: Berkley Books.

This grassroots publication advises consumers on what they can do to limit pesticides in the their diet.

Freudenthal, Ralph I., and Susan Loy Freudenthal. 1991. *Food: Facts and Fictions.* Greens Farms, CT: Hill and Garnett.

This consumer-level book discusses America's food supply, focusing on pesticides, organic foods, natural toxins, regulatory agencies, anti-cancer food ingredients, and consumer responsibility. Although dated, it is very easy to read and has a good glossary of terms.

Water

Barzilay, Joshua I., Winkler Weinberg, and William Eley. 1999. *The Water We Drink: Water Quality and Its Effects on Health.* Piscataway, NJ: Rutgers University Press.

The authors provide readers with practical information on the health issues relating to water quality and suggests ways to improve the quality and safety of drinking water. Featured are summaries of drinking water contaminants and their known health effects, a review of purification technologies for public and private supplies, including bottled water, and a discussion of government regulations. The book has a glossary of terms and a bibliography of additional agencies, books, and Web sites to consult for more information.

Gustafson, David I. 1997. *Pesticides in Drinking Water.* New York: John Wiley.

This comprehensive resource guide brings together historical data, trends in scientific thought, regulatory guidelines, and future technical strategies to examine questions such as what types of pesticides are in drinking water, how they get there, and what is being done to remedy the problem. Suitable for chemists, biologists, environmental consultants, engineers, farmers, and regulators, as well as students.

Texts

Cliver, Dean O., and Hans Riemann. 2000. *Foodborne Infections and Intoxications.* 3rd ed. San Diego: Academic Press.

The principles of foodborne disease and its causes, transmission, and control are presented in a comprehensive reference for students and professionals in food science and public health. It examines basic concepts and practices of epidemiology as related to foodborne disease; the nature, detection, prevention, and control of foodborne infections; intoxications of microbial origin; and techniques for the safe processing and preservation of foods.

Hemminger, Jane. 2000. *Food Safety: A Guide for What You Really Need to Know*. Ames, IA: Iowa State University Press.

The purpose of this manual is to help food service managers put into practice safe food handling techniques. Each chapter contains learning objectives and study questions. Topics covered include food hazards, foodborne illness, preparation and serving, cleaning and sanitation, facilities and equipment, and pest control. Appendices contain useful HACCP and other forms.

Jay, James M. 2000. *Modern Food Microbiology*. 6th ed. Gaithersburg, MD: Aspen Publishers.

This text for advanced students explores the fundamental elements affecting the presence, activity, and control of microorganisms in food. It covers the history of microorganisms in food; the taxonomy, role, and significance of microorganisms in foods; and intrinsic and extrinsic parameters of foods that affect microbial growth.

McSwane, David, Nancy Rue, and Richard Linton. 2000. *Essentials of Food Safety and Sanitation*. 2nd ed. Upper Saddle River, NJ: Prentice Hall.

This easy-to-read manual is based on the Food Code and is designed to serve as a workplace reference guide to safe food handling procedures. It can be used to prepare for one of the national certification exams or as a teaching tool for training on the basics of food safety. An instructor's manual and study guide with additional exercises are also available, as are slides for preparing presentations.

Cliver, Dean O., and Hans Riemann. 1999. *Foodborne Diseases*. 2nd ed. San Diego: Academic Press.

This technical work surveys diseases transmitted by food and examines the evidence linking the "lifestyle" diseases, such as cancer and heart disease, to diet on a chapter-by-chapter basis. It includes chapters on organizing a safe food supply system and other issues in food safety.

Marriott, Norman G. 1999. *Principles of Food Sanitation*. 4th ed. Gaithersburg, MD: Aspen Publishers.

This text serves as a reference for students and food industry personnel, teaching principles necessary to ensure safe food handling practices. It covers contamination, cleaning compounds, sanitizers, cleaning equipment, waste disposal, pest control, and monitoring sanitation. Students learn how to apply these sanitation basics to various food processing and food preparation facilities.

Kinneer, James W. 1998. *Managing Food Protection*. Dubuque, IA: Kendall/Hunt.

This large-print, easy-to-read resource on food safety includes key concepts, case studies, and review questions. The 190-page text is based on HACCP principles and the 1997 FDA Model Food Code. Checklists and graphic visuals will enhance learning and be of practical use to the food service manager.

National Assessment Institute. 1998. *Handbook for Safe Food Service Management*. 2nd ed. Upper Saddle River, NJ: Prentice Hall.

This textbook for food service workers is part of the food service certification course offered by Experior Assessments, LLC. It covers all aspects of safe food handling and person hygiene for the food service worker. Also comes in Spanish.

Seperich, George J. 1998. *Food Science and Safety*. Danville, IL: Interstate Publishers.

This text for high school and community college students covers careers and disciplines within the food science and safety fields, applications of food safety principles in industry, food marketing, and world food problems. A teacher's edition is also available.

Walkins, Joyce K. and Javier Heras. 1998. *Safe-at-the-Plate*. Palo Alto: Safe-at-the-Plate.

This easy-to-read explanation of food safety principles is written in a conversational style with many illustrations. The text covers microbiology, personal hygiene, the flow of food with HACCP explanations, sanitation, pest control, and health regulations. In addition, a chapter titled How to Teach Others proves especially helpful. The combination of information applied to the food establishment as well as the home setting makes this text appealing to every reader. Also available in Spanish as, *A Salvo en el Plato*.

Garbutt, John. 1997. *Essentials of Food Microbiology*. London: Arnold.

This introductory text assumes no previous knowledge of microbiology and treats microbiological principles within a food context. It is heavily illustrated, written to be user-friendly and interesting, and is appropriate for those interested in food and food safety who do not have a technical background.

Shibamoto, Takayuki. 1993. *Introduction to Food Toxicology*. San Diego: Academic Press.

An introductory text for undergraduate students, this book is aimed at students who do not have a strong background in toxicology or food science, but who do have a solid science background. It covers the important principles of food toxicology-risk assessment, pesticides, microbial toxins, food additives, naturally occurring toxins, and toxins formed during food processing.

NEWSLETTERS

Food Biotechnology

AgBioForum
Illinois Missouri Biotechnology Alliance
Web site: Available full-text at http://www.agbioforum.missouri.edu/
Cost: Free
Description: AgBioForum is a quarterly online magazine devoted to the economics and management of agricultural biotechnology. Its focus is on the interactions of agro-biotechnology with economics and with sociopolitical processes. AgBioForum publishes short, nontechnical articles on current research, providing a space where academics, private- and public-sector analysts, and decision makers can present timely scientific evidence to enrich the ongoing public debate regarding the economic and social impacts of agricultural biotechnology.

AgBiotech Reporter
Freiberg Publishing Company
2302 West 1st Street
Cedar Falls, IA 50613-9800
Telephone: 800-959-3276, Fax: 319-277-3783
Email address: bmcchane@cfu-cybernet.net
Web site: http://www.bioreporter.com/
Cost: $465/year
Description: This monthly publication covers the business and technical aspects of agricultural biotechnology, and includes notices of publications, a calendar of events, reports of meetings, interviews, and international news stories.

Agri-Food BioGram
Bowditch Group
75 Sunnyside Ave.
Arlington, MA 02474-3820
Telephone: 718-316-8180, Fax: 718-316-8179
Email address: info@bowditchgroup.com.
Web site: Available full-text at http://www.bowditchgroup.com/index2.htm
Cost: Call for prices
Description: The BioGram is an online weekly newsletter intended to provide information on the commercialization of agricultural biotechnology. The sponsors are a management consulting firm serving agribusiness, the food industry, and some segments of the chemical industry.

Biolink
Agricultural Biotechnology Support Project
Agriculture Hall, Michigan State University
East Lansing, MI 48824-1039
Telephone: 517-353-2290, Fax: 517-353-1888
Email address: absp@pilot.msu.edu
Web site: Available full-text at http://www.iia.msu.edu/absp/biolink.html
Cost: Free
Description: Biolink, the quarterly newsletter of the Agricultural Biotechnology for Sustainable Productivity Project, supports that organization's mission of improving the capacity and policy environment for the use, management, and commercialization of agricultural biotechnology in developing countries and transition economies.

Campaign for Food Safety News
Campaign for Food Safety/Organic Consumers Association
6114 Hwy 61
Little Marais, MN 55614
Telephone: 218-226-4164 or 236-6165, Fax: 218-226-4157
Web site: Available full-text at http://www.purefood.org/
Cost: Free
Description: This monthly online newsletter provides information on the state of genetically modified (GM) foods around the world, the dangers of GM foods, how to avoid them, and how to become politically active in the cause against GM foods.

GM-FREE
KHI Publications
Beacon House
Woodley Park, Skelmersdale
Lancashire, UK WN8 6UR
Telephone: 01695 50504, Fax: 01695 731394
Email address: gmfree@cableinet.co.uk
Web site: Available full-text at http://wkWeb4.cableinet.co.uk/pbrown/index.htm
Cost: Free
Description: This biannual online newsletter strongly opposes genetically modified foods and covers the topics: risks to health and environment, bad science and big business, government and industry cover-ups, research, the organic alternative, how to avoid GM foods, and consumer information.

Iowa Biotech Educator
Iowa State University
Office of Biotechnology
1210 Molecular Biology Bldg.
Ames, IA 50011-3260
Telephone: 515-294-9818, Fax: 515-294-4629
Email address: biotech@iastate.edu
Web site: Available full-text at http://www.biotech.iastate.edu/publications/IA_biotech_educator/
Cost: Free
Description: This roughly quarterly newsletter is geared towards educators who are incorporating biotechnology into their curriculums. One copy of the Iowa Biotech Educator is mailed to each Iowa school.

New Scientist
New Science Publications
IPC Magazines Ltd.
Kings Reacg Tower, Stamford Street
London SE1 9LS, England
Telephone: 020 7261 5000, Fax: 020 7261 6464
Web site: http://www.newscientist.com/gm/
Description: These selections from this weekly science journal all focus on issues surrounding genetically modified crops. Articles are available full-text online, and there are links to other biotechnology resources.

Food Safety Regulations

Food Environmental Weekly
Food Industry Environmental Network (FIEN)
33 Falling Creek Court
Silver Spring, MD 20904
Telephone: 301-384-8287, Fax: 301-384-8340
Email address: JLC@fien.com
Web site: http://www.fien.com
Cost: Fee varies, check with editor
Description: This online weekly newsletter serves as an alert service for the food and agricultural industry on policy, regulatory, and legislative developments concerning food safety, biotechnology, pesticides, hazardous substances, agricultural research, and other environmentally related issues. It is available by email or fax.

HACCP and Food Compliance News
FCN Publishing, CRC Press
1725 K St. N.W., Suite 506
Washington, DC 20006-1401
Telephone: 888-732-7070, Fax: 202-887-6337
Email address: newsdiv@crcpress.com
Web site: http://www.fcnpublishing.com/
Cost: $457
Description: This 12-page newsletter contains practical guidance on writing and implementing compliance plans, early warnings on enforcement actions, alerts of what areas regulators are targeting, notification of specific violations by suppliers, tips on passing rigorous inspections, and notification of food product recalls.

Heads Up for HACCP
National Meat Association
1970 Broadway, Suite 825
Oakland, CA 94612
Email address: jeremy@nmaonline.org
Web site: Available full-text at http://www.nmaonline.org
Cost: Free
Description: The purpose of Heads Up for HACCP is to provide straightforward technical information about HACCP and the scientific principles on which it is based so that company and regulatory employees can better understand the inspection system changes that have been implemented.

General Food Safety for Consumers

FDA Consumer
U.S. Food and Drug Administration
Order from Superintendent of Documents
P.O. Box 371954
Pittsburgh, PA 15250-7954
Telephone: 202-512-2250, Fax: 202-512-1800
Web site: Available full-text at http://www.fda.gov/fdac/
Cost: $12

Description: Although not specifically for food safety topics, this monthly consumer magazine often has food safety-related stories. Issues with a food safety focus are: Sept/Oct 1997, Nov/Dec 1997, Sept/Oct 1998, Sept/Oct 1999, Jan/Feb 2000, Jan/Feb 2001, and March/April 2001.

Food Allergy News
Food Allergy Network
10400 Eaton Place, Suite 107
Fairfax, VA 22030-2208
Email address: fan@worldweb.net
Web site: http://www.foodallergy.org/newsletter.html
Cost: Free to members of FAN
Description: The Food Allergy News is a bimonthly newsletter distributed to all members of The Food Allergy Network. Each issue includes feature articles and the latest information about food allergies and food allergy research.

Food Insight
International Food Information Council Foundation (IFIC)
1100 Connecticut Ave., NW, Suite 430
Washington, DC 20036
Email address: foodinfo@ific.health.org
Web site: http://ificinfo.health.org/
Cost: Free
Description: This bimonthly consumer newsletter covers such food safety topics as food allergies, additives, irradiation, food biotechnology, and general food safety. Available full-text from the above Web site.

On the Plate
National Consumer Coalition's Food Group by Consumer Alert
Web site: Available full-text at http://www.consumeralert.org/pubs/OnthePlate/index. htm
Cost: Free
Description: The mission of this online newsletter is to evaluate current policies and new proposals relating to food issues on the basis of sound science, risk assessment, and their impact on consumers.

Quality For Keeps
University of Missouri, Outreach and Extension
St. Charles County Extension Center
260 Brown Rd.
St. Peters, MO 63376
Telephone: 636-970-3000
Web site: Available full-text at http://www.outreach.missouri.edu/stcharles/qualitykeeps/index.html
Description: Quality For Keeps is an online newsletter for individuals who produce and preserve food; published April through October.

General Food Safety for Educators and Food Professionals

Best Practices: The Professional's Guide to Food Safety and Sanitation
International Food Safety Council
Web site: http://www.foodsafetycouncil/org/orderform.htm
Cost: $50
Description: Geared towards the restaurant and retail food service professional, this quarterly publication contains profiles of exemplary food safety practices, food safety updates from the industry's top food safety experts, and training tips from leading industry trainers.

Cryptosporidium Capsule
F.S. Publishing
976 McLean Ave., Suite 213
Yonkers, NY 10704
Telephone: 212-439-7203, Fax: 212-439-7231
Email address: crypcap@fspubl.com
Web site: http://www.fspubl.com/
Description: This newsletter solely devoted to *Cryptosporidium* includes information on the news, research, outbreaks, epidemiology, clinical studies, water treatment methods, and microbiological assays pertaining to *Cryptosporidium.* Although publication of Cryptosporidium Capsule ended with the October 1999 issue (Volume 4, Issue 12), a CD-ROM containing all of the issues is available. The CD-ROM includes searchable text of all published issues from November 1995 to October 1999. Approximately 3,000 searchable citations of the published literature on *Cryptosporidium* from 1995 to 1999 are included on the CD-ROM.

EdNet-National Food Safety Educator's Network
Food and Drug Administration, Food Safety and Inspection Service, Centers for Disease Control and Prevention
Email address: Subscribe by sending the command "*'subscribe Ednet-L Your Name'" to listserv@foodsafety.gov*
Web site: Available full-text at http://www.foodsafety.gov/~fsg/ednet.html

Cost: Free
Description: EdNet is a monthly online newsletter from the Food and Drug Administration, Food Safety and Inspection Service, and the Centers for Disease Control and Prevention, providing updates on food safety activities to educators and others concerned about food safety.

Emerging Infectious Diseases
Centers for Disease Control and Prevention (CDC)
To subscribe: EID Editor, CDC/NCID/MS D61
1600 Clifton Road NE
Atlanta, GA 30333
Email address: eideditor@cdc.gov.
Web site: Available full-text at http://www.cdc.gov/ncidod/eid/index.htm
Cost: Free
Description: Emerging Infectious Diseases is a peer-reviewed journal established by CDC to promote the recognition of new and reemerging infectious diseases around the world and to improve the understanding of factors involved in disease emergence, prevention, and elimination. Issued from four to six times per year.

Food Chemical News
FCN Publishing, CRC Press
1725 K St. N.W., Suite 506
Washington, DC 20006-1401
Telephone: 888-732-7070, Fax: 202-887-6337
Email address: newsdiv@crcpress.com
Web site: Available online for a fee at http://www.fcnpublishing.com/
Cost: $1,295
Description: This weekly update of news in food regulation, additives, microbiology, and contaminants covers food-related news from government, industry, and academia.

FOOD Environment News Digest
National Environmental Health Association
NEHA/FOOD e.n.d. Subscriptions
720 S. Colorado Blvd., Suite 970-S
Denver, CO 80246-1925
Telephone: 303-756-9090, Fax: 303-691-9490
Email address: staff@neha.org
Web site: http://www.neha.org/
Cost: $17.50
Description: Although this monthly journal covers the whole field of environmental science, many of the stories are on food and water safety topics.

FoodNet News
Centers for Disease Control and Prevention (CDC)
1600 Clifton Rd, NE, Mialstop A-38
Atlanta, GA 30333
Web site: Available full-text at http://www.cdc.gov/foodnet
Cost: Free
Description: This quarterly newsletter reports on FoodNet activities, accomplishments, and plans for future directions. FoodNet is an active surveillance system for foodborne diseases and related epidemiologic studies designed to help public health officials better understand the epidemiology of foodborne diseases in the United States.

Food Protection Report
Pike and Fischer, Inc
1010 Wayne Ave., Suite 1400
Silver Spring, MD 20910-5600
Email address: food@imaxx.net
Cost: $135
Description: This easy-to-read monthly newsletter offers reports of current developments in food safety including news stories, outbreaks, resources, and interviews with leaders in the food safety field from government, academia, and industry.

Food Safety Concerns Bulletin
Leatherhead Food Research Association
Randalls Road
Surrey, UK KT22 7RY
Telephone: +44-01372376761, Fax: +44-01372386228
Email address: help@lfra.co.uk
Web site: Available online for a fee at http://www.lfra.co.uk
Cost: Call for pricing information
Description: The Food Safety Concerns Bulletin is a comprehensive monthly compilation of articles on food safety issues as reported in the U.K. daily press. The bulletin highlights topical issues and subjects of continuing concern, both in the United Kingdom and worldwide.

Food Safety Educator
USDA Food Safety and Inspection Service (FSIS)
Food Safety Education, Room 2942
South Bldg., FSIS/USDA
Washington, DC 20250
Fax: 202-720-9063
Email address: fsis.outreach@usda.gov

Web site: Available full-text at http://www.fsis.usda.gov/oa/educator/educator.htm
Cost: Free
Description: This quarterly publication from FSIS is geared towards food safety educators but would also be of interest to consumers. The newsletter contains stories about research, resources, interviews with food safety experts, conferences, and more.

Food Safety and Hygiene
Food Science Australia
Web site: Available full-text at http://www.foodscience.afisc.csiro.au/fshlist.htm
Cost: Free
Description: Although originating in Australia and geared towards the Australian food industry, this quarterly online newsletter contains articles of interest to consumers and food service personnel in the United States too.

Food Safety Issues
The Food Institute
Box 972, 28-12 Broadway
Fair Lawn, NJ 07410
Telephone: 201-791-5570, Fax: 201-791-5222
Email address: food1@foodinstitute.com
Web site: http://www.foodinstitute.com/
Cost: Free to members
Description: Food Safety Issues, prepared by the law firm of Olsson, Frank and Weeda, P.C. and The Food Institute, is a monthly publication providing insights on food safety issues that shape the food industry.

Food Safety News
Kansas State University, Research and Extension
Animal Sciences and Industry
216 Call Hall
Manhattan, KS 66506
Telephone: 785-532-1672
Email address: kpenner@oz.oznet.ksu.edu
Web site: Available full-text at http://www.oznet.ksu.edu/pr_fsaf/Newsletter/foodsafetynews_.htm
Cost: Free
Description: This bimonthly newsletter for educators features field-to-fork information and resources on a variety of food safety topics.

food-safety-news.com
Food-safety.com.au
13 Campbell Street
Scarborough, Redcliffe, Queensland 4020
Telephone: +61 (7) 3880-4432, Fax: +61 (7) 3880-4804
Email address: info@food-safety.com.au
Web site: http://food-safety-news.com
Description: This monthly online newsletter produced by food-safety.com.au is geared towards the retail food industry, e.g., restaurants, fast food outlets, hotels, motels, cafeterias, etc. Available full-text at the above Web site.

Food Safety Professional
Chartered Institute of Environmental Health
Web site: http://www.cieh.org.uk
Cost: Free to members of The National Registry of Food Safety Professionals.
Description: This quarterly magazine for those who work in the food industry contains feature articles, advice on food safety in the workplace, interviews, news, views, letters, reviews, facts, figures, anecdotes and competitions.

Food Safety and Security
PJ Barnes and Associates
P.O. Box 200
Bridgewater, TA7 0YZ England
Telephone: +44-1823698973, Fax: +44-1823698971
Email address:sales@pbarnes.demon.co.uk
Web site: http://www.pbarnes.demon.co.uk/foodsafety.htm
Cost: $332
Description: Geared towards the food and drinks industry, this international monthly newsletter offers the latest information and advice on security, safety, and hygiene. Regular topics include tampering and contamination, research focus, processing, microbiological hazards, chemical hazards, and consumer and regulatory issues.

Food Safety Report
Bureau of National Affairs, Inc
1231 25th St. NW
Washington, DC 20037
Telephone: 202-452-4200
Email address: icustrel@bna.com
Web site: Available online for a fee at http://www.bna.com/
Cost: $795
Description: Food Safety Report is a weekly notification service that covers requirements of the Hazard Analysis and Critical Control Point programs, research of food technologies and safety measures, emerging pathogens, irradiation, pesticides, enforcement, recalls, and more.

Food Safety Today
Leatherhead Food Research Association
Randalls Road
Surrey, UK KT22 7RY
Telephone: +44 01372 376761, Fax: +44 01372 386228
Email address: help@lfra.co.uk
Web site: Available online for a fee at http://www.foodsafetytoday.com
Cost: Call for pricing information
Description: Food Safety Today is a regular Web publication providing up-to-date news about food safety for the food industry and anyone with a professional interest in the subject.

The HACCP Practitioner
Chartered Institute of Environmental Health (CIEH)
Chadwick Court, 15 Hatfields
London, UK SE1
Web site: http://www.cieh.org.uk/
Description: This quarterly technical publication gives detailed coverage of legislation, good practice, and legal issues of the complex and developing field of HACCP, looking at implementation in the United Kingdom and abroad.

International Food Safety News
Research Information Ltd
222 Maylands Avenue
Tel: +44 0-1813282470, Fax: +44 0-1442259395
Hemel Hempstead
Herts, UK HP2 7TD
Email address: info@resinf.co.uk
Web site: http://www.foodsafetynews.com/
Cost: $198
Description: This newsletter, published 10 times a year, provides concise, comprehensive information on important current issues, legislation, recent outbreaks, and events involving food safety from around the world.

Microbiology Newsletter
Leatherhead Food Research Association
Randalls Road
Surrey, UK KT22 7RY
Telephone: +44 01372376761, Fax: +44 01372386228
Email address: help@lfra.co.uk
Web site: http://www.lfra.co.uk
Cost: Call for pricing information
Description: This monthly newsletter keeps food microbiologists in touch with the latest developments in the field. It includes an editorial, legislation news, a digest of recent news stories from the media, and an extensive section of literature abstracts covering all aspects of food microbiology.

Morbidity and Mortality Weekly Report (MMWR)
Centers for Disease Control and Prevention
MMS Publications
C.S.P.O. Box 9120
Waltham, MA 02254
Telephone: 800-843-6356
Web site: Available full-text at http://www.cdc.gov/mmwr
Cost: $130
Description: The MMWR publishes data on specific diseases as reported to CDC by state and territorial health departments. Of interest to food safety professionals are case studies and foodborne illness statistics.

On Tap
National Drinking Water Clearinghouse
West Virginia University
P.O. Box 6064
Morgantown, WV 26506-6064
Telephone: 800-624-8301, Fax: 304-293-3161
Email address: webmaster@mail.estd.wvu.edu
Web site: http://www.estd.wvu.edu/ndwc/DiscussionFrame.html
Description: This quarterly newsletter is aimed at keeping community leaders, water industry professionals, and others interested in environmental issues informed about drinking water regulations, products, technologies, health, finance, and management issues relevant to America's small communities.

Thought for Food Safety Monthly
CFBE Publishing
P.O. Box 81161
Phoenix, AZ 85069-1161
Email address: FoodSafety@aol.com
Web site: http://expage.com/page/foodsafety
Cost: $39.95
Description: This monthly publication is dedicated to providing useful information on the risks from foods that occur every day. Written for food professionals and nonprofessionals alike.

Pesticides

Agrichemical and Environmental News
Washington State University Cooperative Extension
Web site: Available full-text at http://www2.tricity.wsu.edu/aenews/
Cost: Free
Description: This monthly online newsletter reports on environment and pesticide related topics, including pesticide residues, produce safety, and other food safety topics.

Pesticide and Toxic Chemical News
FCN Publishing, CRC Press
1725 K St. N.W., Suite 506
Washington, DC 20006-1401
Telephone: 888-732-7070, Fax: 202-887-6337
Eail address: newsdiv@crcpress.com
Web site: http://www.fcnpublishing.com/
Cost: $957
Description: A weekly report on the regulation, legislation, and other general issues concerning pesticides and toxic substances.

Pesticide Report
Darcey Publications
3918 Oglethorpe St.
Hyattsville, MD 20782
Telephone: 301-864-3088, Fax: 301-864-3089
Email address: sdarcey@erols.com
Cost: $299
Description: Pesticide Report is a biweekly 12-to-14-page print newsletter covering pesticide regulations/legislation, IPM, pesticide adverse effects, and risk assessment.

Pesticide Research Updates
Pesticide Action Network North America
49 Powell St., Suite 500
San Francisco, CA 94102
Email address: panna@panna.org
Web site: Available full-text at http://www.panna.org/
Cost: Free
Description: Pesticide Research Updates is an online quarterly newsletter providing up-to-date summaries of recent scientific articles covering epidemiological and toxicological studies of pesticides as well as medical case reports.

Chapter 9

Internet Web Sites and Electronic Media

Web sites listed in this chapter are stand-alone sites that either belong to an organization whose main presence is through its Web site or to an organization that has as its main focus, something other than food safety. Readers should also look at the organizations in chapter 10, as they all have Web sites not listed in this chapter. Web sites are divided into the following categories (sites that offer a wide variety of food safety information are listed under General Food Safety):

Food Allergy
Food Biotechnology
Food Preservation
Food Professionals' Web Sites
General Food Safety
Microbiology
Miscellaneous
Pesticides
Risk Assessment
Water Quality

The databases range from very broad to very specific. Those just beginning their research or those with access to a well-connected public or school library could begin with the general reference and resource databases. These typically have full-text items of interest from news sources, popular magazines, encyclopedias, and other general references. The bibliographic databases tend to draw materials from technical, peer-reviewed journals. They offer citations of books, journal articles, reports, and proceedings, but generally do not have the full-text of these works. Libraries are able to obtain these items through interlibrary loan. The more specialized databases are for those wishing to broaden their knowledge within specific subject areas. The databases are divided into:

General Reference and Resource Databases
General Bibliographic Databases
Databases with Data on Additives, Pesticide and Drug Residues, Toxins
Water Quality Databases
Miscellaneous Databases

After databases are listed:

E-mail Discussion Groups
E-mail News Distribution Groups
Reference Tools

A distinction is made here between e-mail discussion groups and e-mail news distribution groups. The former allows the subscriber to interact and have two-way "discussions" with other members of the group. It is an excellent way to exchange information with others interested in the same topic. E-mail news distribution groups offer only one way communication, from the owner of the list to the subscriber. These function more like a newspaper in that they condense news and other events on a food safety topic. To subscribe to either type of group visit the Web sites indicated. All of the e-mail groups are free. Many reference tools that in the past were paper editions are now available on the Internet or on CD-ROM. This offers the advantage of searchability, usually by keyword, date, author, etc.

INTERNET WEB SITES

Food Allergy

Aspartame Toxicity Information Center
Web site: http://www.holisticmed.com/aspartame/
Sponsor: Mark D. Gold
Description: This site links to scientific and general information resources regarding the toxicity of Nutrasweet, Equal, Diet Coke, Diet Pepsi, and other aspartame-containing items. It includes reports of acute and chronic toxicity due to long-term ingestion.

Food Allergy News for Kids
Web site: http://www.fankids.org/
Sponsor: Food Allergy Network
Description: This kid-oriented Web site covers the basics of food allergies, and includes school projects ideas, tips for managing food allergies, and activities.

Online Resources for People with Food Allergies and Intolerances.
Web site: http://www.skyisland.com/OnlineResources/
Sponsor: Michelle Peterson
Description: This site contains links to sites of interest to those with food allergies and intolerances, including cookbooks, a chat room, food additives, hidden ingredients, and links to other sites.

PeanutAllergy.Com
Web site: http://www.peanutallergy.com/
Sponsor: Owned and run by and for people with peanut allergy
Description: One of the goals of this Web site is to make it as easy as possible for everyone to find the peanut allergy community. It has bulletin boards, news articles, e-mail alerts, book lists, a list of peanut-free businesses, and anaphylaxis-related products.

Food Biotechnology

Ag BioTech InfoNet
Web site: http://www.biotech-info.net/
Sponsor: A consortium of scientific, environmental, and consumer organizations Ag BioTech InfoNet.
Description: Ag BioTech InfoNet covers all aspects of the application of biotechnology and genetic engineering in agricultural production and food processing and marketing. The focus is on scientific reports and findings and technical analysis, although the site also covers emerging issues

of widespread interest, policy developments, and media coverage. Offers coverage on both sides of the issue.

AgBiotechNet
Web site: http://www.agbiotechnet.com/
Sponsor: CABI developed AgBiotechNet with the Agricultural Biotechnology Support Project based at Michigan State University.
Description: AgBiotechNet publishes current information about agricultural biotechnology and biosafety for researchers and policy makers world-wide. The site provides access to research developments in genetic engineering and updates on economic and social issues. Included is information on patents, emerging issues, technology transfer, biosafety, research briefs, journal articles, and more. The site also has information on the issues involved in biotech for the general public.

Agricultural Biotechnology Web site
Web site: http://www.aphis.usda.gov/biotechnology/
Sponsor: USDA Animal and Plant Health Inspection Service (APHIS)
Description: This site contains frequently asked questions (FAQs) about agricultural biotechnology; information about laws, rules, and regulations pertaining to the subject; research reports; and links to other sites.

Alliance for Better Foods
Web site: http://betterfoods.org/
Sponsor: Alliance members are primarily from industry trade associations
Description: The Alliance for Better Foods Web site supports modern food biotechnology and the significant benefits it offers to consumers and to those that produce and process foods. The alliance is committed to helping people understand those benefits as well as the safety of using biotechnology in foods. The site contains a news archive of food biotechnology stories and a calendar of biotech events.

Biosafety Web Pages
Web site: http://www.icgeb.trieste.it/biosafety/
Sponsor: International Centre for Genetic Engineering and Biotechnology (ICGEB)
Description: The Biosafety Web Pages seeks to promote the safe use of biotechnology world-wide, with special regards to the need of the developing world. The site maintains a scientific bibliographic database on biosafety studies that is updated monthly and contains scientific articles published in international scientific journals since 1990. ICGEB sponsors workshops on biosafety and risk assessment. Genetically modified organisms and food security are major topics on the site

Biotechnology Information Resource
Web site: http://www.nal.usda.gov/bic/
Sponsor: National Agricultural Library
Description: This site provides access to a variety of information services and publications covering many aspects of agricultural biotechnology. Included are issue papers, reports, speeches, meetings, patents, bibliographies, links to other agricultural biotechnology sites, and more.

Biotechnology in Our Food Chain
Web site: http://www.jic.bbsrc.ac.uk/exhibitions/bio-future/index.htm
Sponsor: Institute of Food Research
Description: Biotechnology in Our Food Chain is a 1998 Web-based U.K. Schools' Project on food production and consumption, now and in the future. Two schools participated in the project with 16- to 17-year-old students researching how biotechnology is used in the food chain. They investigated how biotechnology is increasingly becoming part of farming practice and food production and its role in improving food quality and safety. They also looked at environmental and consumer issues, taking note of the various viewpoints that exist.

Canadian Citizen's Conference on Food Biotechnology
Web site: http://www.acs.ucalgary.ca/~pubconf/
Sponsor: University of Calgary
Description: The purpose of this citizen conference, held March 5–7, 1999, was to bring together divergent views on food biotechnology using a public participation mechanism. A panel of lay citizens set an agenda and discussed with a panel of experts matters they found important to influence the direction of food biotechnology in Canada. This site contains background papers, suggested reading, educational materials, FAQs, and links to sites that are both critical of and supportive of agricultural biotechnology.

foodfuture
Web site: http://www.foodfuture.org.uk/
Sponsor: Food and Drink Federation

Description: The foodfuture program aims to improve public understanding of genetic modification. The program facilitates wider discussion of the technology, the perceived benefits and disadvantages, and the ethical and moral concerns. It provides a clear and comprehensible explanation of the benefits that GM technology could bring to our food supply.

gmIssues
Web site: http://www.gmissues.org/
Sponsor: The Genetic Modification and Biosafety Assessment Research Group of the John Innes Centre, Norwich. UK.
Description: gmIssues provides a balanced public information resource on the science of genetically modified crops and related issues. It collects and posts documents, reports, and informed commentary relating to the scientific research application, regulation, socioeconomic, and environmental implications of genetically modified crops.

Information Systems for Biotechnology (ISB)
Web site: http://www.nbiap.vt.edu/
Sponsor: Virginia Polytechnic Institute and State University in Blacksburg, Virginia
Description: ISB resources are designed to serve the agricultural and environmental biotechnology community at large, including scientists, regulators, teachers, administrators, and the interested public. Through its affiliation with a land-grant university and funding through the Research, Education, and Extension arm of USDA, ISB provides a balanced view of the potential benefits and concerns of this powerful technology. The focus of ISB activities is to provide value-added information in a readily accessible form.

Transgenic Crops: An Introduction and Resource Guide
Web site: http://www.colostate.edu/programs/lifesciences/TransgenicCrops/
Sponsor: Colorado State University
Description: The goal of this Web site is to provide balanced information and links to other resources on the technology and issues surrounding transgenic crops (also known as genetically modified or GM crops). The site's authors are engaged in plant genetics research and teaching at Colorado State University. They receive no funds from companies involved in transgenic crop development, nor are they affiliated with groups campaigning against such crops.

Food Preservation

Food Safety and Food Preservation
Web site: http://www.foodpres.com/
Sponsor: Shirley VanGarde, co-author of the book Food Preservation and Safety
Description: This site assists consumers in determining whether the food in their household is safe to consume or should be discarded. It is also a good place for information on custom-preserving foods. This site is written by two Ph.D.s who specialize in food safety and food preservation issues. Science-based information on canning, freezing, making jerky, pickling, salvaging flooded kitchens, and much more is available.

How Stuff Works-Food Preservation
Web site: http://www.howstuffworks.com/food-preservation.htm
Sponsor: Marshall Brain. BYG Publishing, Inc.
Description: Offers short description of major food preservation technologies, including refrigeration and freezing, canning, irradiation, dehydration, freeze drying, salting, pickling, pasteurizing, fermentation, carbonation, and chemical preservation. The site also has section on how refrigerators and microwaves work.

Food Professionals' Web Sites

Cyberchefs Electronic Union
Web site: http://www.geocities.com/TheTropics/3348/
Sponsor: Chef Mars
Description: This site is a communications platform for chefs, cooks, and all others intrigued by the mysteries of food and the kitchen. It provides users with the opportunity to communicate and exchange ideas and information with other professionals. See the online Kitchen Training Manual for food safety training.

FoodHACCP.com
Web site: http://foodhaccp.com
Sponsor: Dr. D.Y.C. Fung and Dr. D. H. Kang
Description: This web site for food professionals contains sections on current news, recalls, journal abstracts, detection methods, pathogens, education, and hot topics.

Food Online
Web site: http://www.foodonline.com
Sponsor: VerticalNet, Inc
Description: Food Online is an Internet resource for the food processing industry. The site is directed to plant engineers, production managers, manufacturing engineers, processing technicians, operations supervisors, and business managers involved in the food processing industry. It provides daily news updates and reports on business and technology trends. Food Online also covers quality control and quality assurance systems, information management systems, process control systems and equipment, as well as clean-in-place systems, inspection equipment, measurement systems, sanitation systems, and X-ray equipment.

Foodservice.com
Web site: http://foodservice.com/
Sponsor: Foodservice.com
Description: Foodservice.com was created for the food service professional. Food safety resources include HACCP information, a moderated food safety forum, links to other sites, product recalls, posters, and articles.

Integrated Food Safety Information Delivery System (IFSIDS)
Web site: http://www.profoodsafety.org/
Sponsor: Food and Consumer Safety Bureau of the Iowa Department of Inspections and Appeals
Description: This Web site serves the needs of food safety regulators by providing factual information and educational materials for use with local food establishment operators. Materials are available in English and thirteen foreign languages.

National Food Safety Education Month
Web site: http://www.restaurant.org/nfsem/
Sponsor: International Food Safety Council
Description: This site contains training materials for food service workers and promotional materials related to National Food Safety Education Month, which is September.

General Food Safety

Alliance for Food and Fiber
Web site: http://www.foodsafetyalliance.org/
Sponsor: Alliance for Food and Fiber
Description: An educational clearinghouse to inform the public on the issues of food safety and crop protection that impact the production, processing, and distribution of food and fiber products. The site has sections on produce safety and pesticide residues, the Food Quality Protection Act, and consumer tips for safe food handling.

Centers for Disease Control and Prevention (CDC)
Web site: http://www.cdc.gov/foodsafety/
Sponsor: Centers for Disease Control and Prevention
Description: This food safety Web site by CDC is geared towards consumers and offers general food safety information with an extensive FAQ section.

Egg Nutrition Center
Web site: http://www.enc-online.org/
Sponsor: American Egg Board and United Egg Producers
Description: Although most of this site is dedicated to egg nutrition, it does have a growing section of egg safety for consumers and food service professionals.

European Commission Web Site on Food Safety
Web site: http://europa.eu.int/comm/food
Sponsor: European Commission
Description: This Web site from the European Commission covers animal health, animal feed safety, pesticides, safety of food products, food labeling, international food safety issues, food biotechnology, and more.

Fight BAC! Food Safety Campaign
Web site: http://www.fightbac.org/
Sponsor: Partnership for Food Safety Education
Description: This public-private partnership, created to reduce the incidence of foodborne illness by educating Americans about safe food handling practices, maintains a Web site with consumer food safety messages; tools for educatorsl and ordering information for games, kits, magnets, mugs, puppets, T-shirts, aprons, bookmarks, posters, and patches with the Fight BAC! logo.

Foodlink
Web site: http://www.foodlink.org.uk/index.htm
Sponsor: Food and Drink Federation
Description: This site hosts the U.K. National Food Safety Week, which provides a focus for communicating messages designed to help people understand and initiate basic precautions that

can be taken to reduce the risk of food poisoning. National Food Safety Week provides participants with activities and materials to raise awareness of food poisoning in a fun and effective way.

FoodNet
Web site: http://foodnet.fic.ca/
Sponsor: Food Institute of Canada
Description: This site links to product recalls (it is also possible to receive product recalls by email), HACCP materials and other food safety training materials, food regulations, and agencies involved in food processing and safety.

Foodsafe Program
Web site: http://foodsafe.ucdavis.edu/
Sponsor: University of California, Davis
Description: The most unique aspect of this site is the food safety music, adaptations of popular songs to food science and food safety themes. Other sections include hot topics and a directory of experts for the state of California.

Foodsafety.gov—The Gateway to Government Food Safety Information
Web site: www.foodsafety.gov
Sponsor: Centers for Disease Control and Prevention, Environmental Protection Agency, Food and Drug Administration, USDA Food Safety and Inspection Service
Description: Contains a wealth of information from federal and state agencies pertaining to food safety for consumers, educators, and food industry professionals. This is the main link to federal food safety information.

Food Safety Campaign Group's Education Pages
Web site: http://www.safefood.net.au/
Sponsor: Australian Food Safety Campaign Group
Description: Although written by a group in Australia, the food safety information is relevant to consumers in the United States too. The site has a children's section, home food safety tips, fact sheets on pathogens, and more.

Food Safety Information Retrieval System
Web site: http://www.ces.ncsu.edu/depts/foodsci/agentinfo/
Sponsor: North Carolina State University Cooperative Extension
Description: The goal of this Web site is to promote food safety education via the Internet, providing a gateway to information that is already available on the Internet while also including new information. In addition to consumer information, there is also information specific to extension educators such as program materials, resources, and general information.

Food Safety Project
Web site: http://www.exnet.iastate.edu/Pages/families/fs/homepage.html
Sponsor: Iowa State University Cooperative Extension
Description: The goal of the Food Safety Project is to develop educational materials that give the public the tools they need to minimize their risk of foodborne illness. It contains research-based, unbiased information on food safety and quality for consumers, educators, and students.

Food Safety Throughout the System
Web site: http://foodsafety.cas.psu.edu
Sponsor: Penn State Department of Food Science
Description: This site has sections for educators, consumers, retail food service, food processors, and those interested in food preservation.

Food Safety Web
Web site: http://www.okstate.edu/OSU_Ag/fapc/fsw/fswmain.htm
Sponsor: Oklahoma State University
Description: Geared more towards the educator and/or food safety professional, this site contains sections on food microbiology, outbreaks, HACCP, resources, and methods of analysis.

Food Science Australia
Web site: http://www.csiro.au/
Sponsor: Food Science Australia is an unincorporated joint venture between CSIRO and the Australian Food Industry Science Centre (AFISC).
Description: This Web site contains a consumer section with fact sheets and media stories, plus a wide selection of technical information for food industry personnel. From main CSIRO site, look under directories, select food science and food processing.

Home Food Safety . . . It's in Your Hands
Web site: http://www.homefoodsafety.org/
Sponsor: American Dietetic Association and the ConAgra Foundation
Description: This consumer education program communicates the important role consumers play in preparing foods safely in their own homes. The

Web site has an interactive kitchen food safety quiz, FAQ site, tips for safe food preparation, and links to food safety news stories and Web sites.

Hospitality Institute of Technology and Management Web Site
Web site: http://www.hi-tm.com/
Sponsor: Pete Snyder, Hospitality Institute of Technology and Management
Description: This site contains informative writings on such food safety topics as handwashing, growth of microorganisms, and HACCP for both consumers and those in the retail food market.

Kansas State University Research and Extension Food Safety Page
Web site: http://www.oznet.ksu.edu/foodsafety/
Sponsor: Kansas State University
Description: This Web site has consumer food safety tips, the full-text version of the Kansas Food Code, links to food safety and food science sites, and an online newsletter for food safety educators.

NSW Multicultural Health Communication Service
Web site: http://mhcs.health.nsw.gov.au
Sponsor: South Eastern Sydney Area Health Service
Description: This service translates health-related documents into other languages. The site has consumer-level food safety documents in Arabic, Chinese, Croatian, English, Italian, Khmer/Cambodian, Korean, Macedonian, Portuguese, Russian, Spanish, Thai, Turkish, and Vietnamese.

Restaurant Health Inspection Scores on the Web
Web site: http://www.restaurantsafety. com/inspections.html
Sponsor: The Restaurant Management Resources Network
Description: Links to health inspection scores from those jurisdictions in the United States that have them available online.

Safefood.org
Web site: http://www.safefood.org/
Sponsor: National Food Processors Association
Description: This site provides consumers with information to safely handle, prepare, and store foods. Sections include frequently asked questions; fact sheets on food safety topics; a flowchart of how products are processed and packaged, featuring a different product each month; a history of processed foods; and links to other sites.

SafetyAlerts.com
Web site: http://www.safetyalerts.com/
Sponsor: Started by a private citizen concerned about access to safety recall notices in the United States
Description: This site lists food recalls and other consumer-level food safety information.

Tacoma-Pierce County Health Department Food and Community Safety Program
Web site: http://www.healthdept.co.pierce.wa.us
Sponsor: Tacoma-Pierce County Health Department
Description: In this excellent state health department site users can find handwashing lessons for children, consumer food safety bulletins on hot topics of the day, and information for the retail food industry all with colorful, well-done graphics and layout.

Thermy Campaign
Web site: http://www.fsis.usda.gov/thermy/
Sponsor: USDA Food Safety and Inspection Service
Description: This is the Web site for the USDA campaign to encourage the use of food thermometers, centered around the character Thermy. The site contains Thermy campaign artwork, resources for kids and educators, consumer fact sheets, and background research information on thermometers.

Microbiology

Bugs in the News
Web site: http://falcon.cc.ukans.edu/~jbrown/bugs.html
Sponsor: John (Jack) C. Brown, University of Kansas, Lawrence, Kansas
Description: This Web site aims to provide information on microorganisms to the general public in a reader-friendly format. The "What the Heck is" section includes *E. coli*, food allergy, mad cow disease, genetic engineering, and viruses.

Bugs on the Web
Web site: http://bugs.uah.ualberta.ca/webbug/index.htm
Sponsor: Microbiology and Public Health for Northern Alberta

Description: This Web site features articles on various facets of bacteria, viruses, and parasites. Included are pages on *E. coli* O157:H7 and *Cyclospora cayetanensis.*

E. Coli Help Organization-Eric's Echo
Web site: http://www.ericsecho.org/
Sponsor: Rainer Mueller
Description: This site is maintained by the father of Eric Jackson Mueller, who died after eating an *E.Coli* O157:H7–contaminated hamburger. The site contains links to many different sources of *E. coli* information.

Infection Detection Protection
Web site: http://www.amnh.org
Sponsor: American Museum of Natural History
Description: This interactive children's site teaches about the microbial world. It has several games, and includes a section on bacteria in the cafeteria.

Microbe World
Web site: http://www.microbeworld.org/
Sponsor: American Society for Microbiology
Description: Microbe World is full of learning activities and teaching resources. This excellent site is divided into two areas: Stalking the Mysterious Microbe for elementary students and The Microbial Literacy Collaborative (MLC) for older students and science teachers. Although not geared towards just foodborne microbes, they are included in some areas. Also contains a career section.

Outbreak!
Web site: http://www.nbif.org/outbreak/
Sponsor: National Biotechnology Information Facility (NBIF), New Mexico State University
Description: Outbreak! is an online interactive teaching tool for use by students and science educators. Players must use microbial identification techniques to identify the causative agent of an illness outbreak.

Miscellaneous

FoodNet
Web site: http://www.cdc.gov/foodnet/
Sponsor: Centers for Disease Control and Prevention (CDC), Foodborne and Diarrheal Diseases Branch, Division of Bacterial and Mycotic Disease, National Center for Infectious Diseases
Description: This is the main access page for the Foodborne Diseases Active Surveillance Network (FoodNet) project, a program for active surveillance of foodborne diseases and related epidemiology designed to help public health officials better understand the nature of foodborne diseases in the United States. Yearly surveillance report, a newsletter, and a detailed explanation of FoodNet are on the site.

Healthy School Meals Resource System (HSMRS)
Web site: http://www.nal.usda.gov:8001/index.html
Sponsor: USDA Food and Nutrition Information Center, National Agricultural Library
Description: The Healthy School Meals Resource System (HSMRS) is a searchable Web site developed as a component of the USDA Team Nutrition to implement the School Meals Initiative. It provides information to persons working in USDA Child Nutrition Programs. Food safety highlights on the site include full-text of the training kit, "Serving it Safe: A Manager's Tool Kit" and links to other food safety resources useful to this audience.

Official Mad Cow Disease Home Page
Web site: http://www.mad-cow.org/
Sponsor: Sperling Biomedical Foundation
Description: This Web site contain 6,000+ article and abstracts on mad cow disease and Creutzfeldt-Jakob disease (CJD), prions, bovine spongiform encephalopathy (BSE), scrapie, and other transmissible spongiform encephalopathies.

Seafood Network Information Center
Web site: http://www-seafood.ucdavis.edu/
Sponsor: The California Sea Grant College Program, University of California Cooperative Extension, and Food Science and Technology, University of California, Davis
Description: This seafood safety site contains sanitation and HACCP information for industry, as well as consumer seafood safety information. It is also home to the Seafood Mailing List.

www.food-irradiation.com
Web site: http://www.irradiation-information.com/
Sponsor: Foundation for Food Irradiation Education (FFIE)
Description: The purpose of this Web site is to provide factual information and to improve communications about food irradiation to the public, the industry, media, and academia so that consumer choices, media coverage, and industry de-

cisions can be made rationally and beneficially through access to full information. The goal is to provide information leading to the adoption of food irradiation when it would improve the quality of life through increased food safety, technical or marketing improvements, enhanced agriculture production, or food security; assist food trade and food availability to consumers; and/or provide an environmentally more suitable process.

Pesticides

EXtension TOXicology NETwork (EXTOXNET)
Web site: http://ace.ace.orst.edu/info/extoxnet/
Sponsor: EXTOXNET is a cooperative effort of University of California-Davis, Oregon State University, Michigan State University, Cornell University, and the University of Idaho.
Description: The EXTOXNET InfoBase provides a wealth of information about pesticides and is written in an unbiased form that the nonexpert can understand. Contains fact sheets, FAQs, information briefs, news, resources, and technical information. The FAQ section on food safety is particularly useful.

Pesticide Information Center On-Line (PICOL)
Web site: http://picol.cahe.wsu.edu/
Sponsor: Washington State University
Description: This site contains information on the Food Quality Protection Act, plus the Pesticide Tolerance/Label Database, the Pesticide Impact Assessment Program, and other information related to pesticides.

Risk Assessment

Food Safety Network
Web site: http://www.plant.uoguelph.ca/safefood/
Sponsor: University of Guelph, Agri-Food Risk Management and Communication Project
Description: This site is about applying risk communication theory to issues of food safety and agricultural biotechnology, integrating scientific knowledge with public perceptions, and addressing the cultural and societal implications of new technologies as they relate to the food supply. Included are basics about risk management and communication; crisis response and communication; course information for a science, technology, and risk course; and links to risk communication issues for food safety, plant agriculture, and animal agriculture.

Food Safety Risk Analysis Clearinghouse
Web site: http://www.foodriskclearinghouse.umd.edu/
Sponsor: Joint Institute for Food Safety and Applied Nutrition (JIFSAN)
Description: The aim of this site is to assist people involved with any of the many aspects of risk analysis as it pertains to food safety. It provides tools and links to numerous sources of information, including terminology, risk assessments, events, links, databases, and consumer information.

Water Quality

Drinking Water Outbreaks
Web site: http://water.sesep.drexel.edu/outbreaks
Sponsor: Professor Charles N. Haas
Description: This site collects information on outbreaks of infectious disease in drinking water, and related topics. Links to, or files with, information from the popular press, as well as primary source information are included.

Water Online
Web site: http://www.wateronline.com
Sponsor: VerticalNet, Inc
Description: Water Online serves the information needs of engineers, planners, operational and financial managers, business executives, consultants, elected officials, government personnel and others who are involved in the municipal water supply industry, and the municipal and industrial wastewater treatment field. It provides technical, operational, product, management, and regulatory information available for the water industry.

DATABASES

General Reference and Resource Databases

Combined Health Information Database (CHID)
Sponsor: National Institutes of Health
Description: CHID is a bibliographic database produced by health-related agencies of the federal government. This database provides titles, abstracts, and availability information for health information and health education resources.
Web: http://chid.nih.gov/

General Reference Center
Sponsor: Gale Group
Description: This general reference tool, available in many school and public libraries, provides access to full-text general interest magazines, children's magazines, almanacs, encyclopedias, dictionaries, reference books, maps, historical images, and newspaper articles. Of particular interest to those studying food safety are: Asimov's Chronology of Science and Discovery, FDA Consumer, Issues in Science and Technology, Popular Science, Science Digest, and Science News.
Web site: http://www.galegroup.com/

InfoTrac
Sponsor: Gale Group
Description: InfoTrac K-12 Student Edition is the one-stop, multisource general reference center designed especially for school libraries. It provides a combination of indexing abstracts, images, and full-text for general interest periodicals, maps, reference books, and thousands of newspaper articles.
Web site: http://www.galegroup.com/

OCLC FirstSearch Electronic Collections Online
Sponsor: OCLC
Description: This powerful electronic journals service offers Web access to a growing collection of more than 2,300 titles including most of the major publications covering food issues.
Web site: http://www.oclc.org/firstsearch

SIRS Discoverer and SIRS Researcher
Sponsor: SIRS Mandarin, Inc.
Description: SIRS Discoverer provides young researchers with a wealth of information on topics of high interest. Articles and graphics from more than 1,200 U.S. and international magazines, newspapers, and U.S. government documents are carefully selected for their educational content, interest, and level of readability.

SIRS Researcher is a general reference database that contains thousands of full-text articles exploring social, scientific, health, historic, economic, business, political, and global issues. Articles are selected from more than 1,500 domestic and international newspapers, magazines, journals, and U.S. government publications and may be accessed instantaneously. Articles are archived from 1989 to the present. Many articles are accompanied by graphics, including charts, maps, diagrams, and illustrations.
Web site: http://www.sirs.com/

Student Resource Center
Sponsor: Gale Group
Description: The Student Resource Center provides one-stop cross-curricular access to resource for schools and libraries. It is a comprehensive Web-based resource containing an archive of 41,000 primary source documents, up to 1.7 million full-text periodical and newspaper articles that are updated daily, and more than 82,000 biographies, essays, overviews, dictionaries, encyclopedias, magazines, and newspapers.
Web site: http://www.galegroup.com/

Bibliographic Databases

AGRICOLA
Sponsor: USDA National Agricultural Library
Description: AGRICOLA (AGRICultural On-Line Access) is a database of 3.5 million bibliographic records from 1970 to the present. The records describe publications and resources encompassing all aspects of agriculture and allied disciplines, including plant and animal sciences, forestry, entomology, soil and water resources, agricultural economics, agricultural engineering, agricultural products, alternative farming practices, and food and nutrition. Auxiliary subjects that support NAL's Information Center activities, such as agricultural trade and marketing, rural information, animal welfare, and food safety are also included.
Web site: http://www.nal.usda.gov/ag98/

Biotechnology and Bioengineering Abstracts
Sponsor: Cambridge Scientific Abstracts
Description: This database provides bibliographic coverage of groundbreaking research, applica-

tions, regulatory developments, and new patents across all areas of biotechnology and bioengineering, including agricultural, antibiotics, genetic engineering, food production, and food safety.
Web site: http://www.csa.com/

Epidemiology Information System
National Library of Medicine
Description: The Epidemiology Information System (EIS) file, built and maintained by the FDA Center for Food Safety is a subfile of the National Library of Medicine's TOXLINE. The file includes citations to literature on the distribution and health effects of food contaminants, including natural toxicants in foods. It was developed to provide FDA with a computerized, indexed information system referring to literature related to the health effects of food contaminants. Citations in the file are predominantly from published literature such as journal articles, reports, books, and conference proceedings. Dates of publication of the citations in the file are from 1940 to 1988.
Web site: http://www.nlm.nih.gov/pubs/factsheets/toxlinfs.html

Food Science and Technology Abstracts (FSTA)
Sponsor: International Food Information Service
Description: To produce FSTA, specialists monitor approximately 1,800 journals and other regular publications and many other types of literature (books, conference proceedings, theses, patents, standards, legislation, etc.) published in more than 40 languages, and select the items relevant to the food sector. Each month nearly 2,000 records, covering every subject related to food and drink, are added to the 510,000 records already in the database.
Web site: http://www.ifis.co.uk/index.html

Medline
Sponsor: National Library of Medicine
Description: Medline is the National Library of Medicine's premier bibliographic database covering the fields of medicine, nursing, dentistry, veterinary medicine, the health care system, and the preclinical sciences. The database contains records from 4,300 journals dating from 1966 to the present.
Web site: http://www.nlm.nih.gov/databases/databases.html

Databases with Data on Additives, Pesticide and Drug Residues, Toxins

Codex Alimentarius: Maximum Limits for Pesticide Residue in Foods
Sponsor: Food and Agriculture Organization of the United Nations
Description: This database contains Codex Maximum Residue Limits for Pesticides and Extraneous Maximum Residue Limits adopted by the Codex Alimentarius Commission up to and including its Twenty-second Session (June 1997).
Web site: http://apps.fao.org/CodexSystem/pestdes/pest_ref/pest-e.htm

Codex Alimentarius: Veterinary Drug Residues in Food
Sponsor: Food and Agriculture Organization of the United Nations
Description: This database contains Maximum Residue Limits for Veterinary Drugs (MRLVDs) adopted by the Codex Alimentarius Commission up to and including its Twenty-second Session (July 1997) based on the advice of the Codex Committee on Residues of Veterinary Drugs in Foods.
Web site: http://apps.fao.org/CodexSystem/vetdrugs/vetd_ref/vetd-e.htm

EAFUS: A Food Additive Database
Sponsor: U.S. FDA Center for Food Safety and Applied Nutrition (CFSAN)
Description: This is an informational database maintained under an ongoing program known as the Priority-based Assessment of Food Additives (PAFA). It contains administrative, chemical, and toxicological information on more than 2,000 substances directly added to food, including substances regulated by FDA as direct, "secondary" direct, color additives, generally recognized as safe (GRAS), and prior-sanctioned substances. The more than 3,000 total substances together comprise an inventory often referred to as Everything Added to Food in the United States (EAFUS).
Web site: http://vm.cfsan.fda.gov/~dms/eafus.html

Food Additive and Preservative Allergy and Intolerance Database (FAP-AID)
Sponsor: Zing Solutions
Description: Published in 1998, this database is a diagnostic aid that indicates what foods, additives, or preservatives can cause allergies or adverse reactions. It describes background

information and reported reactions to foods, additives, preservatives, molds, fungi, and naturally occurring substances. A demo of the database is available online.
Web site: http://zingsolutions.com/food/

Food Animal Residue Avoidance Databank (FARAD)
Sponsor: USDA, Cooperative State Research, Education, and Extension Service
Description: FARAD is a computer-based decision support system designed to provide livestock producers, extension specialists, and veterinarians with practical information on how to avoid drug, pesticide, and environmental contaminant residue problems. Also has a telephone hotline: 1–888–US-FARAD.
Web site: http://www.farad.org/

National Milk Drug Residue Database
Sponsor: U.S. FDA and the National Conference on Interstate Milk Shipments
Description: The National Milk Drug Residue Data Base is a voluntary industry reporting program. It includes information on the kind and extent of the animal drug residues identified and the amount of contaminated milk, including whether it was disposed of properly for nonhuman use. The database is operated by an independent third party, under contract to the FDA.
Web site: http://vm.cfsan.fda.gov/~ear/p-mis.html

Pesticide Analytical Behavior Data
Sponsor: U.S. Food and Drug Administration (FDA)
Description: Pestrak and Pestdata files provide information about pesticides of interest to the U.S. Food and Drug Administration because of their potential for use on foods. Data include names, molecular formulas, and references to Code of Federal Regulations sections that list food tolerances.
Web site: http://vm.cfsan.fda.gov/~frf/pestdata.html

Pesticide Program Pesticide Monitoring Database
Sponsor: U.S. Food and Drug Administration (FDA)
Description: The downloadable data files represent samples from more than 90 countries that are analyzed under the regulatory monitoring component of FDA pesticide programs. Yearly updates are available on the Web.
Web site: http://vm.cfsan.fda.gov/~lrd/pestadd.html

TOXNET (Toxicology Data Network)
Sponsor: National Library of Medicine (NLM)
Description: Toxnet is a cluster of databases on toxicology, hazardous chemicals, and related areas. Included is factual information related to the toxicity and other hazards of a wide variety of chemicals, including pesticide residues, bibliographic information with citations to the scientific literature, data on the estimated quantities of chemicals released into the environment, and chemical information. Available for free from the NLM Web site.
Web site: http://sis.nlm.nih.gov/sis1/

Water Quality Databases

EPA Information Collection Rule Federal Database
Sponsor: U.S. Environmental Protection Agency
Description: This database contains information on pathogens in drinking water sources (lakes, reservoirs, etc.), indicators of fecal contamination, the amount of disinfectant present, the presence of disinfection by-products in treated drinking water, and the effectiveness of certain treatment technologies. The data are used to help assess the potential health risks of pathogens, disinfectants, and disinfection by-products, and to guide future regulatory and public health decisions.
Web site: http://www.epa.gov/OGWDW/icr.html

Ground Water On-Line
Sponsor: National Ground Water Association
Description: Ground Water On-Line is a database containing more than 78,000 groundwater literature citations with key words, abstracts, chemical compounds, biological factors, geographic locations, authors, titles, publication source names, and more. Each citation may contain up to 25 fields of information. Documents that are indexed include scientific, technical, and trade journals; newsletters; books; government documents; university reports; dissertations and theses; state publications; and proceedings of national and international conferences and symposia.
Web site: http://www.ngwa.org/gwonline/index.html

National Drinking Water Contaminant Occurrence Database (NCOD)
Sponsor: U.S. Environmental Protection Agency
Description: In 1996 Congress mandated that drinking water quality data be made available to EPA decision makers and the public. The purpose of the database is to support EPA's decisions related to identifying contaminants for regulation and subsequent regulation development. NCOD contains occurrence data from public water systems and other sources on physical, chemical, microbial, and radiological contaminants. There are some summary statistics, but no actual analysis of the data is provided. Instead, NCOD is used to build a set of data that can be downloaded and analyzed offline. It is updated quarterly.
Web site: http://www.epa.gov/ncod/
This site has links to more consumer-friendly resources about safe drinking water.

Registry of Equipment Suppliers of Treatment Technologies for Small Systems (RESULTS)
Sponsor: National Drinking Water Clearinghouse
Description: RESULTS is a searchable public reference database containing information about water treatment technologies in use at small water systems around the country. Searchable by contaminant, technology, manufacturer, and state, the database also contains general information about the technology and manufacturer, state official, and system contact information.
Web site: Searchable online at http://www.estd.wvu.edu/ndwc/

Safe Drinking Water Information System / Federal Version (SDWIS/FED)
Sponsor: U.S. Environmental Protection Agency (EPA), Office of Ground Water and Drinking Water
Description: SDWIS/FED is a database designed and implemented by EPA to meet its needs in the oversight and management of the Safe Drinking Water Act (SDWA). The database contains data submitted by states and EPA regions in conformance with reporting requirements established by statute, regulation, and guidance. Users may search the database to find reported violations of the SDWA in their local area.
Web site: http://www.epa.gov/OGWDW/sdwisfed/sdwis.htm

Miscellaneous Databases

Foodborne Illness Educational Materials Database
Sponsor: USDA/FDA Foodborne Illness Education Information Center
Description: The Foodborne Illness Educational Materials Database is a compilation of consumer and food worker educational materials developed by universities; private industry; and local, state, and federal agencies. This includes computer software, audiovisuals, posters, games and teaching guides for elementary and secondary school education; training materials for the management and workers of retail food markets, food service establishments and institutions; and more.
Web site: http://www.nal.usda.gov/foodborne/

HACCP Training Programs and Resources Database
Sponsor: USDA/FDA Foodborne Illness Education Information Center
Description: The Hazard Analysis Critical Control Points (HACCP) Training Programs and Resources Database provides up-to-date listings of HACCP training programs and resource materials. Its intended users are educators; trainers; field staff in Extension; Food Safety and Inspection Service (FSIS) personnel; FDA personnel; private sector food processing plants and organizations; and others interested in identifying HACCP training resources.
Web site: http://www.nal.usda.gov/foodborne/

USDA Current Research Info System (CRIS)
Sponsor: USDA Cooperative State Research, Education, and Extension Service
Description: CRIS serves as the USDA documentation and reporting system for publicly supported agricultural, food and nutrition, and forestry research in the United States. The database contains the information on ongoing and recently completed projects sponsored or conducted primarily within the USDA and state university research system. Some 30,000 project summaries, including latest progress reports and lists of recent publications coming out of the research are maintained in the file on an ongoing basis.
Web site: http://cris.csrees/usda.gov

EMAIL DISCUSSION GROUPS

Biotechnology in Food and Agriculture Electronic Forum
Sponsor: Food and Agriculture Organization of the United Nations
Description: The forum will operate a series of email conferences on specific topics that will be discussed for a limited two-month time period only. The topics all have biotechnology as the core subject and may cover themes such as biosafety, public/private agricultural research, biodiversity, capacity-building, food safety, poverty alleviation, benefit sharing, intellectual property rights, and food production. The site also contains a glossary of biotechnology and bioengineering terms.
Web site: http://www.fao.org/biotech/forum.htm

Cryptosporidium Discussion Group
Sponsor: Macquarie University, Sydney Australia
Description: This discussion group is composed of people interested in discussion of news and ideas on *Cryptosporidium* and sharing resources for research on *Cryptosporidium*.
Web site: http://www.bio.mq.edu.au/Cryptosporidium/

Drinking Water Discussion Forum
Sponsor: National Drinking Water Clearinghouse (NDWC)
Description: This online discussion group is for professionals and other individuals with an interest in small community drinking water issues. This forum is open to anyone wishing to post drinking water-related questions and receive feedback.
Web site: http://www.estd.wvu.edu/ndwc

Food-Law Listserve
Sponsor: Institute of Food Technologists and Division and the Food Science Department at the University of Minnesota
Description: The Web site is a forum for the exchange of information on issues relating to food laws and regulations.
Web site: http://www.ift.org/divisions/food_law/flr_list.htm

Food Quality Protection Act Discussion Group
Sponsor: National Pesticide Telecommunications Network
Description: This unmoderated forum is dedicated to the discussion of the Food Quality Protection Act (FQPA) of 1996, focusing mainly on pesticides and how they are regulated under the act. The FQPA discussion group is operated and maintained by the National Pesticide Telecommunications Network, a cooperative effort of Oregon State University and the U.S. Environmental Protection Agency.
Web site: http://ace.orst.edu/info/nptn/fqpalist/fqpalist.htm

Foodsafe
Sponsor: USDA/FDA Foodborne Illness Education Information Center
Description: Foodsafe is an electronic discussion group to link professionals interested in food safety issues. Searchable archives of all past postings are maintained on the Web site.
Web site: http://www.nal.usda.gov/foodborne

Food Safety Discussion Forum
Sponsor: Foodservice.com
Description: This moderated online discussion group focuses on food safety topics for food industry professionals.
Web site: http://foodservice.com/

Foodserv Listserve
Sponsor: Michigan State University
Description: The Foodserv Listserve is designed to be a world-wide forum for issues of concern in the food service industry. Advertising is discouraged; education is encouraged.
Web site: http://list.msu.edu/archives/foodserv.html

HACCP System for Retail Food Safety Listserve
Sponsor: University of Arizona
Description: This electronic discussion group focuses on HACCP concerns in retail food establishments.
Web site: http://listserv.arizona.edu/lsv/www/haccp.html

Seafood Mailing List
Sponsor: University of California at Davis Sea Grant Extension Program
Description: The purpose of this discussion list is to provide information about the Hazard Analysis and Critical Control Points (HACCP) system of

food safety control in the seafood industry, and to facilitate information sharing among seafood researchers; industry; and regulatory, extension, and academic personnel.
Web site: http://seafood.ucdavis.edu/listserv/listinfo.htm

Speak Out Watershed Information Group
Sponsor: U.S. Environmental Protection Agency (EPA)
Description: In an effort to gain more public participation in discussing water quality issues, EPA created an information exchange for citizens and managers interested in watershed-based environmental protection. Discussion topics include drinking water issues, source water assessment and protection programs, watershed lessons learned, and biological assessment.
Web site: http://www.epa.gov/watershed/speak/

EMAIL NEWS DISTRIBUTION GROUPS

Agnet
Sponsor: Doug Powell, University of Guelph, Ontario, Canada, Agri-Food Risk Management and Communication Project
Description: The Agnet daily electronic news service covers material related to plant agriculture-food biotechnology, chemical hazards, productivity, and sustainability.
Web site: Information on subscribing and accessing the archives is at: http://www.plant.uoguelph.ca/safefood/

AnimalNet
Sponsor: Doug Powell, University of Guelph, Ontario, Canada, Agri-Food Risk Management and Communication Project
Description: The AnimalNet daily electronic news service covers material related to animal agriculture-including new diseases, sustainability, and animal welfare.
Web site: Information on subscribing and accessing the archives is at: http://www.planr.uoguelph.ca/safefood/

Biotechnology Outreach
Sponsor: Monsanto
Description: This news list by Monsanto, a leader in biotechnology products, informs readers of new developments and current news in the field of food biotechnology. To subscribe send an email to: biotechoutreach@monsantolist.com with "subscribe" in the subject bar and your email address in the body of the message.
Web site: http://www.monsanto.com/monsanto/

FSIS Constituent Update
Sponsor: USDA, Food Safety and Inspection Service (FSIS)
Description: FSIS provides a weekly FSIS Constituent Update, which is communicated via fax and is available online through the FSIS Web page. The update provides information regarding FSIS policies, procedures, regulations, Federal Register notices, FSIS public meetings, recalls, and any other types of information that could affect or would be of interest to constituents/stakeholders. The constituent fax list consists of industry, trade, farm groups, consumer interest groups, allied health professionals, scientific professionals, and other individuals that have requested to be included. For more information and to be added to the constituent fax list, fax your request to the Office of Congressional and Public Affairs, at 202-720-5704.
Web site: http://www.fsis.usda.gov

Fsnet
Sponsor: Doug Powell, University of Guelph, Ontario, Canada, Agri-Food Risk Management and Communication Project
Description: The Fsnet daily electronic news service covers material related to food safety topics such as microbial hazards, new technologies, and outbreak information.
Web site: Information on subscribing and accessing the archives is at: http://www.oac.uoguelph.ca/riskcomm/index.html

Pesticide Action Network Updates Service (PANUPS)
Sponsor: Pesticide Action Network North America
Description: The Pesticide Action Network Updates Service (PANUPS) is a biweekly online international email news service covering the latest pesticide research, regulatory and other policy decisions, and pesticide- and agriculture-related activism. Some issues of PANUPS are Resource Pointers, which briefly describe new books, re-

ports, and other resources related to pesticides, sustainable agriculture, and genetic engineering.
Web site: http://www.panna.org/

Program for Monitoring Emerging Diseases (ProMED)
Sponsor: Federation of American Scientists
Description: ProMed sends out reports on infectious diseases and outbreaks around the world. Many international foodborne illnesses are reported on ProMed.
Web site: http://fas.org/promed/

Radfood
Sponsor: Public Citizen
Description: Subscribers to this list receive information, updates, and action alerts regarding food irradiation. To subscribe to the radfood list send an email to cmep@citizen.org with the words "subscribe radfood" in the subject.
Web site: http://www.citizen.org/cmep/rad-food/radfoodindex.htm

REFERENCE TOOLS

Bad Bug Book (aka Foodborne Pathogenic Microorganisms and Natural Toxins)
Sponsor: Food and Drug Administration
Description: The premier guide for information on foodborne and waterborne bacteria, parasitic protozoa, worms, viruses, and natural toxins. Each entry includes links to CDC for outbreak information, to NIH for definition of terms, and to other pertinent resources.
Web site: http://vm.cfsan.fda.gov/~mow/intro.html

BioTech's Biotechnology Dictionary
Sponsor: Indiana University and University of Texas
Description: BioTech is a free, searchable online dictionary of biology, chemistry, and biotechnology terms. It aims to serve everyone from high school students to professional researchers. BioTech is intended to be a learning tool that will attract students and enrich the public's knowledge of biology issues in the world today. At the same time, BioTech is also a research tool for Web site: http://biotech.icmb.utexas.edu/

Electronic Guide to Food Regulations, 1999
Sponsor: Written by Tracy Altman. Published by John Wiley
Description: This CD-ROM provides access to actual texts of federal rules with an in-depth analysis of the legal and regulatory requirements affecting the production, packaging, and sale of meat, poultry, seafood, dietary supplements, and other food products. Included are detailed analyses of FDA, USDA, and EPA rules; compliance diagrams that summarize complex rules in concise charts; text of the U.S. Code of Federal Regulations and Federal Register.

Food Chemicals Codex
Sponsor: Published by Chapman and Hall/CRC in cooperation with National Academy Press.
Description: This is a searchable CD-ROM version of the Food Chemical Codex, the accepted standard for defining the quality and purity of food chemicals. It is frequently referenced by the FDA and other international food regulatory authorities. Entries include a description of substances and their use in foods, tolerable levels of contaminants, appropriate tests to determine compliance, packaging and storage guidelines, and more. The Codex will be of interest to producers and users of food chemicals, including processed-food manufacturers, food technologists, quality control chemists, research investigators, teachers, students, and others involved in the technical aspects of food safety.

Food Quality and Safety Compliance Information Manager
Sponsor: J. J. Keller and Associates
3003 W. Breezewood Lane
P.O. Box 368
Neenah, Wisconsin USA 54957–0368
Phone: 1–800–327–6868
Fax: 1–800–727–7516
Description: This Windows-based program provides immediate access to the full-text of food-related FDA and USDA regulations, explanatory text of key compliance topics, and related government documents to further explain the regulations. Topic explanations, applicable regulations, and related key words from the government documents are cross-referenced throughout the program. Extensive search capabilities allow the user to search by key words, phrases, or regulation numbers. A quarterly update service is available, which eliminates the need

to review the Federal Register for regulatory changes. The changes are highlighted within the applicable sections and a list of changes is kept for convenient tracking.
Web site: http://www.jjkeller.com/

Outreach Resource Guide: A Directory of Small Community Drinking Water Information

Sponsor: National Drinking Water Clearinghouse
Description: This resource guide includes descriptions of more than 80 federal agencies, national organizations, and programs that have interests in drinking water-related issues. It helps users learn about an organization's mission and its water-related activities, publications, programs, and contact information.
Web site: Available full-text at http://www.estd.wvu.edu/ndwc/NDWC_eduprod.html

Regulatory Fish Encyclopedia (RFE)

Sponsor: U.S. Food and Drug Administration, Center for Food Safety and Applied Nutrition
Description: The RFE is a compilation of data in several formats that assists with the accurate identification of fish species. It was developed by FDA's RFE Team to help federal, state, and local officials and purchasers of seafood identify species substitution and economic deception in the marketplace. Included for each species are market name, common name, and scientific name; high-resolution photographs of whole fish and their marketed product forms (including fillets, steaks, or whole crustaceans) that may be used for visual comparison to a whole fish in question; and species-characteristic biochemical patterns that may be compared to patterns obtained by an appropriate laboratory analysis of the fish specimen in question.
Web site: http://vm.cfsan.fda.gov/~frf/rfe0.html

CHAPTER 10

EDUCATIONAL MATERIALS

The 149 items in this chapter are intended to be teaching tools. Formats include games; manuals; videos; whole curriculums with teacher's and student guide, activities, and tests; software packages; posters; interactive CD-ROMs; coloring books; science experiments; even popular songs "remixed" to provide food safety themes.

Methods of teaching and types of materials needed vary depending on who is being taught. The materials are categorized mostly into for whom they are intended and their subject area if it is other than general food safety principles. The sections are as follows:

Children—General Food Safety
Children—Biotechnology, Pesticides, Additives
Consumers—General Food Safety
Consumers—Biotechnology, Pesticides, Additives
Consumers—Seniors
Food Service Workers—General Food Safety
Food Service Workers—HACCP
Handwashing
Providers at Child Day Care Centers and Institutions
School Food Service
Volunteers at Picnics, Church Suppers, Fairs, Food Banks

Tools for teaching children obviously need to be on a different level than those for adults. Many of the children's materials are designed to be taught at school. Materials for both children and consumers tend not to become out of date because they teach the basics, which don't change. Food service worker training materials that are based on the FDA Food Code can become outdated as various provisions, such as recommended temperatures, change. Some of the training materials for food service workers teach the very basics of food safety, while others teach according to a Hazard Analysis and Critical Control Points system. Handwashing is so crucial to food safety that the teaching aids are broken down into their own category, whether they be for children, adult consumers, or food service workers.

Some groups have special circumstances that necessitate special types of training materials. Seniors fall into this group since they are more vulnerable to foodborne illness. Many seniors receive packaged meals delivered to their homes, which are a potential source of food safety problems if not handled properly. Providers at day care or adult care centers are dealing with very vulnerable populations, and have a special set of circumstances in which they are preparing and serving food. Often the kitchens they use are not as well-equipped as a kitchen in a restaurant would be. School food service has its own set of circumstances that affects the safety of food—namely the population, the kitchen facilities, and the need for extremely quick service. Finally, volunteers working at church suppers, picnics, outside venues, and food banks also have a very special set of circumstances. The facilities may be primitive, sometimes even lacking a sink or proper refrigeration. The workers typically are not professional food service workers, even though they may be feeding large groups of people, and in some cases vulnerable populations.

Unless otherwise directed, materials may be ordered from the producers listed (lists are arranged alphabetically by producer). Some materials, especially those geared towards training food professionals, are relatively expensive, while others, particularly those geared towards teaching children or consumers, are fairly inexpensive. Many of these materials can be borrowed from the National Agricultural Library (NAL) through interlibrary loan. Readers should contact their public or organization librarian to inquire if the item is in the NAL collection.

CHILDREN—GENERAL FOOD SAFETY

Be Safe Around Food
Altschul Group Corporation
1560 Sherman Ave., Suite 100
Evanston, IL 60201
Telephone: 800-421-2363 Fax: 847-328-6706
Email address: agcmedia@starnetinc.com
Web site: http://www.agcmedia.com/
Date produced: 2000 Cost: $195
Description: This 12-minute video with facilitator's guide, designed for children ages three to five, teaches the importance of washing hands, rinsing fruit, not sharing dishes, packing a lunch, putting food in the refrigerator, and cleaning up. Facilitator's guide has discussion and follow-up activities Also available in Spanish.

Adventures with Mighty Egg
American Egg Board
1460 Renaissance Dr.
Park Ridge, IL 60068
Telephone: 847-296-7043 Fax: 847-296-7007
Email address: aeb@aeb.org
Web site: http://www.aeb.org/
Date produced: 1999 Cost: $9, extra posters and stickers can be ordered for $3.50; for quantity copies kits are $5 each. Add shipping and handling.
Description: This integrated curriculum unit for use with students in grades kindergarten through three features a hands-on approach. It was designed to encourage students to want to know more about eggs and other subjects as they develop math, science, language arts, creativity, and other skills. Safe handling of eggs is integrated in some of the lessons. Curriculum includes stickers, poster, activities, recipes, eight lesson plans, and reading list.

The Incredible Journey from Hen to Home
American Egg Board
1460 Renaissance Dr.
Park Ridge, IL 60068
Telephone: 847-296-7043 Fax: 847-296-7007
Email address: aeb@aeb.org
Web site: For related food safety information from this producer: http://www.aeb.org/
Date produced: 1998 Cost: Single copies $9, for quantity orders $5, extra gameboard/poster or bookmarks can be ordered for $3.50
Description: This cross-curricular educational unit has been designed for use with youth in grades four through six. Lessons include real-life problems that help teach not only the basic skills of language arts, math, science, nutrition, food safety, and consumer education, but also enrichment skills using logic puzzles, cooking, economic decision making, and creativity.

Throughout the 30- to 40-minute lessons, the class or group will be learning how to learn by comparing, contrasting, analyzing, and evaluating. Each lesson is designed to encourage active participation in the learning process. Curriculum includes game, poster, book marks, teacher's guide with plans for seven lessons, activities, and reading list.

Food Safety at Home, School and When Eating Out
Chef and Child Foundation
American Culinary Federation
10 San Bartola Drive
St. Augustine, FL 32086
Telephone: 904-824-4468 ext. 104
Fax: 904-825-4758
Date produced: Undated Cost: $8 per 50 coloring books
Description: This is a coloring book for elementary school children. Available full-text at: http://www.foodsafety.gov/~dms/cbook.html

Creating Informed Citizens For Tomorrow's Food Safety Decisions
Colorado State University
Department of Food Science and Human Nutrition
Fort Collins, CO 80523
Telephone: 970-491-5798 Fax: 970-491-7252
Email address: wilken@condor.cahs.colostate.edu
Date produced: 1994 Cost: $20; also available on disk in WordPerfect for $10 with purchase of one manual
Description: Geared for classroom use for teachers of middle and junior high school students, this complete curriculum covers the following topics in food safety: food safety overview, microbial contamination, food irradiation, pesticides, animal antibiotics and hormones, food additives, fat and sugar substitutes, and biotechnology. It could be used as a full-semester food safety course or as a supplement to ongoing curricula. Curriculum has eight chapters. Each chapter includes lesson outline, background references, student activities, discussion questions with answers, glossary of key words, student test questions.

SLIC: Secondary Level Interdisciplinary Curriculum
Creative Enterprises
576 Severn Dr.
State College, PA 16803
Telephone: 814-237-8711 Fax: 814-237-0892
Email address: starpenn@juno.com
Date produced: 1997 Cost: $90
Description: The food safety part of this curriculum is suitable for teaching in biology, microbiology, American history, and environmental science classes. Lessons include *E. coli* in undercooked hamburger; toxins and pesticides in our food supply; and the historic and future role of the government, the manufacturer, and the consumer in assuring a safe food supply. Designed for students in grades nine through 12.
Comments: PA high school teachers can receive a free copy of SLIC. Contact NET program for a copy (717-783-6557). Teachers out of state may be able to borrow a copy from their own state NET coordinator. (NET is part of the Department of Education in each state.)

Alexander, The Elephant Who Couldn't Eat Peanuts
Food Allergy Network
Web site: http://www.foodallergy.org
Date produced: 1994 Cost: $15
Description: This video combines the animated story of an elephant who is allergic to peanuts with interviews of children who have food allergies. It's designed to show children that they aren't alone, and to discuss the feelings that go along with having food allergies.

Childcare and Preschool Guide to Managing Food Allergies
Food Allergy Network
Web site: http://www.foodallergy.org
Date produced: 1994 Cost: $75
Description: This comprehensive program, endorsed by the American Academy of Allergy Asthma and Immunology and the American Academy of Pediatrics, is designed to educate caregivers of children under age five. Included are two videos, *It Only Takes One Bite* and *Alexander the Elephant Who Couldn't Eat Peanuts*, a binder filled with vital information, an EpiPen trainer, a laminated sheet of "How to Read a Label," cards, and a food allergy awareness poster.

Science and Our Food Supply
Food and Drug Administration and National Science Teachers Association
Web site: http://www.nsta.org
Date Produced 2000 Cost: Free
Description: The goal of this curriculum is to develop a science-based education program for middle and high school students that incorporates the farm-to-table food safety continuum. The primary components of this project include a

stand-alone introductory videotape and a print-based version of the curriculum, resources, and other materials. Order from JMH Communications, foodsafety@jmhcomm.com, Fax: 212-924-3052.

In Good Taste: Careers in Food Science
Institute of Food Technologists
221 North LaSalle S., Suite 300
Chicago, IL 60601
Telephone: 312-782-8424 Fax: 312-782-0045
Email address: careers@ift.org
Web site: http://www.ift.org/careers/
Cost: $29.95
Description: This 14-minute video, teaching guide, and poster highlights career opportunities in food science. Schools may request a free copy of the video on "permanent loan," by calling IFT's Career Guidance Department (312-782-8424) or writing to IFT for a Video Request Form. Requests should specify the grade level (7–9 or 10–12) for appropriate collateral materials.

The Great Food Fight
Institute of Food Technologists
221 North LaSalle S., Suite 300
Chicago, IL 60601
Telephone: 312-782-8424 Fax: 312-782-0045
Cost: $29.95
Description: This video presents food safety information for students in grades four through 12. It introduces students to foodborne illnesses, various related microorganisms, and proper food handling. Schools may request a free copy of the video on permanent loan, by calling IFT's Career Guidance Department (312-782- 8424) or writing to IFT for a Video Request Form.

Microbiology in Food Systems Experiments
Institute of Food Technologists
221 North LaSalle S., Suite 300
Chicago, IL 60601
Telephone: 312-782-8424 Fax: 312-782-0045
Cost: Single copies are free; additional copies are $1 each (or the booklet may be copied).
Description: This 67-page booklet contains four food science experiments related to food microbiology and fermentation for use in middle and high school science classes. It contains teacher information, sample data tables, student activity guides, and visual masters for copying.

Operation Risk
Michigan State University Extension
103 Human Ecology Building
East Lansing, MI 48824
Telephone: 517-355-6586
Date produced: 1993
Cost: Notebook and learning materials $60, Risk Raiders computer game $30, Handwashing Rap $5; videotape $25
Description: Operation Risk is a curriculum designed to assist in teaching the hows and whys of safe food handling. Through this curriculum, kids explore ways to ensure their own health by learning what they can do to prevent foodborne illness. Kids assume the role of detectives as they work through this multimedia program with fun-to-solve cases, missions to complete at home with an adult, and a variety of learning activities designed to challenge problem solvers in grades three through five. Curriculum includes four lessons (15–25 minutes each), teacher/leader guide, activities, videocassettes, poster, Handwashing Rap audiocassette tape, and an interactive computer software game called Risk Raiders (for Macintosh computers and Windows).
Order from MSU Bulletin Office, 10B Agriculture Hall, MSU, East Lansing, MI 48824-1039.

Project Food Safety—Educational Units for the Middle Level Science Classroom
Montana State University Extension Service
Extension Publications
Rm 115, Culbertson Hall, MSU
Bozeman, MT 59717
Telephone: 406-994-3273
Date produced: 1992
Cost: Workbooks are $5 each; set of workbook and video are $25 each.
Description: Project Safety consists of three different modules for middle school youth. The eighth-grade unit is about food irradiation, the seventh-grade unit focuses on pesticides, and the sixth-grade unit topic is microbial contamination. The units can be purchased together or separately. The units were designed to be easily incorporated into the present science curriculum at each grade level. Supplemental videocassettes instruct the teacher on how to prepare and conduct the science experiments. These cassettes are ordered separately from the workbooks. Curriculum includes three teacher's guides with lesson plans, pre- and post-test, activities.

Food Safety Bingo
NASCO
901 Janesville Ave., PO Box 901
Fort Atkinson, WI 53538-0901
Telephone: 920-563-2446 Fax: 920-563-8296

Email address: info@nascofa.com
Cost: $18.50
Description: Although the primary resource for this bingo game was Preventing Foodborne Illness: A Guide to Safe Food Handling, by the USDA, Home and Garden Bulletin Number 247, 1990, there are several misleading statements used, such as "Most foodborne illness grows in temperatures of 60 to 125 degrees F." These could be changed by the user.

Food Safety Folding Display
NASCO
901 Janesville Ave.
PO Box 901
Fort Atkinson, WI 53538-0901
Telephone: 920-563-2446 Fax: 920-563-8296
Email address: info@nascofa.com
Web site: To see a picture of this display go to: http://www.nascofa.com/
Cost: $74.95
Description: This is a visual aid for teaching about foodborne illnesses, the effects of temperature on bacterial growth, common bacteria *(Clostridium botulism, Clostridium perfringens, Campylobacter, Salmonella, Escherichia coli, Listeria*, and *Staphylococcus)*, and safe food handling procedures. Colorful, accordion-fold display measures 58" W × 22" H. Grades six and up. Shipping weight 13 lbs.

Safe Food Journey
National Cattlemen's Beef Association
444 North Michigan Ave. Suite 1800
Chicago, IL 60611
Telephone: 800-368-3138 Fax: 800-368-3136
Email address: cows@beef.org
Web site: To see a picture of this poster go to http://www.beefnutrition.org/resources/
Date produced: 1996 Cost: $1.50
Description: This curriculum introduces children in grades two through four to food safety principles by showing foods as they journey from farm to table. Refrigeration, labeling, handwashing, and safe food handling concepts are taught. Curriculum includes poster, activity sheets, lesson plan.
Order from above address. CODE #17-516. Qualified 2nd–4th grade teachers can get this free. See http://www.teachfree.com/

Food Safety Can Be Fun
Ontario Agri-Food Education Inc.
P.O. Box 460, 8560 Tremaine Rd.
Milton, Ontario, Canada L9T 4Z1
Telephone: 905-878-1510 Fax: 905-878-0342
Email address: resource@oafe.org
Web site: http://www.oafe.org/index.htm
Date produced: 1996 Cost: $15 Canadian
Description: Food Safety Can Be Fun is an episode of "Street Cents," the popular CBC (Canadian Broadcasting Corporation) consumer television series. The episode consists of segments in which different aspects of food safety are highlighted. The video serves as a motivator to introduce food safety concepts into the classroom or a youth group gathering. The accompanying guide develops the concepts introduced in the video through specific activities and additional information. Students are encouraged to involve the family in food safety awareness and even gather data in the home. The video is geared towards students in grades seven to 10 (ages 12 to 17).

Fight BAC! Presenter's Guide
Partnership for Food Safety Education
API/Fight BAC! and API/BAC Store
4550 Forbes Blvd.
Lanham, MD 20706
Telephone: 301-731-6100 Fax: 301-731-6101
Email address: fightbac@mindpsring.com
Web site: http://www.fightbac.org/
Date produced: 1998 Cost: $12
Description: Developed for community educators, this program teaches young children in grades kindergarten through three about the importance of safe food practices. The kit includes two story and song scripts, reproducible masters of songs and poems for the children, a food safety fact sheet for parents, full-color Safe Food National Park Family Vacation Game (10 games per kit), and a pattern for constructing a paper bag or sox puppet.

Your Game Plan for Food Safety
Partnership for Food Safety Education
API/Fight BAC! and API/BAC Store
4550 Forbes Blvd.
Lanham, MD 20706
Telephone: 301-731-6100 Fax: 301-731-6101
Email address: fightbac@mindpsring.com
Web site: http://www.fightbac.org/
Date produced: 1999 Cost: $15
Description: Your Game Plan for Food Safety is a food safety education program for students in grades four through six. The program includes teacher's guide, video, student activities, 60 "BAC Catcher" games, and two classroom posters.

Bacterial Contamination of Foods
Pennsylvania State University
Department of Food Science
203B Borland
University Park, PA 16802
Telephone: 814-863-3973 Fax: 814-863-6132
Email address: f9a@psu.edu
Date produced: 1996 Cost: $30, discount for quantity purchases
Description: This curriculum is geared towards grades seven through 10 and is multidisciplinary, encompassing lessons for science, math, home economics, and social studies classes. Each lesson is designed for a 30-minute class period. General study areas are bacterial contamination of food, food ingredients, genetic engineering, and chemical residues. Curriculum contains 18 lessons with objectives, teacher preparation, activities, test, transparency masters, and the videos "Mystery of the Poisoned Panther Picnic" and "Dirty Dining."
Order from Ag Publications, Penn State University, College of Agricultural Sciences, 112 Ag Administration, University Park, PA 16802, telephone 814-865-6713

Food Ingredients
Pennsylvania State University
Department of Food Science
203B Borland
University Park, PA 16802
Telephone: 814-863-3973 Fax: 814-863-6132
Date produced: 1999
Description: This curriculum, geared towards students in middle and high school, focuses on ingredients of food as they relate to food allergies. Topics covered include where ingredients come from, how they are handled, and how they are indicated on food labels.
Order from Ag Publications, Penn State University, College of Agricultural Sciences, 112 Ag Administration, University Park, PA 16802, telephone (814-865-6713)

Students Serving It Safe
Pennsylvania State University
5 Henderson Building
University Park, PA 16802
Telephone: 814-865-7054 Fax: 814-865-5870
Email address: ssis@psu.edu
Date produced: 1998 Cost: $24.95, quantity discount and site license available
Description: This interactive CD-ROM program was designed specifically for middle school students. The student user explores different areas of a food service operation, learning basic food safety techniques and strategies along the way. The program includes a presenter's manual, various short quizzes, and provides immediate feedback.

Kitchen Safety Game
Pineapple Appeal, Inc.
P.O. Box 197
Owatonna, MN 55060
Telephone: 507-455-3041
Date produced: 1995 Cost: $19.95
Description: Designed for children in grades six through nine, this game covers kitchen safety, food safety, emergency techniques, cleaner is safer, and common sense in the kitchen.
Order from Learning Zone Express, 130 W. Main, PO Box 1022, Owatonna, MN, 55060, 888-455-7003, fax 507-455-3380.

Meeting the Food Safety Needs of Bilingual and Low Literacy Youth
Purdue University Cooperative Extension Service
Purdue University
1264 Stone Hall
West Lafayette, IN 47904-1264
Telephone: 765-494-8539 Fax: 765-494-0674
Email address: masona@cfs.purdue.edu
Date produced: 1995 Cost: $50
Description: This curriculum for students in grades four through six consists of the 13-minute video "The Mystery of the Poisoned Panther Picnic" in both English and Spanish (the Spanish video is a dubbed version of the English version), two audiocassettes (Panther Picnic and the rap song Path-O-Gens Are on Your Path), teacher's guide, and student handouts.
Order from Media Distribution Center, 301 South 2nd St., Lafayette, IN 47901-1232, 765-494-6794, fax 765-496-1540.

The Mystery of the Poisoned Panther Picnic
Purdue University Cooperative Extension Service
Purdue University
1264 Stone Hall
West Lafayette, IN 47904-1264
Telephone: 765-494-8539 Fax: 765-494-0674
Email address: masona@cfs.purdue.edu
Date produced: 1992 Cost: $20
Description: This curriculum was developed to help fourth, fifth, and sixth graders see how they fit into the food safety system. The curriculum consists of five sequential lessons along with an optional field trip activity, overhead transparency

masters, game cutout sheets, background fact sheets.
Order from Media Distribution Center, 301 South 2nd St., Lafayette, IN 47901-1232, 765-494-6794, fax 765-496-1540.

Operation Food Safety: Grades 9–12 and Prekindergarten—Grade 4
University of Arkansas
Department of Poultry Science
Fayetteville, AR 72701
Telephone: 501-575-4409 Fax: 501-575-8775
Email address: awaldro@comp.uark.edu
Date produced: 1999 Cost: Free
Description: These curricula were developed in response to legislation requiring food safety education in Arkansas public schools. For the prekindergarten through grade four curriculum each grade consists of three units: (1) Handwashing—stresses the importance of personal hygiene in the prevention of foodborne illness, (2) Keeping Things Clean—focuses on the importance of cleanliness in the kitchen and the dangers of cross-contamination, and (3) Keeping Food Hot or Cold—teaches students time and temperature guidelines critical to food safety. The grades—nine through 12 curriculum is divided into four units: (1) the problem of foodborne illness, (2) handwashing, (3) cross-contamination, and (4) keeping food hot or cold. Units contain pre-test, terms, Internet activities, lab activities, and handouts. Curricula include lesson goal, objectives, materials needed, procedures, background information for teachers, plenty of activities for students, and tests.

Let's Have a Killer Cookout—NOT
University of Florida, Home Economics Department
Gainesville, FL 32611-0365
Web site: http://www.foodsafety.org/train.htm
Date produced: 1997 Cost: $70
Description: This interactive CD-ROM teaches youth about food safety from the grocery store to the kitchen. A student evaluation package allows teachers to track student's progress and learning.
Order from Lighthouse Education and Design Inc., 825 23rd Ave., Suite 1-B, Gainesville, FL 32609, telephone 352-378-4888

Discovering Food Safety—Detective Mike Robe's Fantastic Journey
University of Rhode Island Cooperative Extension Service
Food Science and Nutrition Department, University of Rhode Island
530 Liberty Lane
West Kingston, RI 02892
Telephone: 401-874-2972 Fax: 401-874-2994
Email address: pivarnik@uriacc.uri.edu
Date produced: 1992 Cost: $65
Description: This curriculum was designed for second and third graders. It consists of a 10-minute video, a science experiment, coloring book, and outlines for other activities and word games relating to food safety. There is also a curriculum by the same name designed for preschool through first grade.
Order from Food Safety Education Program, Department of Food Science and Nutrition, 21 Woodward Hall, University of Rhode Island, Kingston, RI 02881; 401-792-2960.

Food Safety Education. A Program Using the Community Service Learning Model to Teach Youth Food Safety
University of Rhode Island Cooperative Extension Service
Food Science and Nutrition Department, University of Rhode Island
530 Liberty Lane
West Kingston, RI 02892
Telephone: 401-874-2972 Fax: 401-874-2994
Email address: pivarnik@uriacc.uri.edu
Date produced: 1999
Description: This curriculum is geared towards use in a community service learning program. The teacher's guide instructs Family and Consumer Sciences teachers how to teach high school students about food safety. The high school students then use this information to teach food safety principles to preschool and elementary school children. Curriculum includes teacher's guide, student activities.
Order from Food Safety Education Program, Department of Food Science and Nutrition, 21 Woodward Hall, University of Rhode Island, Kingston, RI 02881.

Food Safety House
University of Rhode Island Cooperative Extension Service
Food Science and Nutrition Department, University of Rhode Island
530 Liberty Lane
West Kingston, RI 02892
Telephone: 401-874-2972 Fax: 401-874-2994
Email address: pivarnik@uri.edu
Date produced: 2000

Description: This curriculum is divided into two parts, one for first grade through third grade, and the other for fourth grade through sixth grade. Each lesson includes student activities and background information and goals for the teacher. There are six units overall that teach students the basics of food safety. Curriculum includes teacher's guide and flip chart to be used in classroom.

Order from Food Safety Education Program, Department of Food Science and Nutrition, 21 Woodward Hall, University of Rhode Island, Kingston, RI 02881; 401-792-2960.

The Danger Zone

USDA, Food Safety and Inspection Service (FSIS)

Web site: http://www.fsis.usda.gov/

Cost: $43.97. Add $5 for shipping and handling.

Description: This video teaching package is designed for science, health, and home economics teachers at the secondary level. Students join a class that encounters Fester, a villain who encourages them to eat food that has been in the Danger Zone too long. Upon completion of the program students will be able to describe the role of bacteria in contaminating food; demonstrate how time, temperature, and cleanliness affect bacterial growth; identify the four major types of bacteria that cause foodborne illness and in what foods they are commonly found; and discuss how to control growth of bacteria to prevent foodborne illness. Curriculum includes videocassette (25 minuntes), teacher's guide with reproducible learning activities, colorful poster, post-test.

Contact FSIS at 202-720-3897 or fsis.webmaster@usda.gov for ordering information.

Bill Nye the Science Guy: Insects and Germs

Walt Disney Education Productions
105 Terry Dr., Suite 120
Newtown, PA 18940
Telephone: 800-295-5010
Date produced: 1995 Cost: $49.95

Description: This video plus teacher's guide contains two lessons-one on insects and one on germs. Each is 26 minutes in length.

Get a Jump on Germs: Making Food Safer

Washington State University
Cooperative Extension
Department of Food Science and Human Nutrition
Pullman, WA 99164-6376
Telephone: 509-335-2970 Fax: 509-335-4815
Email address: hillersv@wsu.edu
Web site: http://foodsafety.wsu.edu/
Date produced: 1997 Cost: $15

Description: This curriculum provides hands-on exploratory science activities for youth to learn about food safety. The University of California SERIES (Science Experiences and Resources for Informal Education Settings) science education curriculum was used as the model. Originally geared towards grades three through five, it is also suitable for older or younger audiences. Curriculum includes activities, teaching guides, background information.

CHILDREN—BIOTECHNOLOGY, PESTICIDES, ADDITIVES

Cut the Fat and Keep the Flavor

Iowa State University
Extension Distribution Center
119 Kooser Drive
Ames, IA 50011
Telephone: 515-294-5247
Email address: pubdist@exnet.iastate.edu
Date produced: 1999 Cost: $4

Description: This food biotechnology curriculum of activities and resources for middle and high school students focuses on LoSat Soy oil that was developed at ISU and is now available nationally in the school's commodity program.

Dining on DNA: An Exploration of Food Biotechnology. A Food Biotechnology Unit for High School Students and Teachers

Montana State University Extension Service

Web site: The entire curriculum can be downloaded from http://www.accessexcellence.com/AB/BA/DODpub/

Date produced: 1996

Description: This student guide investigates food biotechnology with laboratory exercises and additional classroom activities. The unit is designed for incorporation into the high school biology and social science classrooms, as it explores both the scientific principles and social issues associated with food biotechnology.

Can be ordered from: http://www.montana.edu/wwwpub/pubscatalog.html

Fields of Genes: Making Sense of Biotechnology in Agriculture
National 4-H Council
Families, 4-H and Nutrition, CSREES/USDA
Stop 2225, 1400 Independence Ave SW
Washington, DC 20250-2225
Telephone: 202-720-2908
Email address: 4h-usa@reeusda.gov
Web site: http://www.4h-usa.org/
Date produced: 1996 Cost: $5
Description: This curriculum provides challenging activities to help youth develop critical thinking skills while gaining knowledge about biotechnology and agriculture. The leader's guide introduces and extends the concepts of life, from the smallest one-celled protozoa to the multi-billion-celled human. It also helps youth and leaders understand topic areas of cells, ecological systems, and the past and future of genetics. It can be used with participants aged five to 18.
Order from National 4-H Supply Service, telephone 301-961-2934, 4hstuff@fourhcouncil.edu, http://www.fourhcouncil.edu/4hstuff/

Genetic Engineering and Plant Food Production
Pennsylvania State University
Department of Food Science
203B Borland
University Park, PA 16802
Telephone: 814-863-3973
Fax: 814-863-6132
Date produced: 1998
Description: This biotechnology curriculum is designed for students in grades eight through 12 and undergraduate university. The 16 lessons include background information, learning objectives, and activities relating to genetic engineering in plants.
Order from Ag Publications, Penn State University, College of Agricultural Sciences, 112 Ag Administration, University Park, PA 16802, 814-865-6713.

Sweet as You Are
Teacher-Scientist Network, the John Innes Centre, and the Y Touring Theatre Company
John Innes Centre
Norwich Research Park
Colney, Norwich, UK NR4 7UH
Telephone: +4401603452571
Email address: ts.network@bbsrc.ac.uk
Web site: http://www.tsn.org.uk/TSNnewsite/news/saya.html
Date produced: 1999
Description: This drama and debate project for young people addresses concerns about genetically engineered crops. The aim is not to convince participants to hold different views. Rather, it is to encourage consideration of the factors that influence our attitudes, to assess information more objectively, and to recognize that decision making can involve trying to reconcile conflicting views, discussing issues, and recognizing that reaching consensus must take into account varying views and values. The play, "Sweet as You Are," is a story of love and genetically modified tomatoes. It is a funny, thought provoking love story that explores social, moral, and scientific issues raised by current developments in biotechnology.

Biotechnology and Food; Additives and Food; Pesticides and Food
University of California
Web site: Available full-text at http://mollie.berkeley.edu/~outreach/ whif.htm
Date produced: 1994
Description: Designed for children 11 to 14 years old, these curricula contain instructor information and six to eight lessons with student hands-on activities. Students are encouraged to use problem-solving skills and critical and creative thinking to make informed decisions about their food. Part of the What's in Food (WHIF) food safety education program, each curriculum can be purchased separately. There is also a trainers' manual.
Order from: DANR Publications, 800-994-8849, fax: 510-643-5470.

CONSUMERS—GENERAL FOOD SAFETY

Prime Time Live Kitchen Safety Segments
ABC News
New York, NY
Telephone: 800-913-3434
Date produced: 1995-96 Cost: $30 plus $5 shipping and handling.
Description: Videos from two "Prime Time Live" segments on bacteria in home kitchens are available for purchase. The first, "Hot Villain," aired November 1, 1995. The second, "Killer Kitchens," aired June 26, 1996. Both deal with bacteria and cross-contamination in the home kitchen.

Food: Keep It Safe to Eat, 2nd edition
Alfred Higgins Productions, Inc.
6350 Laurel Canyon Blvd.
North Hollywood, CA 91606
Telephone: 800-766-5353 Fax: 818-762-8223
Date produced: 1997 Cost: $245
Description: This 15-minute video alerts viewers to the risk and dangers of foodborne illnesses by addressing common methods of food contamination and revealing how simple cleaning techniques can eliminate most of them.

Ask Sofia Safe About Food Safety
Altschul Group Corporation
1560 Sherman Ave., Suite 100
Evanston, IL 60201
Telephone: 800-421-2363 Fax: 847-328-6706
Email address: agcmedia@starnetinc.com
Web site: http://www.agcmedia.com/
Date produced: 1996 Cost: $295
Description: Sofia Safe, newspaper advice columnist and the Dear Abby of safe food handling, responds to readers who write in and ask questions about food safety in this 12-minute video. Through Sofia's responses the dangers of *Salmonella, E. coli*, and other foodborne illnesses are uncovered, and ways to avoid them are shown. Other topics include freshness dates, choosing meats, storing food effectively, avoiding cross contamination, the importance of cleanliness, how long to keep leftovers, proper ways of cooking and reheating, and picnic safety.

Food Allergies
American Academy of Allergy, Asthma and Immunology
611 East Wells St.
Milwaukee, WI 53202
Telephone: 414-272-6071 Fax: 414-272-6070
Web site: http://www.aaaai.org/
Date produced: 1999 Cost: $25
Description: This 15-minute video and brochure describe how true food allergy differs from food intolerance, common foods known to trigger symptoms, avoidance and treatment of serious allergic reactions (anaphylaxis), and proper handling of food allergy in school and other child care settings.

Dirty Little Secrets
Food and Drug Administration
200 C St. SW, HFS-555
Washington, DC 20204
Fax: 202-401-3532
Web site: http://vm.cfsan.fda.gov/list.html
Date produced: 1996 Cost: $8.95
Description: This nine-minute video conveys basic home food safety lessons to consumers in short, but contains entertaining scenes.
Order from: Interface Video Systems, PO Box 57138, Wash., DC, 20037, telephone 202-861-0500, Fax 202-296-4492

Pearls of Wisdom for Oyster Lovers
Food and Drug Administration, Florida District Office
7200 Lake Ellenor Dr., Suite 120
Orlando, FL 32809
Telephone: 407-855-0900 Fax: 407-648-6881
Date produced: 1997 Cost: Free
Description: This curriculum is designed to teach consumers about oysters and the potential dangers of eating them raw. Curriculum contains slides with talking points, camera-ready brochure, press releases.

Drinking Water Source Assessment and Protection Workshop Guide
The Groundwater Foundation
P.O. Box 22558
Lincoln, NE 68542-2558
Telephone: 800-858-4844 Fax: 402-434-2742
Email address: info@groundwater.org
Web site: http://www.groundwater.org/
Date produced: 1998 Cost: Free
Description: This detailed workshop guide includes overheads and handouts that may be used by individuals sponsoring a workshop. Anyone with an interest in groundwater, surface water, and drinking water quality/quantity can use this guide to present a workshop in their community.

Media Guide on Food Safety and Nutrition
International Food Information Council
1100 Connecticut Avenue NW, Suite 430
Washington, DC 20036
Telephone: 202-296-6540 Fax: 202-296-6547
Email address: foodinfo@ific.health.org
Web site: For related food safety information from this producer: http://ificinfo.health.org/infofsn.htm
Date produced: 1998 Cost: $90 plus $5.95 shipping and handling
Description: These materials, updated every two or three years, provide definitions of scientific terms and concepts; tips on evaluating research reports; names and phone numbers of academic, government, and health experts; responsibilities of governmental agencies and organizations that

protect the food supply; and contacts for additional food safety and nutrition information.

Understanding Food Allergy
International Food Information Council Foundation and American Academy of Allergy and Immunology
Date produced: 1994 Cost: $19.95
Description: Based on a satellite videoconference, this two-hour video is designed to provide an overview on food allergy and food intolerance. Leading medical experts highlight important information on proper diagnosis and management of food allergy. Special topics include prevention, recognition, and treatment of anaphylaxis.
Order from the International Food Information Council

Babies, Children and Food Allergy
J.A. Hall Publications
Health Sciences Publisher
Suite 502-9500 Erickson Dr.
Burnaby, British Columbia, V3J 1M8 Canada
Telephone: 888-993-6133
Email address: info@hallpublications.com
Date produced: 1999
Description: This educational resource by Janice Vickerstaff Joneja is designed for those who counsel mothers of children from birth to five years. The curriculum consists of a manual with handouts for mothers, audiotapes, and videocassette.

Food Safety
The Learning Seed
330 Tesler Rd.
Lake Zurich, IL 60047
Telephone: 800-634-4941
Date produced: 1994 Cost: $89
Description: Designed for adult consumers, the objective of this 24-minute video and teaching guide is to encourage safe food handling and storage of food so as to minimize the risk of foodborne illness. It teaches about the major causes of food poisoning, the danger signals, and how to prepare and handle food safely. A "poison investigator" shows a video of a meal that was prepared in an unsafe manner. Then she goes over the errors that were made and how to correct them. The video is closed captioned.

Food Safety: What You Don't Know Can Hurt You CD-ROM
Meridian Education Corporation
236 E. Front St.
Bloomington, IN 61701
Telephone: 800-727-5507 or 309-827-5455
Fax: 309-829-8621
Email address: meridian@ice.net
Web site: http://www.meridianeducation.com/main.asp
Date produced: 1999 Cost: $79
Description: Using live-action video, this interactive CD-ROM program teaches viewers about the dangers present in everyone's kitchen. It guides the user through a series of learning objectives and interactive testing to make sure the information is absorbed. After each section of the video, pertinent questions are asked. If viewers give the wrong answer, they will automatically be taken back to review the video component containing the answer. When they are finished, users can print out a certificate of completion that can be turned in to the course instructor. An older version of the program in video is also available, with user's guide.

Keep Food Safe—Safe Quantity Food Production for Migrant Farm Families
Ohio State University Extension Service
Department of Human Nutrition and Food Management, Ohio State University
1787 Neil Ave., 315 Campbell Hall
Columbus, OH 43210-1295
Telephone: 614-292-2699 Fax: 614-292-8880
Email address: medeiros.1@osu.edu
Date produced: 1996 Cost: $22
Description: The primary audience for this curriculum is Spanish-speaking migrant farm workers and their families. The secondary audience is English-speaking individuals with limited resources and their families. Each of the five lessons can be presented as a mini-lesson format, lasting about five minutes, or a full lesson format, lasting about an hour. Each lesson also includes an evaluation instrument. Food safety basics that pertain to situations and foods that migrant workers encounter are presented in the lessons. Curriculum includes five lessons that contain fact sheets, overheads, handouts, activities, thermometer, water bottle, magnet.
Order from Ohio State University Extension Publication Office, 385 Kottman Hall, 2021 Coffey Rd., Columbus, OH 43210-1044, 614-292-1607, fax 614-292-2270.

Dr. Sal Monella's Safe Food Prescriptions
Oregon State Extension
Western Rural Development Center, Oregon State University
Ballard Extension Hall, Room 307
Corvalis, OR 97331-3607
Telephone: 503-737-3621 Fax: 503-737-1579
Email address: wrdc@ccmail.orst.edu
Cost: $25
Description: A late-night radio talk show format is used in which callers ask for advice on refrigerated food storage and handling, leftovers, and handwashing. Curriculum includes slides (80), script, audiocassette (15 minutes).

Are You Making Your Family Sick?
Pug Dog Enterprises
Home Food Safety
303 NE 4th St.
Battle Ground, WA 98604
Telephone: 360-666-0218
Email address: eatsafe@aol.com
Web site: http://www.homefoodsafety.com
Date produced: 1996 Cost: $20 plus $4 shipping and handling
Description: This 40-minute video takes consumers through a step-by-step inspection of a home kitchen, while supplying them with everything they need to do their own home examination. Aspects of food safety covered are handwashing; refrigeration; proper food handling; safe chemical and food storage; proper sanitizing techniques; temperatures for thawing, cooking, and cooling; and everything in between. Associated test materials included are chlorine test strips, a dishwasher thermometer test strip, brochures on common foodborne illnesses, and a handy temperature reference guide.

Barbecues, Picnics and Potlucks
Pug Dog Enterprises
Home Food Safety
303 NE 4th St.
Battle Ground, WA 98604
Telephone: 360-666-0218
Email address: eatsafe@aol.com
Web site: http://www.homefoodsafety.com
Date produced: 1996 Cost: $20 plus $4 shipping and handling
Description: Consumers journey to a family barbecue to learn the principles of planning, packing, transporting, cooking, and serving. Disposable T-strip thermometers for measuring hamburger temperature and a safety handbook are included with this 45-minute video.

Happy, Healthy Holidays
Pug Dog Enterprises
Home Food Safety
303 NE 4th St.
Battle Ground, WA 98604
Telephone: 360-666-0218
Email address: eatsafe@aol.com
Web site: http://www.homefoodsafety.com
Date produced: 1996 Cost: $20 plus $4 shipping and handling
Description: This 41-minute video looks at special foods prepared during the holidays and the problems that can go with them. An actual turkey dinner is prepared, served, and cleared. Dressing, casseroles, potatoes, gravy, and many other traditional foods are discussed. Included with the video are a holiday hot sheet outlining safe temperature recommendations, safe serving hints, hot and cold holding advice, a holiday meal planning form.

Cleaning the Kitchen: Things My Parents Never Told Me
The School Company
P.O. Box 5379
Vancouver, WA 98668
Telephone: 360-696-3529
Date produced: 1993 Cost: $39.95
Description: This 10-minute video focuses on cleaning the home kitchen. A chef teaches what to clean pans with, how to avoid cross-contamination, the difference between cleaning and sanitizing and how to do both, and the importance of keeping hands clean.
Order from Cambridge Educational, P.O. Box 2153, Charleston, WV, 25328-2153, 800-468-4227, fax 304-744-9351.

Safe Food Storage: I Thought It Would Last Forever
The School Company
P.O. Box 5379
Vancouver, WA 98668
Telephone: 360-696-3529
Date produced: 1993 Cost: $39.95
Description: This 10-minute video discusses safe food storage in the home kitchen. A chef teaches about safe storage temperatures and how to monitor temperatures to avoid the danger zone, washing and storing produce, freezing foods, rotating foods, proper refrigeration storage, and avoiding cross-contamination.
Order from Cambridge Educational, P.O. Box 2153, Charleston, WV, 25328-2153, 800-468-4227, fax 304-744-9351.

Be Food Safe!: Curriculum Unit for Nutritional Education Assistants
University of California
Date Produced: March 2000 Cost: $35
Description: Be Food Safe! is a self-teaching, train-the-trainer food safety curriculum unit developed for nutrition educators teaching adult consumers. The unit includes 133 pages of background information, appendices, lesson plans, and hands-on activities; a 20-page supplement with references and ordering information for additional materials; 124 pages of camera-ready materials; and a 24" × 18" laminated, color poster to use with the lesson plans. The materials were developed for use with low-income, low-to-moderate literacy adults but can be used with any adult consumers. Order from ANR Communication Services, 800-994-8849, Fax: 510-643-5470.

Food Safety Music
University of California, Davis
Web site: http://foodsafe.ucdavis.edu/
Date produced: 1998, 1999
Description: Associate extension food toxicologist Dr. Carl Winter explores his musical side by recording and performing musical parodies of popular songs with a food safety/science twist on these three CD-ROMs. The songs are also available for listening or downloading from the Web site.

Don't Get Bugged by a Foodborne Illness
University of Nebraska-Lincoln Cooperative Extension
444 Cherrycreek Rd.
Lincoln, NE 68528-1507
Telephone: 402-441-7180
Fax: 402-441-7148
Email address: cnty5021@unlvm.unl.edu
Web site: http://ianrwww.unl.edu/ianr/lanco/family/buggame.htm
Date produced: Updated 1998 Cost: $14
Description: This game is a quiz game of food safety questions. The program package includes master copies of all materials needed to play the game, including materials to help market, present, and evaluate the program.

Safe Food for Outfitters
University of Wyoming, Cooperative Extension Service
University of Wyoming, CES
P.O. Box 3354
Laramie, WY 82071-3354
Telephone: 307-766-5375 Fax: 307-766-3379
Date produced: 1994 Cost: $25
Description: This 26-minute video and manual addresses food safety challenges not faced by typical commercial food services. Packing foods for trips, keeping perishable foods cold using coolers, meal options, keeping foods away from animals, avoiding cross contamination while cooking out, washing dishes in the outdoors, water purification, and personal hygiene in a camping setting are covered. Video is closed captioned.

Get With a Safe Food Attitude
USDA, Food Safety and Inspection Service (FSIS)
Web site: http://www.fsis.usda.gov/
Date produced: 1995 Cost: $27. Add $5 for shipping and handling.
Description: This is a video about safe food handling for moms-to-be developed by the U.S. Department. of Agriculture. It was produced to appeal to a young, diverse audience. The video follows four pregnant women, who make up the fictionalized rap group "The 2-B Moms," as they learn about food safety and prevention of foodborne illness. The video is suitable for viewing in a waiting room or classroom, or during one-on-one counseling sections. The tape is made up of nine segments, each less than five minutes long, which may be viewed individually or as a group.
Contact FSIS at 202-720-3897 or fsis.webmaster@usda.gov for ordering information.

CONSUMERS—BIOTECHNOLOGY, PESTICIDES, ADDITIVES

A Growing Appetite for Information
Food Biotechnology Communications Network (FBCN)
1 Stone Road West, Fourth Floor, NW
Guelph, Ontario, N1G 4Y2 Canada
Telephone: 877-FOOD-BIO
Fax: 519-826-3441
Email address: info@foodbiotech.org
Web site: http://www.foodbiotech.org
Date produced: 1999 Cost: Free

Description: This 16-page booklet, available in English and French, is intended to be bias-free, providing a basic introduction to food biotechnology in Canada. It includes a look at products on the market, products being developed, how products are approved in Canada, some science, and a resource list.

Food Safety: Pesticides, Antibiotics, Hormones, Food Additives, and Biotechnology
Health Science Institute
PMB 206
1350 Beverly Rd, 115
McLean, VA 22101-3917
Telephone: 800-474-6211 Fax: 703-917-1593
Web site: http://www.healthscienceinstitute.com/
Date produced: 1997 Cost: $29.95
Description: Intended for lay audiences at the postsecondary level of education, this curriculum provides contemporary research data from the scientific literature. It is peer-reviewed by research scientists and health professionals. Curriculum contains a teacher's guide and video (15 minutes).

Food Biotechnology: A Communications Guide to Improving Understanding
International Food Information Council
1100 Connecticut Ave. NW, Suite 430
Washington, DC 20036
Telephone: 202-296-6540 Fax: 202-296-6547
Web site: For more information on this topic, visit http://ificinfo.health.org
Date produced: 2000 Cost: $19.95 plus $2.50 shipping and handling.
Description: This speaker's manual provides food, agricultural, academic, and government professionals with an informative resource guide to effectively and informatively speak to the growing confusion regarding foods produced using biotechnology. It features a summary of key food biotechnology issues, a discussion guide for speakers, a power point presentation, background materials, media summaries, a "who's who" guide on the issues, Web site suggestions, a list of national and regional resources, camera-ready and reproducible handouts, and guidelines for interacting with the media.

Understanding Food Safety and Irradiation Technology in the Meat Industry
Iowa State University Extension, Iowa Pork Industry Center
Extension Distribution Center
119 Kooser Dr.
Ames, IA 50011-3171
Telephone: 515-294-5247 Fax: 515-294-2945
Date produced: 1996 Cost: $35
Description: This curriculum examines issues surrounding the irradiation of food. Topics covered are irradiation's strengths and limitations, the regulatory environment under which it is approved and must be utilized, and the rationale for its use. Curriculum includes background materials, overhead templates, educator's guide, video.

Food Science Technology
Meridian Education Corporation
236 E. Front St.
Bloomington, IN 61701
Telephone: 800-727-5507 or 309-827-5455 Fax: 309-829-8621
Email address: meridian@ice.net
Web site: http://www.meridianeducation.com/main.asp
Date produced: 1997 Cost: $89
Description: This 23-minute video and user's guide teaches consumers basic food characteristics and illustrates how foods can be controlled or changed through preparation and storage.

Investigating Food Additives
Meridian Education Corporation
236 E. Front St.
Bloomington, IN 61701
Telephone: 800-727-5507 or 309-827-5455 Fax: 309-829-8621
Email address: info@meridianeducation.com
Web site: http://www.meridianeducation.com/main.asp
Date produced: 1997 Cost: $79
Description: This 23-minute video and user's guide identifies common food additives and describes their use as flavor enhancers, preservatives, thickeners, texturizers, and nutritional supplements. It also discusses government regulation of additives.

Is It Safe to Eat? Part I and II
Oklahoma Cooperative Extension Service
OSU Ag Communications
Room 116 PIO Building
Stillwater, OK 74078-6041
Telephone: 405-744-4050 Fax: 405-744-5739
Email address: clkeig@okway.okstate.edu
Web site: http://agweb.okstate.edu/pearl/video/healthy.htm
Date produced: 1991 Cost: $24.95 each

Description: Consumer concerns about the safety of plant and animal foods treated with pesticides, antibiotics, and hormones are addressed. Also discussed are the options and responsibilities of the consumer in maintaining a safe, wholesome food supply. Part I focuses on foods from plants, part II focuses on foods from animals. Each video is 60 minutes.

Biotechnology: A Better Understanding
University of California
Date produced: 1993 Cost: $15
Description: The potential benefits of new biotechnology techniques are presented as analogous to traditional practices of plant selection and breeding. Areas of consumer interest and concern are specifically addressed in this 10-minute video. Includes written materials.
Order from DANR Publications, 800-994-8849, fax: 510-643-5470

Pesticides, Food Safety, and Science
University of California
Date produced: 1990 Cost: $15
Description: This 30-minute video presents the science surrounding the issue of pesticide residues in food, some of the limitations of the science, and the relative risks of pesticide residues in our diet.
Order from DANR Publications, 800-994-8849, fax: 510-643-5470

What's Up in Biotechnology?
University of California
Department of Plant Biology
Berkeley, CA 94720
Cost: $50 plus shipping and handling.
Description: This generic talk and slide set was developed to fill the need for individuals to be able to speak knowledgeably about various aspects of biotechnology: what is in the biotechnology pipeline and how does biotechnology differ from classical methods of genetic manipulation? These information materials are being expanded to cover emerging topics in biotechnology, e.g., animal, plant, and environmental diagnostics; food safety; animal biotechnology; plants and human health; and environmental biotechnology.
Slides and talk may be downloaded from http://plantbio.berkeley.edu/~outreach/slide.htm, or ordered from the same Web site address.

Biotechnology and Food: A Public Issue for Extension Education
University of Wisconsin Cooperative Extension
Web site: Written materials available full-text at http://www.biotech.wisc.edu/PDF/BiotechFood.pdf
Date produced: 1994
Description: This curriculum focuses on ways to teach and communicate with the community about issues and opportunities of biotechnology and food. Includes case studies of CHY-MAX chymosin, bovine growth hormone/bovine. Curriculum includes leader and participant guide, video (120 minutes).
Order from Cooperative Extension Publications, Rm. 170, 630 W. Mifflin St., Madison, WI 53703, telephone 877-947-7827. Can also be downloaded from http://www.biotech.wisc.edu/PDF/BiotechFood.pdf

Allergic to Biotech?
University of Wisconsin-Extension
Date produced: 1996 Cost: $19.95 plus shipping and handling
Description: Carol Koby discusses issues relating to genetic engineering and food allergies with UWEX Biotechnology Education specialist Tom Zinnen and UW Hospitals allergist Dr. Robert Bush. Zinnen describes biotechnology and its use in food. Bush explains food allergies, particularly those relating to biotechnology.
Order from Picture of Health, 800-757-4354.

CONSUMERS—SENIORS

To Your Health! Food Safety for Seniors
Food and Drug Administration
200 C St. SW, HFS-555
Washington, DC 20204
Date produced: 2000
Description: This 16-minute video and brochure cover food safety issues that are of concern to older persons. The brochure is in large type with color photos.

Food Safety for Seniors
Texas Woman's University
Dept of Nutrition and Food
P.O. Box 425888
Denton, TX 76204
Date produced: 1997 Cost: $8.95
Description: The video depicts senior consumers in a home setting, grocery store, restaurant, and

Meals on Wheels delivery situation and stresses 10 guidelines for food safety.

Food Safety for Older Adults
University of Arkansas
P.O Box 391
Little Rock, AR 72203
Telephone: 501-671-2108
Fax: 501-671-2294
Email address: pbrady@uaex.edu
Date produced: 1997
Description: This curriculum contains materials aimed at helping older adults make informed, responsible decisions related to food safety and quality issues. All client materials are printed in large type to facilitate use by older adults. Lesson plans with suggested activities are included for the instructor. Curriculum includes six lessons including participant handouts, learning activities, pre-/post-test, newsletters.

FOOD SERVICE WORKERS—GENERAL FOOD SAFETY

Case History Series
Altschul Group Corporation
1560 Sherman Ave., Suite 100
Evanston, IL 60201
Telephone: 800-421-2363 Fax: 847-328-6706
Email address: agcmedia@starnetinc.com
Web site: http://www.agcmedia.com/
Date produced: 1985 Cost: $245 for each video
Description: Each 10-minute video covers a specific pathogen: *Staphylococcus aureus* (from sauces), Hepatitis A, *Staphylococcus aureus* (from meats), *Bacillus cereus*, *Salmonella* (from eggs), *Campylobacter*, *Clostridium botulinum*, *Salmonella* (from meat). Scenarios take place in a restaurant with background narration. The series also includes the following titles: Food Service Facilities and Equipment, Receiving and Storage, Microbiology for Food Service Workers, and Housekeeping and Pest Control. Videos demonstrate what went wrong and how the problem could have been avoided.

Food Handler's Sanitation Interactive CD-ROM
American Culinary Federation, Inc.
10 San Bartola Dr.
St. Augustine, FL 32086
Telephone: 800-624-9458
Fax: 904-825-4758
Email address: acf@aug.com
Web site: http://www.acfchefs.org/
Date produced: 1998 Cost: $75 plus shipping and handling. Quantity discounts available.
Description: This program has been approved by the American Culinary Federation as an eight-hour refresher course for renewal. Program takes participant approximately two-and-a-half hours to complete.
Order from ACF Accounting Dept at above address, 800-624-9458 ext. 113.

The Eggs Games
American Egg Board
1460 Renaissance Dr.
Park Ridge, IL 60068
Telephone: 847-296-7043 Fax: 847-296-7007
Email address: aeb@aeb.org
Web site: For related food safety information from this producer: http://www.aeb.org/
Date produced: 1999 Cost: $10 includes shipping, handling and tax. Only prepaid orders accepted.
Description: Booth announcers for the Egg Safety National Championships "sporting events" illustrate proper and improper techniques for egg handling and safety in this 18-minute video.
Order from above address. Call, fax, or email producer to receive a video ordering form.

Food Hygiene
ASI Food Safety Consultants
7625 Page Blvd.
St. Louis, MO 63133
Telephone: 800-477-0778 Fax: 314-727-2563
Email address: asi@asifood.com
Web site: http://www.asifood.com
Cost: Call for prices, discounts for quantities
Description: The first of these two videos deals with the start of the food poisoning chain: sources of food poisoning bacteria, cross-contamination, protecting high-risk foods, symptoms of food poisoning with particular emphasis on personal hygiene, and hand-washing. The second video emphasizes what can happen with a breakdown in temperature control. It uses a dramatic reconstruction and investigation by two intrepid detectives into refrigeration abuse as a teaching tool. Also available in Bengali, Hindi, Cantonese, Punjabi, Gujarati, Urdu.

Danger! Underworld!
AVA Scheiner AG

Neugasse 6
8005 Zurich, Switzerland
Telephone: 004114482070
Fax: 004114482075
Email address: info@ava-scheiner.ch
Cost: Call for prices
Description: This curriculum teaches about cleaning and disinfecting at the workplace and in the food processing plant (or the kitchen) in general. Curriculum includes slides (also available as videocassette), course manual for four lessons, questionnaire, and stickers. Also available in German, French, Spanish, Italian.

The Uninvited Guests
AVA Scheiner AG
Neugasse 6
8005 Zurich, Switzerland
Telephone: 004114482070
Fax: 004114482075
Email address: info@ava-scheiner.ch
Cost: Call for prices
Description: In this introduction into basic microbiology and training in personal hygiene, humorous cartoons appear as "uninvited guests" for which one must constantly be on guard. Curriculum includes videocassette (18 minutes), course manual for three lessons (45 minutes each), questionnaire, stickers. Also available in German, French, Spanish, Italian, Portuguese, Dutch, Danish, Serbo-Croatian, Polish, Hungarian, Greek, Turkish, Arabic, Tamil, Chinese, Thai.

Preventing Foodborne Illness
Colorado Department of Public Health and Environment
Disease Control and Environmental Epidemiology Division
4300 Cherry Creek Dr. South
Denver, CO 80222-1530
Telephone: 303-692-2700 or 692-3620
Fax: 303-782-0338
Email address: pkendall@lamar.colostate.edu
Date produced: revised 1999 Cost: Free
Description: This 10-minute video for food service workers emphasizes washing one's hands before handling food, after using the bathroom, sneezing, touching raw meats and poultry, and before and after handling foods such as salads and sandwiches. Safe food temperatures and cross-contamination are explained. Also available in Spanish.

Personal Hygiene CD-ROM Program
Cornell University Distance Education Program
247 Warren Hall
Ithaca, NY 14853
Telephone: 607-253-3227 Fax: 607-254-5122
Date produced: 1996 Cost: $125
Description: This interactive computer-based training program for retail store associates combines video, audio, graphics, and animation to explain why personal hygiene is important and how to practice good personal hygiene. The total time to complete the training will range from 30 to 45 minutes. Testing and tracking features allow management to monitor the training progress of associates.

Food Safety First!
Drexel University
Food Safety First!
One Drexel Plaza, 3001 Market St.
Philadelphia, PA 19104-2875
Telephone: 215-895-2055 Fax: 215-895-2153
Web site: http://www.foodsafetyfirst.com
Date produced: 1998 Cost: $149 plus $5 shipping and handling. Quantity discounts available.
Description: These five 10-minute video segments cover key topics in a unique style, guaranteed to get and keep workers' attention. The topics covered are: The Top Ten Causes of Foodborne Illness (Introduction and Overview); Personal Hygiene and Handwashing; Cleaning and Sanitation; Preventing Cross-contamination; and Avoiding Time and Temperature Abuse. Reading level of printed materials is sixth grade. Curriculum includes videocassette (50 minutes), handout photocopy masters, pre- and post-tests, training log, trainer's guide. Also available in Spanish.
Order from Food Safety First! PO Box 189, Moab, UT 84532, 800-842-6622, in Canada 800-634-0770, Email: moabking@citlink.net

Food Safety Showdown!
The Educational Foundation of the National Restaurant Association
250 S. Wacker Dr., Suite 1400
Chicago, IL 60606-5834
Telephone: 800-765-2122 Fax: 312-715-0331
Web site: http://www.edfound.org/
Date Produced: 2000 Cost: $59
Description: This interactive game has been revised and updated to reflect the 1999 FDA Model Food Code.

SERVSAFE Food Safety and Sanitation Training Program
The Educational Foundation of the National Restaurant Association
250 S. Wacker Dr., Suite 1400
Chicago, IL 60606-5834
Telephone: 800-765-2122 Fax: 312-715-0807
Web site: http://www.edfound.org/
Cost: Call for prices.
Description: This complete food safety training program for food service workers comes in a variety of formats-videos, CD-ROM, instructor guides, employee workbooks, slides, Food Safety Showdown game, posters, signs. Many materials are also available in Spanish.

Focused on Food Safety Training Resource Binder
Food Safety Resources, Inc.
P.O. Box 231780
Encinitas, CA 92023
Telephone: 877-475-6468 Fax: 760-942-7246
Email address: mikestes@cts.com
Web site: http://www.foodsafetyresources.com or http://www.haccp-compliant.com
Date produced: 1999 Cost: $99.95 retail plus 6.95 shipping
Description: This set of 20 food safety posters are modeled after the 1999 FDA Food Code and are laminated with English on one side, Spanish on the other.

Food Safety and Sanitation
The Grossbauer Group
PO Box 2001
Chesterton, IN 46304-2001
Telephone: 219-926-2883 Fax: 219-929-1502
Email address: sgbauer@grossbauer-group.com
Web site: http://www.grossbauer-group.com/train
Date produced: 1996 Cost: $169 plus $9 shipping and handling
Description: Designed for in-service food service workers, this curriculum covers getting to know foodborne bacteria, introduction to HACCP, understanding sanitation, cleaning and sanitizing, dealing with complaints about foodborne illness, hygiene, and cooling. Each lesson should take 30 minutes. Based on the 1997 FDA Food Code. Curriculum includes learning objectives, presentation outline, background information for presenter, transparencies, handout masters, pre- and post-tests, training tips.

More Food Safety and Sanitation
The Grossbauer Group
PO Box 2001
Chesterton, IN 46304-2001
Telephone: 219-926-2883 Fax: 219-929-1502
Email address: sgbauer@grossbauer-group.com
Web site: http://www.grossbauer-group.com/train
Date produced: 1998 Cost: $169 plus $9 shipping and handling
Description: Designed for in-service training, topics are: hygiene, cleaning kitchen equipment, what to do when the inspectors come, pests, heating and cooling, egg safety, and microwave cooking.

Food Safety 2000
Highfield Publications
'Vue Pointe,' Spinney Hill
Sprotbrough, Doncaster
South Yorkshire, United Kingdom DN5 7LY
Telephone: 01302850007 Fax: 01302311112
Email address: jayne@highfieldpublications.com
Web site: http://www.highfieldpub.u-net.com/
Date produced: 1999 Cost: Call for prices, discounts for quantities
Description: This interactive CD-ROM training package contains 15 modules, which take approximately six to nine hours to complete. Learning is enhanced as food handlers work through the colorful screens, watch the video clips, take part in the interactive games, and complete the test at the end of each module.

A Clean Sweep
Highfield Publications
'Vue Pointe,' Spinney Hill
Sprotbrough, Doncaster
South Yorkshire, United Kingdom DN5 7LY
Telephone: 01302850007 Fax: 01302311112
Email address: jayne@highfieldpublications.com
Web site: http://www.highfieldpub.u-net.com/
Cost: Call for prices, discounts for quantities
Description: This 16-minute video takes staff through the following stages: (1) What is Cleaning?, (2) The Need for Cleaning, (3) How to Clean, (4) When to Clean, (5) Chemicals Used for Cleaning, (6) Caring for Cleaning Equipment, and (7) Tips to Ensure Cleaning and Disinfecting Is Successful.

A Case of Ignorance
Highfield Publications
'Vue Pointe,' Spinney Hill
Sprotbrough, Doncaster
South Yorkshire, United Kingdom DN5 7LY

Telephone: 01302850007 Fax: 01302311112
Email address: jayne@highfieldpublications.com
Web site: http://www.highfieldpub.u-net.com/
Cost: Call for prices, discounts for quantities
Description: This 20-minute video uses a Sherlock Holmes adventure to expound the principles of food poisoning prevention. The program consists of two linked parts. The first is a screenplay, filmed in authentic historical settings to a scenario that faithfully follows the style of Sherlock Holmes scripts. The plot leads the viewer through the intricate maze of the circumstances that lead to a major food poisoning outbreak. To reinforce this section—but useable as a separate part—the settings revert to the modern day where the experience of Holmes and Watson are updated and the key points of basic food hygiene are visualized.

***E. coli*—The Facts**
Highfield Publications
'Vue Pointe,' Spinney Hill
Sprotbrough, Doncaster
South Yorkshire, United Kingdom DN5 7LY
Telephone: 01302850007 Fax: 01302311112
Email address: jayne@highfieldpublications.com
Web site: http://www.highfieldpub.u-net.com/
Cost: Call for prices, discounts for quantities
Description: This 20-minute video provides essential information about *E. coli* 0157:H7 from pasture to plate.

Sanitation in School Cafeterias
Long Island Productions
106 Capitola Dr.
Durham, NC 27713
Telephone: 800-397-5215 Fax: 919-544-5800
Email address: lipmail@mindspring.com
Web site: http://www.lip-online.com/
Date produced: 1996 Cost: $99.95
Description: This 12-minute video instructs food service employees on how to avoid contaminating food. Included is bacteria control, chemical and metal contaminants, sanitizing vs. cleaning, food storage, pest control, and many kitchen cleanliness tips.

Foodsafe
Magic Lantern Communications, LTD.
10 Meteor Dr.
Toronto, Ontario, Canada M9W 184
Telephone: 416-675-1155 Fax: 416-675-1154
Email address: lmitchell@magiclantern.ca
Date produced: revised, 1994 Cost: $754 for complete package; other options available. Contact source.
Description: Geared towards food service workers, this curriculum is divided into two levels, one basic and one advanced. The basic level is made up of seven sections, the advanced is four sections. Curriculum includes manual, instructor's guide, sample quizzes, slides, videocassette. Selected segments of the basic level have been translated into Cantonese and Punjabi.

Diner Detective—Educational Program for Food Service Employees
Ohio State University
Department. of Food Science and Technology
122 Vivian Hall, 2121 Fyffe Rd
Columbus, OH 43210
Telephone: 614-292-3069
Email address: Ndife.1@osu.edu
Date produced: 1997 Cost: Manual $6.75, video $15, set of five posters $10.75 plus $5 shipping and handling.
Description: This curriculum was designed to train teenage and young adult food service workers. It could also be used for a high school class. Curriculum includes manual, five laminated posters, video.
Order from Ohio State University Extension Publication Office, 385 Kottman Hall, 2021 Coffey Rd., Columbus, OH 43210-1044, 614-292-1607, fax 614-292-2270.

Food Safety: You Make the Difference
Seattle King County Department of Public Health
Public Health Distribution Center
56 South Lucille St.
Seattle, WA 98134
Telephone: 206-296-4766 Fax: 206-296-0185
Web site: http://metrokc.gov/health/foodsfty
Date produced: 1995 Cost: Video $25 plus shipping and handling. Flyers $10
Description: This 28-minute video tackles four major problem areas of food protection: hand-washing, cross-contamination, cooking/heating/cooling, and hot and cold reheating. The program features real food service workers who talk freely about what they do to protect their clientele and how and why they do it. Although the video is available in six languages and in closed caption, an effort has been made throughout to make the hands-on demonstrations language independent. Viewers, even though they might not understand a word of dialogue, can come away with the essentials. Languages are Spanish, Chinese (Cantonese and Mandarin), Korean, Vietnamese, Russian. Eng-

lish version available in open and closed captioning. Booklet available in Tagalog.

Food Service Sanitation/Hygiene
The Training Network, Inc.
1432 Kearney St.
El Cerrito, CA 94530
Telephone: 800-390-8283 Fax: 510-232-5235
Date produced: 1995 Cost: $99
Description: Topics in this 13-minute video are bacteria, chemical and metal contaminants, sanitizing vs. cleaning, food storage and pest control. Also available in Spanish.

Serve It Safely to Seniors
University of Connecticut
43 Marne St.
Hamden, CT 06514
Telephone: 203-789-7865 Fax: 203-789-6461
Date produced: 1994
Description: This curriculum was developed to provide food handlers, those who transport food, and home-delivered meal recipients with the information needed to prevent food-related illness in the elderly population. The modules allow for flexibility of training, depending on needs and time constraints. Curriculum includes manual with course outline, pre-test, handouts, overheads, 10 laminated posters. Suggests use of four videos that are not included with the curriculum.

Safe Food Handling in Community Foodservice Programs
University of Connecticut
43 Marne St.
Hamden, CT 06514
Telephone: 203-789-7865 Fax: 203-789-6461
Date produced: 1997
Description: This curriculum is designed for food handlers, cooks, transportation personnel, and meal site managers in day care, elderly feeding, school lunch, shelters, soup kitchens, and residential homes. Each lesson takes between 15 and 30 minutes. Curriculum includes objectives, handouts, and activities.

The Interactive Food Safety CD
University of Florida, Home Economics Department
Gainesville, FL 32611-0365
Date produced: 1998 Cost: $39.95
Description: The Interactive Food Safety CD-ROM will teach all the essential aspects of sanitation for a food service operation, and runs on both Macintosh and PC computers. This interactive CD-ROM utilizes video demonstrations of proper food handling methods, closed-captioned text that accompanies voice narration for the hearing impaired, and interactive sessions and quizzes. Also has an optional certification mode.
Order from University of Florida, Educational Media and Services, PO Box 110011 Gainesville, FL 32611 800-226-1764. Order #SF15.

Food Protection Video Series
University of Florida, Home Economics Department
Gainesville, FL 32611-0365
Date produced: 1997 Cost: $50
Description: This set of five videos is geared towards training food service personnel about the most important aspects of food safety. The 45-minute training program is formatted in five parts: (1) Food Safety and Personal Hygiene; (2) Receiving, Storing, Record Keeping; (3) Thawing, Cooking, Cooling, Holding Food; (4) Serving; (5) Cleaning and Sanitizing. Also available in Spanish.
Order from University of Florida, Educational Media and Services, PO Box 110011 Gainesville, FL 32611 800-226-1764. Order #SF11 English, SFV12 Spanish.

Food Handling Is a Risky Business
University of Massachusetts Cooperative Extension
202 Chenoweth Laboratory
Amherst, MA 01003
Telephone: 413-545-0552 Fax: 413-545-1074
Date produced: 1992 Cost: $10.50
Description: This is a train-the-trainer curriculum designed to train key staff in human service agencies who in turn will teach a food safety program to other staff and clients. The objective is to increase knowledge and adoption of recommended safe food handling practices of professional and nonprofessional staff in agencies who care for high-risk populations. The program includes information specific to vulnerable groups, food handling, regulations, methods for teaching, and evaluation/administrative materials. The program is intended for food service workers in day care centers, family day care, shelters, resident homes, congregate meal sites, school food service, and soup kitchens. The curriculum is divided into three lessons, each from 20 to 45 minutes and includes lesson plan, camera-ready masters,

resource lists, answer keys, evaluation guidelines, fact sheets, poster. Also available in Spanish.

Microbeman: The Continuing Adventures
University of Tennessee Institute of Agriculture, Agricultural Extension Service
P.O. Box 1071
University of Tennessee, Institute of Agriculture
Knoxville, TN 37901-1071
Telephone: 423-974-7334 Fax: 423-974-7448
Email address: wcmorris@utk.edu
Date produced: 1994 Cost: Call for prices
Description: Program consists of four single-concept 10–15 minute videos designed for low-literacy, inexperienced food service workers: (1) The Case of "La Grande Burgere" (*E. coli* in hamburgers), (2) The Case of Conrad the Egg-Head (the danger zone), (3) The Case of Walley's Salad (cross-contamination), and (4) The Case of the Perfect Pig (personal hygiene). The videos were designed to stand alone, yet make a continuing series with a story line involving a "super-hero" character portrayed as "Microbeman." Professional actors make this a deliciously corny and entertaining way of presenting food safety principles.

Food Safety Is No Mystery
USDA, Food Safety and Inspection Service (FSIS)
Web site: http://www.fsis.usda.gov/
Date produced: 1987 Cost: $43.97. Add $5 for shipping and handling.
Description: This 34-minute video, developed by the U.S. Department of Agriculture, is written in a detective story format. It is geared towards workers at food service establishments. Topics covered include sanitation and personal hygiene, safe food preparation, preventing contamination, and safe cooling and reheating of food. The video shows the how and why behind food safety. The trainer's manual encourages hands-on staff participation through a series of learning activities, which can be used by employees for self-development. Also available in Spanish.
Contact FSIS at 202-720-3897 or fsis.webmaster@usda.gov for ordering information.

Kitchen Care
Vocam S.E. Inc.
7061 Grand National Dr.
Suite 150, Grand National Plaza
Orlando, FL 32819-8379
Telephone: 888-26-VOCAM Fax: 407-363-9001
Date produced: 1997 Cost: $295 for video and manual; $495 includes CD-ROM
Description: Part I of this 19-minute video focuses on food safety issues in the kitchen-personal hygiene, cross-contamination, temperatures, receiving and storage, cleaning and sanitizing, etc. Part II focuses on kitchen safety such as fire, lifting, knives. Videos could be shown in sections. CD-ROM version is interactive with questions. Curriculum includes video, manual with checklists, training tips, script of video; interactive CD-ROM optional. Also available in Spanish, Chinese (Mandarin and Cantonese), German.

FOOD SERVICE WORKERS—HACCP

HACCP Training Videos
Certified Foodservice Consulting
P.O. Box 1401
Mexia, TX 76667
Telephone: 254-765-3172
Email address: haccpchef@mexia.com
Web site: http://www.glade.net/~haccp/
Date of publication: 1997 Cost: $189 plus $10 shipping and handling.
Description: This set of three videos and training guide were originally produced for country clubs, but they are applicable to any food service operation.

HACCP Master!
CHL Associates
Box 4015
Walnut Creek, CA 94553
Telephone: 510-370-7778
Fax: 510-370-6900
Cost: $295 plus #13 for FedEx shipping.
Description: This HACCP software product tracks food products and spots potential hazards from the time they enter the door until they are served to the consumer. Software automatically produces flow charts following the HACCP standards, and an array of forms used in monitoring the food products during their flow through the establishment. Computer output is used for planning, record keeping, and employee training (both primary and remedial), and addresses all elements of HACCP. Designed to be used in a work environment to help employees deliver a safe product.

A Practical Approach to HACCP
The Educational Foundation of the National Restaurant Association
250 S. Wacker Dr., Suite 1400
Chicago, IL 60606-5834
Telephone: 800-765-2122 Fax: 312-715-0807
Web site: http://www.edfound.org/
Cost: All components can be bought separately or in sets; check with the Foundation for prices.
Description: This curriculum teaches how to design, implement, and monitor an HACCP system in food service establishments. Curriculum includes coursebook, instructor's guide, four videos.

HACCP: The Hazard Analysis Critical Control Point Manual
Food Marketing Institute
Publications Sales
800 Connecticut Avenue, NW, Suite 500
Washington, DC 20006-2701
Telephone: 202-429-8298
Fax: 202-429-4529
Web site: http://www.fmi.org/
Cost: Member—$95, Nonmember—$195
Description: This manual is designed for in-store use at the soup and salad bar and deli/restaurant and seafood departments. Complete with damage-resistant flowcharts, this manual is a guide to the dangers of foodborne illness.

HACCP for Food Service—Recipe Manual and Guide
LaVella Food Specialists
332 Halcyon
St. Louis, MO 63122
Telephone: 314-822-0089
Fax: 314-822-9305 Email address: lavella@cyberusa.com
Date of publication: 1998 Cost: $79.95 plus $4.95 shipping and handling.
Description: This manual is a ready-to-use compilation of more than 100 food service recipes, developed for 25, 50, and 100 portions. Recipes and HACCP flow charts are presented side-by-side on each page for ease of use in planning and production. Critical control points are clearly highlighted beginning with receiving and continuing through preparation, storage, and reheating. Includes information sections for general reference and training, plus nutritional analyses for each recipe.

HACCP for Food Service Video Training Series
LaVella Food Specialists
332 Halcyon
St. Louis, MO 63122
Telephone: 314-822-0089 Fax: 314-822-9305
Email address: lavella@cyberusa.com
Date of publication: 1997 Cost: $99.95 plus $7.95 shipping and handling.
Description: This training kit consists of a leader's guide and two 10-minute videos, Hand in Hand-An Introduction to Food Safety and HACCP and The HACCP Game: Scoring Points for Your Team. The videos are also available in Spanish.

The HACCP Cookbook and Manual
Nutrition Development Systems
7312 385th St. E
Eatonville, WA 98328
Telephone: 253-925-6561
Fax: 253-847-2321
Date of publication: 1999 Cost: $59.95 plus $5 shipping and handling
Description: This manual contains 95 quantity recipes that conform to the 1997 Food Code and HACCP guidelines, with HACCP flowcharts and CCPs. Recipes are modified for low-sodium, low-fat, diabetic diets. Includes HACCP manual, food safety guidelines, and temperature record charts.

HACCP Training Kit
Southern Illinois University HACCP Project, Food and Nutrition
Mail Code 4317
Carbondale, IL 62901-4317
Telephone: 618-536-2157
Fax: 618-453-7517
Email address: hlashraf@siu.edu
Web site: http://www.siu.edu/~haccp/
Date of publication: 1998 Cost: $100
Description: The workbook is divided into three parts, and should be used with the training video. Part one covers the basics of HACCP. Critical Control Points are discussed in part two, and part three is a summary of the HACCP system. Each part of the video can be viewed separately or in its entirety. Selected pages from the workbook and a very short video clip are available at the Web site. Curriculum contains video (55 minutes), workbook, posters, magnet, stickers, thermometer, carrying case.

Taking Control: A Guide to the HACCP Food Safety System
TV Journal, Inc.
1414 East Fletcher Ave.

Tampa, FL 33612
Telephone: 813-972-4707
Date of publication: 1998 Cost: $699
Description: Curriculum includes instructor's guide, student workbook, and three videos: (1) Understanding the Basics; (2) Going through the Stages; (3) Cheeseburger the HACCP Way. The first video teaches the seven steps of HACCP and reviews the main causes of foodborne illness. The second video takes workers on a journey through purchasing, receiving, storage, preparation, and service. The last video teaches workers to follow an HACCP flow chart and recipe using actual examples. This program has been approved for one hour of credit per video by the American School Food Service Association.

HANDWASHING

The Literary Classics—A New Kind of Reading Material for Public Restrooms
Allegheny County Health Department
Food Protection Program
3901 Penn Ave., Building #1
Pittsburgh, PA 15224-1318
Telephone: 412-578-8044 Fax: 412-578-8190
Email address: gchristy@county.allegheny.pa.us
Date produced: 1997
Description: This series of posters for display in public restrooms are short stories based on literary classics. Following is an example of one of the stories: "Scarlett O'Hara was not beautiful, but men seldom realized it when caught by her charm as the Tarleton Twins were. Nor did they realize when they grew frightfully ill that it was the touch of her magnolia-white skin that made them so sick. For, disregarding all ladylike behavior, Scarlett had frivolously not washed her hands after attending to her business in the lady's parlor. Her delicate hands, being so unguarded, touched those of the twins, causing the unfortunate spread of an atrocious bacterial disease. Shame was brought upon both families, which was the worst disgrace of all."

Hygiene for Hands
AVA Scheiner AG
Neugasse 6
8005 Zurich, Switzerland
Telephone: 004114482070 Fax:004114482075
Email address: info@ava-scheiner.ch
Cost: Call for prices
Description: This curriculum offers guidelines on proper handwashing and motivating employees to examine their own behavior in order to improve it. Includes poster and two videos-seven minutes and four minutes. Also available in German, French, Spanish, Italian, Polish.

Handwash Motivation Aids
Brevis
3310 South 2700 East
Salt Lake City, UT 84109
Telephone: 800-383-3377 Fax: 801-485-2844
Email address: brbrevis@xmission.com
Web site: http://www.brevis.com/
Cost: Call for prices
Description: Brevis offers a number of different ways of conveying the handwashing idea to consumers, food service workers, and health care workers. Materials for children include the books *Buddy Bear's Handwashing Troubles, The Ten Potato Scrub,* and the *Germ Gang Activity Book.* Includes posters, stickers, pencils, T-shirts, mugs, balloons, buttons.

All Hands on Deck!—True Confessions of a Filthy, Rotten, Disgusting Germ
Brevis
3310 South 2700 East
Salt Lake City, UT 84109
Telephone: 800-383-3377 Fax: 801-485-2844
Email address: brbrevis@xmission.com
Web site: http://www.brevis.com/
Date produced: 1996 Cost: $25
Description: An entertaining look at the proper way to wash hands. The narrator is a hand, who persuades a germ to come clean and tell where germs like to live and how they get around. The reasons for handwashing are outlined and proper technique is demonstrated along with suggestions for avoiding immediate recontamination before even leaving the rest room. This 10-minute video is for food service workers, but there is also a version for health care professionals and one for young people.

Glitter Bug
Brevis
3310 South 2700 East
Salt Lake City, UT 84109
Telephone: 800-383-3377 Fax: 801-485-2844
Email address: brbrevis@xmission.com
Web site: http://www.brevis.com/
Cost: Cost varies from $65 to $245; call Brevis for a brochure

Description: This kit teaches proper handwashing techniques. Students put on powder or potion, wash hands, then put them under the UV light. Powder or potion that remains on hands after washing shows up on hands when put under the UV light. Teaching materials then show proper handwashing techniques. Includes Glitterbug powder or potion, UV light, manual, motivation cards.

Glo Germ
Glo Germ Company
P.O. Box 537
Moab, UT 84532
Telephone: 800-842-6622 Fax: 435-259-5930
Email address: moabking@lasal.net
Web site: http://www.glogerm.com
Cost: Kits are $49.95, $65, or $91.95, depending on the type of lamp
Description: Glo germ is a kit that teaches about handwashing and handwashing techniques. The kit consists of an oil, a powder, and a special fluorescent lamp. The oil and powder contain "germs" and the lamp reveals the germs. Students apply either the oil or the powder and then work through their normal handwashing procedure. The fluorescent lamp is then used to spot the remaining germs.

Safe Hand and Fingertip Washing Video Tape Training System
Hospitality Institute of Technology and Management
830 Transfer Rd., Suite 35
St. Paul, MN 55114
Telephone: 612-646-7077 Fax: 612-646-5984
Date produced: 1995 Cost: $65 English only; $95 English and Spanish
Description: This curriculum provides detailed instruction on the procedures for the double handwash (with fingernail brush) and single handwash for the removal of pathogenic microorganisms, and the appropriate times to use these two washes. The curriculum includes videocassette (14 minutes), fingernail brush, handwash poster, instructor and student materials with test. Also available in Spanish.

Wash Your Hands
LWB Company
13614 Fifty-sixth Ave. NE
Marysville, WA 98271
Telephone: 360-653-9122
Date produced: 1995 Cost: $65 plus shipping. Volume discounts available.
Description: Robert starts to leave a restroom without washing his hands. A Voice from beyond tells Robert that he didn't wash his hands. A frightened Robert washes—but not well enough. The Voice shows Robert the germs on his hand and gives him detailed washing instructions. This five-minute video and accompanying brochure can be used with any age or type of group. Also available in Spanish.

Wash Those Hands!
Marsh Media
PO Box 8082
Shawnee Mission, KS 66208
Telephone: 800-821-3303 Fax: 816-333-7421
Email address: order@marshmedia.com
Web site: http://www.marshmedia.com/
Date produced: 1996 Cost: $69.95
Description: This nine-minute video presents concise information about basic personal hygiene, including a look at germs and how they make people sick. Handwashing techniques are taught. Closed captioned.

Hands Down on Germs
Portland Public Schools Television Services
5210 North Kerby
Portland, OR 97217
Telephone: 503-916-5838 Fax: 503-916-2699
Email address: tv53@pps.k12.or.us
Date produced: 1996 Cost: $40
Description: Geared towards children in grades kindergarten through three, this eight-minute video shows how to wash hands using hand puppets. It seems Bobby is not washing his hands properly, which is giving his hand, Digit, nightmares. Hand puppets teach Bobby that germs can't be seen, the importance of handwashing, and how to wash his hands.

The War on Germs
Portland Public Schools Television Services
5210 North Kerby
Portland, OR 97217
Telephone: 503-916-5838 Fax: 503-916-2699
Email address: tv53@pps.k12.or.us
Date produced: 1997 Cost: $40
Description: This seven-minute video, designed for students in grades four through 12, simulates an investigative news journal in which journalists investigate a rash of illnesses. Lack of handwashing is found to be the culprit. The news team travels to the local hospital where they are instructed in the proper handwashing technique.

PROVIDERS AT CHILD DAY CARE CENTERS AND INSTITUTIONS

The ABC's of Safe and Healthy Child Care
Centers for Disease Control and Prevention
1600 Clifton Rd.
Atlanta, GA 30333
Telephone: 404-639-3682 Fax: 404-639-3039
Web site: For related food safety information from this producer: http://www.cdc.gov/cdc.htm
Date produced: 1995 Cost: $20–$25 for video, $5 for poster, $19 for manual
Description: This 13-minute video, manual, and poster focus on handwashing in a child care setting and on diaper changing. Manual includes information on how disease is spread and recommends policies and practices that should be instituted in child care settings to prevent disease, injury, and environmental exposures. It also includes one- or two-page fact sheets on many common childhood illnesses and conditions, a first aid chart, a resource guide for obtaining additional information (many with 800 numbers), and a list of the poison control centers throughout the United States. Available full-text online at http://www.cdc.gov/ncidod/hip/abc/contents.htm.
Order from The Public Health Foundation (877-252-1200); or the National Technical Information Service (800-CDC-1824).

An Ounce of Prevention: Keeps the Germs Away
Centers for Disease Control and Prevention
1600 Clifton Rd.
Atlanta, GA 30333
Telephone: 404-639-3682 Fax: 404-639-3039
Web site: For more information and for full text of brochure visit http://www.cdc.gov/ncidod/op/materials.htm
Date produced: 1998 Cost: $30
Description: This 30-minute video, brochure, and poster covers the topics: handwashing, cleaning, food, immunization, antibiotics, pets, and wild animals. The video is in a television news magazine format with an anchor and three reporters, all television professionals. Each reporter hosts one segment of the show interviewing disease experts from CDC's National Center for Infectious Diseases and then demonstrating the prevention behaviors in a typical home (handwashing, cleaning/disinfecting, food safety), in a medical care setting (immunizations, antimicrobial resistance), and in dealing with animals (pets, insects, and wild animals). The segments can be used together or individually for waiting area or classroom. Also appropriate for community or secondary school use.
Order by calling 800-41-TRAIN (item number VT009)

Safe Food for Children
Kansas State Univiversity Cooperative Extension Service
Safe Food for Children, Justin Hall 244
Kansas State University
Manhattan, KS 66506-1407
Telephone: 785-532-5782
Web site: http://www.oznet.ksu.edu/pr_fsaf/welcome.htm
Date produced: 1992, Spanish version 1997
Cost: Each item available in quantity and separately. Call or write for pricing information.
Description: This curriculum is designed for parents, other child care providers, and trainers of child care providers. It consists of five lessons of 30 to 45 minutes, each with key lesson concepts, materials needed to teach the lesson, discussion to accompany video, activities for adults and for children, questions and answers, resources, and reproducible masters. The lessons are: (1) Clean Hands for Healthy Children; (2) On Your Mark, Get Set, Go Grocery Shopping; (3) Recipe for Success: Prepare and Serve Food Safely; (4) Microbe Family Get Away! Storing Food Smartly and Safely; (5) Clean Kitchen Savvy. Curriculum includes video for children (46 minutes), video for leader (one hour), five leader's guides (one for each lesson), stickers, magnet, certificate of completion, set of five folding brochures. Video also available in Spanish.

Food Safety for Child Caregivers
Mississippi State University Cooperative Extension Service
Box 9745
Mississippi State, MS 39762-9745
Telephone: 601-325-3080 Fax: 601-325-8407
Date produced: 1993 Cost: Contact source
Description: This training for child care providers is designed to be two-and-a-half hours in length. Lessons are: (1) Foodborne Illness or Food Poisoning, (2) Food Shopping and Storage, and (3) Food Handling and Preparation. Curriculum contains three lessons with lesson plans, learning activities, talking points, transparency masters, and video.

CARE Connection
National Food Service Management Institute
University of Mississippi
PO Drawer 188
University, MS 38677-0188
Telephone: 800-321-3054 Fax: 800-321-3061
Email address: nfsmi@olemiss.edu
Web site: http://www.olemiss.edu/depts/nfsmi
Date produced: 1997 Cost: $45
Description: This curriculum contains 48 lessons developed for use by sponsors of child care homes and child care centers to use in training child care providers. Lessons 26 through 29 focus on food safety and sanitation in child care. Other lessons emphasize nutrition, meal planning, food preparation, and basic program requirements.

Making Food Healthy and Safe for Children
National Maternal and Child Health Clearinghouse
2070 Chain Bridge Rd., Suite 450
Vienna, VA 22182-2536
Telephone: 703-356-1964 Fax: 703-821-2098
Email address: ncemch01@gumedlib.dml.georgetown.edu
Web site: Full text of this document is at http://www.ncemch.org/pubs/default.html
Date produced: 1997 Cost: Free
Description: This manual was written to help child care workers provide children with healthy and safe food, and to meet the nutrition standards in National Health and Safety Performance Standards: Guidelines for Out-of-Home Child Care Programs. Information is presented about all of the nutrition-related standards in chapters divided by the following topics: keeping everything clean, using foods that are safe to eat, planning to meet the children's food needs, promoting pleasant meals and snacks, helping children and families learn about food. The standards referenced are printed to the side of each page. Several chapters contain checklists that summarize key points, including food safety and menu planning.

Preventing Foodborne Illness in Preschoolers and Senior Adults: A HACCP Training for Food Handlers in Child and Elder Care
University of Georgia Cooperative Extension Service
Hoke Smith Annex, Room 204
Athens, GA 30602-4356
Telephone: 706-542-3773 Fax: 706-542-1979
Email address: judyh@uga.cc.uga.edu
Date produced: 1997 Cost: $30
Description: This curriculum looks at food preparation in terms of hazards—microbiological, chemical, and physical. Activities guide participants to recognize hazards and to implement steps to eliminate them. Instruction time is three hours, or it can be used as a correspondence course. Curriculum includes video, instructor's materials with talking points, activities with answers, transparency masters, pre- and post-tests.

Safe Food Healthy Children—A Food Safety Videoconference Workshop for Child Care Providers
University of Georgia Cooperative Extension Service
Hoke Smith Annex, Room 204
Athens, GA 30602-4356
Telephone: 706-542-3773 Fax: 706-542-1979
Email address: judyh@uga.cc.uga.edu
Date produced: 1995 Cost: $40
Description: This curriculum contains the materials used in a teleconference to train child care providers in food safety issues. The program was designed to be four hours in length, but may be broken into shorter segments to accommodate other time schedules. The training consists of short video segments interspersed with participant activities. Curriculum includes facilitator's manual, participant packet, camera-ready copies, video (85 minutes).

Educational Program to Train Foodservice Workers
University of Kentucky, Cooperative Extension Service
233 Scovell Hall
Lexington, KY 40546-0064
Telephone: 606-257-1812 Fax: 606-257-7792
Date produced: 1992
Description: Food service workers who prepare and serve food to high-risk clientele, young children at day care facilities, and the elderly at senior citizen centers are the target audience of this distance learning satellite program. The program is presented in three parts of 90 minutes each. Part one, Mean About Clean: Warfare on Germs, focuses on personal cleanliness and kitchen sanitation. Part two, Clean From Start to Finish: Prepare, Cook and Serve Food Safely, looks at receiving/purchasing food and storing, preparing, and cooking food safely. Part three, Hot or Cold,

But Not In Between: Serving, Transporting and Holding Food, discusses transporting and serving food, home-delivered meals, and controlling pests. Activities to do during break times are included.
Order from Agricultural Communications Services, Scovell Hall, Lexington, KY 40546-0064, telephone 606-257-7218.

Training Foodservice Workers and At-Risk Groups to Reduce Foodborne Illness
University of Kentucky, Cooperative Extension Service
233 Scovell Hall
Lexington, KY 40546-0064
Telephone: 606-257-1812 Fax: 606-257-7792
Date produced: 1994
Description: This project was part of a satellite food safety training program geared towards food service workers at senior citizen centers and child care centers. Posters and flyers for senior citizen centers are included, as is a story for children. Activities for three lessons are included: (1) Handwashing, (2) Calibrating a Thermometer, and (3) Using the Safe Food Checklist for Meal Preparation. Curriculum includes: Safe Food Checklist, guidelines for facilitators, children's story and stickers, posters and handouts for seniors. Curriculum includes safe food checklist, guidelines for facilitators, children's story and stickers, posters and handouts for seniors.
Order from Agricultural Communications Services, Scovell Hall, Lexington, KY 40546-0064, telephone 606-257-7218.

SCHOOL FOOD SERVICE

The School Food Allergy Program
Food Allergy Network
Web site: http://www.foodallergy.org
Date produced: 1995 Cost: $75
Description: This program helps parents and school nurses conduct an in-service about food allergy management to school faculty. It includes a video, binder with more than 100 pages, poster, and EpiPen(r) trainer.

Cold Is Cool—School Milk Handling Workshop
National Dairy Council
10255 West Higgins Rd., Suite 900
Rosemont, IL 60018-5616
Telephone: 800-426-8271
Web site: http://www.nationaldairycouncil. org/
Date produced: 1999
Description: Designed for a one-hour in-service for school food service staff, this video, leader's guide, and poster teaches about milk safety in school feeding programs.

Cooking for the New Generation—Storing, Cooking, and Holding
National Food Service Management Institute
University of Mississippi
PO Drawer 188
University, MS 38677-0188
Telephone: 800-321-3054 Fax: 800-321-3061
Email address: nfsmi@olemiss.edu
Web site: http://www.olemiss.edu/depts/nfsmi
Date produced: 1997 Cost: $25
Description: This 19-minute video and manual on Breakfast Lunch Training (BLT) was designed to be used by district directors and managers to instruct food service assistants in the preparation of multiple-ingredient, processed food products for school food service.

No Time to Train? Lessons on Food Safety and Sanitation
National Food Service Management Institute
University of Mississippi
PO Drawer 188
University, MS 38677-0188
Telephone: 800-321-3054 Fax: 800-321-3061
Email address: nfsmi@olemiss.edu
Web site: http://www.olemiss.edu/depts/ nfsmi
Date produced: 1996 Cost: $3.95
Description: Each of the 15 lessons in this manual was designed to be taught in 10 minutes to food service staff. The lessons are drawn from the NFSMI source, Serving it Safe: A Manager's Tool Kit. As this resource was developed for school food service workers, it emphasizes cafeteria-style service.

Serving It Safe: A Manager's Tool Kit
USDA, Food and Consumer Services
Nutition and Technical Services
3101 Park Center Dr. Room 607
Alexandria, VA 22302
Web site: Full text of this curriculum is available at http://www.nal.usda.gov:8001/Safety/safe.html
Date produced: 1999 Cost: $10

Description: This curriculum was designed as part of the Team Nutrition campaign for use with school food service, but is also applicable to other food service organizations. Consists of eight chapters that include lesson plans, talking points, objectives, overhead masters, and activities. The interactive software can be used separately to reinforce ideas learned in the teaching modules. Curriculum includes lesson plans for eight chapters, group exercises, handouts, overhead masters, job aids, poster, interactive computer software (CD-ROM for Windows or Mac and diskettes for Mac and for Windows).

Limited copies for sale from National Food Service Management Institute. Call 800-321-3054. Order no. FCA-295.

VOLUNTEERS AT PICNICS, CHURCH SUPPERS, FAIRS, FOOD BANKS

An Integrated Media Tutorial for Prepared and Perishable Food Rescue Programs

Chef and Child Foundation
American Culinary Federation
10 San Bartola Drive
St. Augustine, FL 32086
Telephone: 904-824-4468 ext. 104
Fax: 904-825-4758

Date produced: 1996 Cost: $5 per manual, $10 per video. Quantity discount available.

Description: These materials were developed for prepared food programs and community service agencies that distribute and utilize perishable prepared foods to the needy. The workbooks and videos cover food safety issues, nutrition, and menu planning. All written materials are in large type and are easy to read.

Soup Up Food Safety in Your Kitchen

Cornell Cooperative Extension
Department of Food Science
8 Stocking Hall
Ithaca, NY 14853
Telephone: 607-255-7922
Email address: dls9@cornell.edu

Date produced: 1999 Cost: Contact source

Description: These program materials are designed for teaching safe food preparation principles to staff and volunteers who work in soup kitchens. The materials include a comprehensive set of full-color overhead transparencies or 35-mm color slides and a 28-page easy-to-read food safety reference booklet, titled A Soup Kitchen Worker's Guide to Food Safety. The visuals and booklet are also available on a CD-ROM.

Safe Aid—A Food Safety Training Program for Food Banks

Montana State University Extension Service
PO Box 173360
Bozeman, MT 59717-3360
Telephone: 406-994-5702
Email address: lpaul@montana.edu

Date produced: 1998 Cost: $15 plus $3 shipping and handling

Description: This curriculum was designed for food bank directors, staff, and volunteers. Booklet titles are: (1) Food Banks and Foodborne illness; (2) Sanitary Surroundings: Setting Up for Safe Food; (3) Risk Management; (4) Safe Food Handling; and (5) Re-packaging Bulk Food. Curriculum includes five lesson booklets, summary sheets, posters, training manual.

Order from Extension Publications, Rm 115, Culbertson Hall, MSU, Bozeman, MT 59717, telephone 406-994-3273.

Safe Food Handling for Occasional Quantity Cooks

Ohio State University Extension Service
Department of Human Nutrition and Food Management, Ohio State University
1787 Neil Ave., 315 Campbell Hall
Columbus, OH 43210-1295
Telephone: 614-292-2699 Fax: 614-292-8880
Email address: medeiros.1@osu.edu

Date produced: 1994 Cost: Posters and brochures are free; camera-ready masters of fact sheets $10.50; videotape $15

Description: This is a comprehensive curriculum developed to teach volunteer food service workers about preparing and serving food safely. The curriculum addresses practices and responsibilities of food service workers using the HACCP approach. Topics include planning and purchasing; storing food supplies; preparing food; transporting, storing, and serving cooked food; and handling leftovers. Curriculum contains video, fact sheets, overhead transparency masters, trainer's manual, participant's manual, posters.

Order from Ohio State University Extension Publication Office, 385 Kottman Hall, 2021 Coffey Rd., Columbus, OH 43210-1044, 614-292-1607, fax 614-292-2270.

Keep Food Safe: We Wish You Well
Oregon State University
Extension Foods and Nutritionist Specialist
161 Milam Hall
Corvalis, OR 97331-5106
Telephone: 503-737-3211 Fax: 503-737-0999
Date produced: 1995 Cost: $7.50
Description: This kit is designed for use by volunteer workers in food pantry operations. Curriculum contains training guide, numerous handouts, overhead transparency masters, poster, pot holder, magnet, quiz.

Ken McKan the Food Safety Man
Purdue University Cooperative Extension Service
Purdue University
1264 Stone Hall
West Lafayette, IN 47904-1264
Telephone: 765-494-8186
Email address: willie@cfs.purdue.edu
Date produced: 1997 Cost: $10 each or all four videos for $30
Description: Originally designed for emergency feeding programs, the Ken McKan series consists of five videos—a focus on diversity, handwashing, time and temperature control, evaluating incoming foods, and nutrition. A sixth video is a Spanish translation of the nutrition video.
Order from Media Distribution Center, 301 South 2nd St., Lafayette, IN 47901-1232, 765-494-6794, fax 765-496-1540.

Safe Food for the Hungry
Purdue University Cooperative Extension Service
Purdue University
1264 Stone Hall
West Lafayette, IN 47904-1264
Telephone: 765-494-8539 Fax: 765-494-0674
Email address: masona@cfs.purdue.edu
Date produced: 1994 Cost: four-hour version—$20; one-hour version—$10
Description: This four-hour video is from a videoconference on safe food handling specific to nonprofit food distribution organizations. Topics covered include: decreasing food waste, making sure incoming food is safe, redistributing, preparing and serving food safely, avoiding contamination, storing food safely, controlling pests, and special issues related to prepared and perishable foods. A shorter, edited version is also available.
Order from Media Distribution Center, 301 South 2nd St., Lafayette, IN 47901-1232, 765-494-6794, fax 765-496-1540.

S.T.R.E.T.C.H. (Safety Training, Resources, and Education to Combat Hunger)
Purdue University Cooperative Extension Service
Purdue University
1264 Stone Hall
West Lafayette, IN 47904-1264
Telephone: 765-494-8539 Fax: 765-494-0674
Email address: masona@cfs.purdue.edu
Date produced: 1996
Description: This curriculum was designed to assist nonprofit food assistance organizations in evaluating their programs in terms of food safety, nutrition, and volunteer management. The S.T.R.E.T.C.H. program developed a self-evaluation tool which can be self-administered, or utilized with the aid of an Extension professional. Curriculum consists of 18 self-evaluation cards and corresponding fact sheets.
Order from Media Distribution Center, 301 South 2nd St., Lafayette, IN 47901-1232, 765-494-6794, fax 765-496-1540.

Temporary Food Stands: Short Times, Fast Service and Safe Foods
Snohomish Health District
Environmental Health Division
3020 Rucker Ave., Suite 102
Everett, WA 98201-3971
Telephone: 206-339-5250 Fax: 206-339-5216
Date produced: 1993
Description: This 21-minute video is geared towards people who will be operating a food stand in a fair or other temporary gathering. Sections covered include determining whether or not a health permit is needed, requirements of and how to apply for a permit, proper construction of a booth, employee hygiene, equipment needs, supplies, and cooking and storing foods.

Looking for a Safe Harbor: Training Manual for Volunteer Foodservice Workers
University of Vermont
UVM Extension System
HCR 31 Box 436
St. Johnsbury, CT 05819
Telephone: 802-748-8177 Fax: 802-748-1955
Email address: dsteen@clover.uvm.edu
Date produced: 1994 Cost: $25 or pieces can be bought separately
Description: This curriculum is for training volunteer food service workers in temporary food events, such as fairs, church suppers, or community gatherings. There is a Train-the-Trainer curriculum, which is to be used by a professional knowledgeable in safe food handling principles

and practices to train those who are in charge of a temporary event or booth. This program is approximately six-and-a-half hours long. Participants in the Train-the-Trainer program will then use the Train-the-Volunteer materials to train their volunteer food service workers. This training program will take approximately three hours. Curriculum includes training the trainer leader's guide, training the trainer handouts, training the volunteer food service worker leader's guide, training the volunteer food service worker handouts, log book, pretest, video (10 minutes).

Food Safety for Fundraisers
University of Wyoming, Cooperative Extension Service
University of Wyoming, CES
P.O. Box 3354
Laramie, WY 82071-3354
Telephone: 307-766-5375 Fax: 307-766-3379
Date produced: 1994 Cost: $25
Description: This 22-minute video and manual is geared towards people who are not accustomed to handling large quantities of food. The manual is large type with plenty of graphics. Growth of bacteria is explained along with factors necessary for bacteria to multiply. Proper temperature control, cooling foods rapidly, cooking foods thoroughly, keeping thermometers calibrated, sanitizing tables and kitchenware, preventing cross contamination, and personal hygiene are discussed. The concept of HACCP is introduced. Included is a list of potentially hazardous foods.

Cooking for Groups: A Volunteer's Guide to Food Safety
USDA, Food Safety and Inspection Service
Web site:
http://www.fsis.usda.gov/OA/pubs/cfg/cfg.htm. Available full-text.
Cost: Single copies free from the Consumer Information Center, www.pueblo.gsa.gov
Description: This 35-page colorful booklet guides consumers through the steps necessary to safely plan and serve food for a large event. It includes cooking temperatures and storage charts.

CHAPTER 11

ORGANIZATIONS, COOPERATIVE EXTENSION, HOTLINES, STATE AND LOCAL AGENCIES

This chapter aims to capture all those involved in food safety, including government agencies, professional organizations, trade associations, consumer organizations, academic-industry partnerships, academic-government partnerships, research institutes, and some that defy categorization. The format of the chapter is as follows:

Organizations
Cooperative Extension Offices
Food and Drug Administration (FDA) Public Affairs Specialists
Hotlines
State Departments of Health and/or Agriculture
State Meat Inspection Programs

Organizations are listed alphabetically, as it would be difficult to break them down in terms of subject area since so many of them cover a wide range of food safety issues. Cooperative Extension Agents are part of the state land-grant university in each state, with a program leader at the university and agents in the counties. They are a local source for food safety information and materials, and in many cases can teach food safety principles to groups. Some university extension offices are equipped to help the small food processor, especially those that are home-based, to prepare their products safely. FDA public affairs specialists can help consumers locate food safety information on foods that come under FDA jurisdiction.

With the advent of and the increasing access to the Internet, hotlines have declined as a method of information distribution. Compared to a Web site, they are expensive to maintain and can serve only a limited number of individuals. Some organizations are still able to maintain hotlines. For general food safety information, the FDA Food Information Line and the USDA Meat and Poultry Hotline are the best sources. For food safety information on products from food companies, call that company's product hotline. For companies not listed here, look on the food packaging. Most food companies now print their telephone number on their food products.

State health and/or agriculture departments also offer food safety training, or have lists of local trainers. These agencies are responsible for the safety of foods in restaurants, grocery stores, convenience stores, schools, hospitals, prisons, institutions, farmer's markets, fairs, and just about anywhere else food is served. Anyone wanting to sell or produce food will quickly become familiar with these offices. Epidemiologists from these agencies investigate outbreaks of water or foodborne illness.

Some states have their own meat and poultry inspection systems. These programs must be at least equivalent to federal inspection programs. For those states that do have their own inspection programs, these programs are responsible for the safety of meat and poultry products produced in those states.

ORGANIZATIONS

Agricultural Biotechnology Support Project (ABSP)
Agriculture Hall, Michigan State University
East Lansing, MI, 48824-1039
Telephone: 517-353-2290 Fax: 517-353-1888
Email address: absp@pilot.msu.edu
Web site: http://www.iia.msu.edu/absp/
Description: The Agricultural Biotechnology Support Project is the result of a U.S. Agency for International Development grant. Its mission is to take an integrated approach, combining applied research, product development, and policy development in the areas of biosafety and intellectual property rights to assist developing countries in accessing and generating biotechnology, and in using that technology in an environmentally and legally responsible manner. It seeks to improve the capacity and policy environment for the use, management, and commercialization of agricultural biotechnology in developing countries and transition economies.
Publications, reports, or services: Publishes Biolink Newsletter, and the AgBiotechNet Web site.

Alliance for Bio-Integrity
406 W. Depot Ave.
Fairfield, IA, 52556
Email address: info@bio-integrity.org
Web site: http://www.bio-integrity.org/
Description: The Alliance for Bio-Integrity is a nonprofit, nonpolitical organization dedicated to the advancement of human and environmental health through sustainable and safe technologies. The alliance's initial project is to gain a more rational and prudent policy on genetically engineered (GE) foods. This entails (1) educating the public about the unprecedented dangers to the environment and human health posed by the massive enterprise to genetically reprogram the world's food supply; (2) securing a scientifically sound system for safety-testing genetically altered foods; and (3) securing a meaningful system of labeling to protect the right of consumers to avoid such foods.
Publications, reports, or services: Provides background information on GE foods, tracks legislation and lawsuits, advises citizens on how to take part in the debate over GE foods.

Alliance for Food and Fiber
10866 Wilshire Blvd. #550
Los Angeles, CA, 90024
Telephone: 310-446-1827
Fax: 310-446-1896
Web site: http://www.foodsafetyalliance.org/
Description: The alliance is an educational clearinghouse to inform the public and the media on the issues of food safety and crop protection that impact the production, processing, and distribution of food and fiber products.
Publications, reports, or services: Operates National Food Safety Hotline (800-266-0200) where callers can access produce safety information, Web site has food safety information related to produce.

American Academy of Allergy, Asthma and Immunology (AAAAI)
611 East Wells St.
Milwaukee, WI, 53202
Telephone: 414-272-6071 Fax: 414-272-6070
Web site: http://www.aaaai.org/
Description: The American Academy of Allergy, Asthma and Immunology is the largest professional medical specialty organization representing allergists, clinical immunologists, allied health professionals, and other physicians with a special interest in allergy. The mission of the academy is the advancement of the knowledge and practice of allergy, asthma, and immunology:
Publications, reports, or services: Has a brochure and video on food allergies in English and Spanish, operates a hotline for allergy in-

formation and physician referrals: 800-822-2762.

American Academy of Sanitarians (AAS)
c/o James W. Pees
829 Brookside Dr.
Miami, OK, 74354
Telephone: 918-540-2025 Fax: 918-540-2025
Email address: jpees@rectec.net
Description: Open to legally registered sanitarians who possess at least a master's degree in public health, environmental health sciences, or environmental management, the purpose of the American Academy of Sanitarians is to improve the environmental health status of humanity through certification of those sanitarians who have helped or who are helping to achieve this long-range goal.

American Association of Meat Processors (AAMP)
One Meeting Place
P.O. Box 269
Elizabethtown, PA, 17022
Telephone: 717-367-1168 Fax: 717-367-9096
Email address: aamp@aamp.com
Web site: http://www.aamp.com/
Description: The American Association of Meat Processors is North America's largest meat trade organization. Its more than 1,800 medium-sized and smaller meat, poultry, and food businesses include slaughterers, packers, processors, wholesalers, in-home food service businesses, retailers, deli and catering operators, and industry suppliers.
Publications, reports, or services: Services to members include help with regulatory and legislative affairs and meat inspection problem-solving. The association provides workshops and training materials on HACCP, control of *Listeria* in plants, and food service worker sanitation.

American Council on Science and Health, Inc. (ACSH)
1995 Broadway, Second Floor
New York, NY, 10023-5860
Telephone: 212-362-7044 Fax: 212-362-4919
Email address: acsh@acsh.org
Web site: http://www.acsh.org
Description: The American Council on Science and Health is a consumer education consortium of physicians, scientists, and policy advisors concerned with issues related to food, nutrition, chemicals, pharmaceuticals, lifestyle, the environment, and health. It was founded in 1978 by a group of scientists who had become concerned that many important public policies related to health and the environment did not have a sound scientific basis. These scientists created the organization to add reason and balance to debates about public health issues and bring common sense views to the public. Many of their publications are available full-text on their Web site.
Publications, reports, or services: ACSH produces a wide range of peer-reviewed reports, press releases, editorials, and food safety publications including: Eating Safely: Avoiding Foodborne Illness, Facts Versus Fears: A Review of the Greatest Unfounded Health Scares of Recent Times, and consumer-level publications on irradiated foods and food biotechnology.

American Crop Protection Association (ACPA)
1156 Fifteenth St. NW, Suite 400
Washington, DC, 20005
Telephone: 202-296-1585 Fax: 202-463-0474
Web site: http://www.acpa.org/
Description: Organized in 1933, ACPA is the nonprofit trade organization representing the major manufacturers, formulators, and distributors of crop protection and pest control products, including bioengineered products with crop production and protection characteristics. APCA's mission is to further the interest of the general public and ACPA member companies by promoting the environmentally sound use of crop protection and plant biotechnology products for the economic production of safe, high-quality, abundant food, fiber, and other crops.
Publications, reports, or services: Educational resources for children, papers on agricultural issues including food biotechnology.

American Culinary Federation, Inc.
10 San Bartola Dr.
St Augustine, FL, 32086
Telephone: 800-624-9458 Fax: 904-824-4468
Email address: acf@acfchefs.net
Web site: http://www.acfchefs.org/
Description: The American Culinary Federation, a professional, nonprofit organization for chefs, was founded in 1929 with the principal goal of promoting a professional image of the American chef worldwide through education at all levels, from apprentices to the most accomplished certified master chefs. Local chapters exist throughout the United States and Caribbean.

Publications, reports, or services: ACF offers the Certified Master Chef accreditation, sponsors scholarships and apprenticeship programs, and develops food safety training materials, such as the Food Handler's Sanitation Interactive CD-ROM.

American Dietetic Association (ADA)
216 W. Jackson Blvd.
Chicago, IL, 60606-6995
Telephone: 800-877-1600
Email address: infocenter@eatright.org
Web site: http://www.eatright.org/
Description: Founded in 1917, ADA's members help shape food choices and impact the nutritional status of the public. The membership includes dietitians, dietetic technicians, students, and others holding baccalaureate and advanced degrees in nutrition and dietetics.
Publications, reports, or services: ADA issues position papers on food irradiation, food biotechnology, and other food safety issues. It also publishes materials for consumers and professionals on general food safety, food allergies, and other food safety–related topics. Has a scholarship program.

American Egg Board (AEB)
1460 Renaissance Dr.
Park Ridge, IL, 60068
Telephone: 847-296-7043 Fax: 847-296-7007
Email address: aeb@aeb.org
Web site: http://www.aeb.org/
Description: The American Egg Board is the U.S. egg producer's link to the consumer in communicating to the American public about eggs. AEB is funded from a national legislative check-off on all egg production from companies with greater than 75,000 layers.
Publications, reports, or services: Materials include games and curricula for children, consumer egg safety publications, and industry food safety training aids.

American Feed Industry Association (AFIA)
1501 Wilson Blvd., Suite 1100
Arlington, VA, 22209
Telephone: 703-524-0810 Fax: 703-524-1921
Email address: afia@afia.org
Web site: http://www.afia.org/
Description: The American Feed Industry Association is the national organization devoted to representing the business, legislative, and regulatory interests of the animal feed and pet food industries and their suppliers. AFIA closely monitors and influences state and federal legislative and regulatory actions on key industry issues such as genetically modified organisms (GMOs), bovine spongiform encephalopathy (BSE), dioxin, clean water, environmental activism, and industrial ergonomics. Through its work with Congress and federal agencies like EPA, USDA, OSHA, and FDA, as well as state agencies, AFIA seeks to build on the industry's record of producing the safest and most abundant supply of meat, milk, and eggs in the world, at the lowest cost to the consumer.
Publications, reports, or services: Issues summaries and news stories on topics of interest to the industry.

American Frozen Food Institute (AFFI)
2000 Corporate Ridge, Suite 1000
McLean, VA, 22102
Telephone: 703-821-0770 Fax: 703-821-1350
Web site: http://www.affi.com/
Description: The American Frozen Food Institute is the national trade association that represents the interests of the frozen food industry. AFFI maintains a united industry voice for the frozen food industry to government agencies, the retail and food service trade, the technical community, the media, consumers, and in the international arena.
Publications, reports, or services: Publications on frozen foods for consumers, media, and industry.

American Institute of Baking (AIB)
P.O. Box 3999
Manhattan, KS, 66505-3999
Telephone: 785-537-4750 Fax: 785-537-1493
Email address: information@aibonline.org
Web site: http://www.aibonline.org/
Description: AIB is a nonprofit corporation, founded in 1919 as a technology transfer center to "put science to work for the baker." The institute maintains links and working relationships with other groups involved in food safety, food production and equipment, trade development, food legislation, and university food science research programs both in the United States and abroad.
Publications, reports, or services: Develops food safety educational materials and offers onsite and distance learning courses for food safety and sanitation; offers scholarships, professional development, and resume service for students.

American Meat Institute
1700 North Moore St., Suite 1600
Arlington, VA, 22209
Telephone: 703-841-2400 Fax: 703-527-0938
Email address: mwilliams@meatami.org
Web site: http://www.meatami.org/
Description: AMI, a national trade association, represents packers and processors of the nation's beef, pork, lamb, veal, and turkey products and their suppliers throughout America. The institute provides legislative, regulatory, and public relations services; conducts scientific and economic research; offers marketing and technical assistance; and sponsors education programs.
Publications, reports, or services: Industry training materials and guidebooks on sanitation standard operating procedures, recalls, irradiation, and HACCP. Consumer publications on *E. coli, Listeria,* meat safety, and foodborne illness.

American Meat Science Association
1111 North Dunlap Ave.
Savoy, IL 61874
Telephone: 217-356-3182 Fax: 217-398-4119
Web site: http://meatscience.org/
Description: The American Meat Science Association provides credible, science-based information to the industry and facilitates a greater understanding of muscle foods and associated animal products as a major food source. Its unique role is to provide a forum for all interests in meat—commercial, academic, government, and consumer—to come together in a reasoned, scientifically based atmosphere and address issues such as meat safety, processing and marketing, inspection, and nutrition.
Publications, reports, or services: The Role of Microbiological Testing in Beef Food Safety Programs is available from the Web site.

American School Food Service Association (ASFSA)
700 S. Washington St., Suite 300
Alexandria, VA, 22314
Telephone: 703-739-3900 Fax: 703-739-3915
Email address: asfsa@asfsa.org
Web site: http://www.asfsa.org/
Description: As the national association dedicated to protecting and enhancing children's health and well-being through school meals, ASFSA offers school food service workers training in food safety and sanitation as well as in improving the nutritional well-being of students.
Publications, reports, or services: Maintains food service electronic discussion boards for members, offers training in food safety and sanitation around the country, sponsors a credentialing program for school food service and nutrition professionals, provides career development services and scholarship opportunities.

American Society for Healthcare Food Service Administrators (ASHFSA)
One North Franklin, 31 North
Chicago, IL, 60606
Telephone: 312-422-3870 Fax: 312-422-4581
Email address: sarmist1@aha.org
Web site: http://www.ashfsa.org/
Description: The mission of the American Society for Healthcare Food Service Administrators is to advance the practice of health care food service management in a broad range of health care settings. ASHFSA serves individuals with health care food service management responsibilities, educators, suppliers, and consultants to the profession. The sSociety develops products and services that provide education, professional growth, skills building, networking, advocacy, and collaboration with other groups or organizations.
Publications, reports, or services: Food safety is included in educational sessions and at annual meetings and in food service publications. Offers scholarships for undergraduate students and lists job openings.

American Society for Microbiology
1752 N. St. NW
Washington, DC, 20036
Telephone: 202-737-3600
Web site: http://www.asmusa.org/
Description: The American Society for Microbiology is the oldest and largest single life science membership organization in the world. Membership has grown from 59 scientists in 1899 to more than 42,000 members located throughout the world. ASM represents 25 disciplines of microbiological specialization plus a division for microbiology educators.
Publications, reports, or services: Food Safety: Current Status and Future Needs, A Global Decline in Microbiological Safety of Water: A Call for Action, sponsors children's site Microbe World, has a food microbiology division, and a career page on Web site.

American Water Works Association (AWWA)
6666 West Quincy Ave.

Denver, CO, 80235
Telephone: 303-794-7711
Web site: http://www.awwa.org/
Description: The American Water Works Association is an international nonprofit scientific and educational society dedicated to the improvement of drinking water quality and supply. Founded in 1881, AWWA is dedicated to promoting public health and welfare by providing drinking water of unquestionable quality and sufficient quantity.
Publications, reports, or services: Partnership for Safe Water program, legislative updates, white papers and policy statements, conference proceedings, manuals.

Animal Health Institute
1325 G St. NW, Suite 700
Washington, DC, 20005-3104
Telephone: 202-637-2440 Fax: 202-393-1667
Web site: http://www.ahi.org/
Description: The Animal Health Institute is the U.S. trade association that represents manufacturers of pharmaceuticals, vaccines, and feed additives for pet and farm animals. As such it interacts with federal agencies regulating animal health products, monitors global food safety regulations as they relate to trade, coordinates research projects to ensure that safe and effective animal health products are available for modern food production, and shares information with veterinary groups to make sure that animal owners understand how to use animal medicines safely and have access to appropriate products.
Publications, reports, or services: Publications include an antibiotic drug residue in animals information kit, a biotechnology information kit, and the Animal Health Source Book.

Animal Industry Foundation (AIF)
1501 Wilson Blvd., Suite 1100
Arlington, VA, 22209
Telephone: 703-524-0810 Fax: 703-524-1921
Email address: aif@aif.org
Web site: http://www.aif.org/
Description: Established in 1987, the Animal Industry Foundation nonprofit education foundation was established to educate consumers about U.S. animal agriculture and its contributions to the public's quality of life. AIF provides information on modern animal agriculture relating to animal well-being, nutrition, food safety, and the environment, and serves as the national source for animal agriculture education programs. AIF is committed to correcting the misinformation directed at the public by animal rights and other activist groups. It serves as the national umbrella organization through which feed, animal health, livestock, poultry groups, and others with a vested interest in animal agriculture develop and deliver consistent messages to consumers.
Publications, reports, or services: Curricula for different age ranges on animal care and issues.

AOAC International
481 North Frederick Ave., Suite 500
Gaithersburg, MD, 20877-2417
Telephone: 800-379-2622 Fax: 301-924-7089
Email address: aoac@aoac.org
Web site: http://www.aoac.org/
Description: Established in 1884, AOAC International (formerly the Association of Official Analytical Chemists) is an independent association of scientists in the public and the private sectors devoted to advancing the global chemistry and microbiology analytical community by promoting laboratory methods validation and quality measurements. The association's primary focus is coordinating the development and validation of chemical and microbiological analytical methods by expert scientists working in their industry, academic, and government laboratories worldwide.
Publications, reports, or services: FDA Bacteriological Analytical Manual; Classification of Visible Can Defects; Ecology and Management of Food Industry Pests; Principles of Food Analysis for Filth, Decomposition, and Foreign Matter; EPA Manual of Chemical Methods for Pesticides and Devices; FDA Food Additives Analytical Manual.

Aspartame Consumer Safety Network, Inc. (ACSN)
P.O. Box 780634
Dallas, TX, 75378
Telephone: 214-352-4268
Email address: marystod@airmail.net
Web site: http://web2.airmail.net/marystod/
Description: Formed in 1987 by Mary Nash Stoddard following a life-threatening reaction to aspartame, the Aspartame Consumer Safety Network is a coalition of consumers and health care professionals around the world who are concerned about the health effects of aspartame and other similar chemical sweeteners. ACSN takes the stand that carcinogens such as aspartame are potentially toxic and do not belong in the food

supply; they are dedicated to educating others about these hazards.

Publications, reports, or services: Produces the book *Deadly Deception: Story of Aspartame.*

Association of Food and Drug Officials (AFDO)
P.O. Box 3425
2250 Kingston Road, Suite 311
York, PA, 17402
Telephone: 717-757-2888 Fax: 717-755-8089
Email address: afdo@blazenet.net
Web site: http://www.afdo.org/

Description: The Association of Food and Drug Officials is an international nonprofit organization composed of members from local, state, and federal regulatory agencies; regulated industry; and academia. It actively works to improve and protect the nation's health and safety by fostering uniformity in the adoption and enforcement of laws and regulations relating to food, drugs, medical devices, and cosmetics. AFDO promotes the concept of a "fully integrated" national food safety system.

Publications, reports, or services: Sponsors Seafood HACCP training, involved in food safety regulation, and inspection issues. AFDO has a scholarship fund for students preparing for a career of research, regulatory work, quality control, or teaching in an area related to some aspect of foods, drugs, or consumer product safety.

Association of Professional Hospitality Managers (APHM)
P.O. Box 16214
Tallahassee, FL, 32317
Telephone: 850-671-4047 Fax: 850-878-5426
Email address: info@aphm.org
Web site: http://www.aphm.org/

Description: The Association of Professional Hospitality Managers promotes the interests of hotel, restaurant, resort, club, cruise ship, and motel management from around the world. APHM provides a peer-level organization for promoting the educational, professional, and legislative interests of its members.

Publications, reports, or services: Quarterly newsletter with industry updates, best practice ideas, peer communication, and legislative updates. Conducts seminars and continuing education workshops that include food safety issues.

Association of State and Territorial Health Officials (ASTHO)
1275 K St. NW, Suite 800
Washington, DC, 20005-4006
Telephone: 202-371-9090 Fax: 202-371-9797
Web site: http://www.astho.org/

Description: Membership in ASTHO is limited to the executive officer of the department of health of any state or territory of the United States. Because of its membership, ASTHO's and activities reflect the major positions and concerns of the state health departments,influence which include food safety.

Publications, reports, or services: Publishes policy papers and a newsletter that covers public health issues, including food safety.

Association of State Drinking Water Administrators (ASDWA)
1025 Connecticut Ave. NW, Suite 903
Washington, DC, 20036
Telephone: 202-293-7655 Fax: 202-293-7656
Email address: asdwa@erols.com
Web site: http://www.asdwa.org/

Description: The Association of State Drinking Water Administrators (ASDWA) is the professional association serving state drinking water programs. Formed in 1984 to address a growing need for state administrators to have national representation, ASDWA has become a respected voice for state agents with Congress, the United States Environmental Protection Agency (EPA), and other professional organizations.

Publications, reports, or services: The ASDWA Update covers late-breaking regulatory and policy issues of special interest to state drinking water officials. ASDWA also publishes reports on issues related to drinking water quality.

BioDemocracy and Organic Consumers Association
6114 Hwy 61
Little Marais, MN, 55614
Telephone: 218-226-4164 Fax: 218-226-4157
Web site: http://www.purefood.org/

Description: Formerly called the Pure Food Campaign and the Campaign for Food Safety, the BioDemocracy and Organic Consumers Association is a grassroots organization advocating organic, non-irradiated food for human and animal health. It provides information on the following issues: genetic engineering, biotechnology, genetically modified organisms, bovine growth hormone, food labeling, food slander, organic

farming, toxic sludge, food contamination, pesticides, and irradiation.
Publications, reports, or services: Fact sheets, Campaign for Food Safety News electronic newsletter, provides forum for consumer advocacy.

BIOTECanada
130 Albert St., Suite 420
Ottawa, Ontario, K1P 5G4 Canada
Telephone: 613-230-5585 Fax: 613-563-8850
Email address: info@biotech.ca
Web site: http://www.biotech.ca/
Description: BIOTECanada represents the Canadian biotechnology community, providing a unified voice for advocacy, human resources, communications, and services to the community. BIOTECanada is involved in projects that service the biotechnology community. Formerly the Industrial Biotechnology Association of Canada and the Canadian Institute of Biotechnology.
Publications, reports, or services: Publications on biotechnology for industry and consumers, reports on the biotechnology industry in Canada.

Biotechnology Industry Organization (BIO)
1625 K St. NW, Suite 1100
Washington, DC, 20006
Telephone: 202-857-0244 Fax: 202-857-0357
Web site: http://www.bio.org/regularwelcome.html
Description: The Biotechnology Industry Organization (BIO) represents biotechnology companies, academic institutions, state biotechnology centers, and related organizations throughout the United States and in many other countries. The members of BIO apply biological knowledge and techniques to develop products and services for use in health care, agriculture, environmental remediation, and other fields.
Publications, reports, or services: Guide to Biotechnology, Biotechnology brochure for consumers. Web site has large section on food and agricultural biotechnology.

Biotechnology Office at Iowa State University
1210 Molecular Biology Building
Iames, IA, 50011-3260
Telephone: 515-294-9818 Fax: 515-294-4629
Email address: biotech@iastate.edu
Web site: http://www.biotech.iastate.edu/
Description: This university-based center covers research, education, and outreach in the area of biotechnology, much of it agricultural biotechnology. Programs include bioethics, educational programs for teachers and children, and technology transfer.
Publications, reports, or services: Web site includes Biotechnology Update newsletter, bioethics case studies, biotechnology curriculum ideas, and Ag Bioethics Forum.

C.H.I.P.S. (Culinary and Hospitality Industry Publications Services)
10777 Mazoch Road
Weimar, TX, 78962
Telephone: 409-263-5683 Fax: 409-263-5685
Email address: orderdept@chipsbooks.com
Web site: http://www.chipsbooks.com/
Description: This is a one-stop-shopping source for professional books for the food science and technology industry.
Publications, reports, or services: Web site has secure pages for ordering online.

Canadian Food Inspection Agency
59 Camelot Dr.
Nepean, Ontario K1A 0Y9, Canada
Telephone: 613-225-CFIA (2342)
Fax: 613-228-6634
Email address: cfiamaster@em.agr.ca
Web site: http://www.cfia-acia.agr.ca/
Description: This is the main government agency dealing with food safety in Canada. Its mission is to enhance the effectiveness and efficiency of federal inspection and related services for food and animal and plant health to ensure safe food, consumer protection, and market access.
Publications, reports, or services: Canadian inspection documents, HACCP plans, information for industry and consumers.

Canadian Meat Science Association (CMSA)
Dow's Lake Ct.
875 Carling Ave., Suite 410
Ottawa, Ontario, K1S 5P1 Canada
Telephone: 613-729-3911 Fax: 613-729-4997
Email address: info@cmc-cvc.com
Web site: http://cmsa.ca/
Description: Objectives of CMSA are to promote the application of science and technology for the production, processing, packaging, distribution, preparation, evaluation, and utilization of all meat and meat products; to coordinate education and research in meat science and related areas; and to sponsor activities designed to promote the adoption of sound and useful research and educational techniques.

Publications, reports, or services: Training and educational resources on meat science and safety.

Canadian On-Farm Food Safety Program (COFFSP)
Suite 1101, 75 Albert St.
Ottawa, Ontario, K1P 5E7 Canada
Telephone: 613-236-6659 or 236-6165
Fax: 613-236-6165
Email address: programm@istar.ca
Web site: http://www.cfa-fca.ca/engsafe.htm
Description: The Canadian On-Farm Food Safety Program is a partnership between the Canadian government and national producer organizations. It is involved in the research, development, and communication of a national on-farm food safety initiative and provides the necessary tools to educate producers and to initiate on-farm food safety practices.
Publications, reports, or services: Produces An Introduction to On-Farm Food Safety Practices and the On-Farm Food Safety Newsletter.

Center for Consumer Research (CCR)
University of California, Davis
Davis, CA, 95616-8598
Telephone: 530-752-2774 Fax: 530-752-3975
Email address: ccr@ucdavis.edu
Web site: http://ccr.ucdavis.edu/
Description: The Center for Consumer Research focuses on consumer attitudes toward food safety and quality. Projects have focused on consumer attitudes towards new techniques, food safety, food labeling, nutritional issues, and produce quality.
Publications, reports, or services: Web site has sections on food biotechnology and food irradiation.

Center for Food Safety (CFS)
International Center for Technology Assessment
666 Pennsylvania Ave., SE, Suite 302
Washington, DC, 20003
Telephone: 202-547-9359 Fax: 202-547-9429
Email address: office@centerforfoodsafety.org
Web site: http://www.centerforfoodsafety.org/ and http://www.foodsafetynow.org/
Description: The Center for Food Safety is a project of the International Center for Technology Assessment. It was established to carry out vital and historic initiatives in food safety, environmental protection, and sustainable agriculture. The goal of CFS is to preserve organic food, ensure the testing and labeling of genetically engineered foods, and to carry out litigation efforts when the U.S. government fails to act appropriately.
Publications, reports, or services: Initiates petitions and legal actions to safeguard the food supply from bioengineered food products, publishes fact sheets, monitors news sites, sends action alerts to members.

Center for Science in the Public Interest (CSPI)
1875 Connecticut Ave. NW, Suite 300
Washington, DC, 20009
Telephone: 202-332-9110 Fax: 202-265-4954
Email address: cspi@cspinet.org
Web site: http://www.cspinet.org/
Description: The Center for Science in the Public Interest is a nonprofit education and advocacy organization that focuses on improving the safety and nutritional quality of the nation's food supply. CSPI's primary focus is to educate the public and policy makers about the critical importance of nutrition and food safety.
Publications, reports, or services: Food safety activities include the Recipe for Safe Food legislative campaign, The Food Safety Report Card for Congress, Outbreak Alert!, testimony before Congress, press releases, and reports such as Dine at Your Own Risk.

Centers for Disease Control and Prevention (CDC)
Foodborne and Diarrheal Diseases Branch
1600 Clifton Rd., MS C-09
Atlanta, GA, 30333
Email address: dbmdnet@cdc.gov
Web site: http://www.cdc.gov/ncidod/dbmd/foodborn.htm and http://www.cdc.gov/foodsafety
Description: The Foodborne and Diarrheal Diseases Branch of the CDC focuses on the control and prevention of bacterial foodborne and diarrheal diseases. The branch conducts surveillance; investigates outbreaks; and consults with state health departments, food safety regulatory agencies, and health authorities around the world. It identifies causes and sources of bacterial foodborne and diarrheal illness to develop new prevention and control methods in collaboration with other public health agencies.
Publications, reports, or services: Consumer-level fact sheets on foodborne pathogens, FoodNet surveillance program, PulseNet program, very extensive Web site.

Chartered Institute of Environmental Health (CIEH)
Chadwick Ct.
15 Hatfields
London, UK, SE1
Web site: http://www.cieh.org.uk/
Description: The Chartered Institute of Environmental Health was founded in 1883 and is an entirely independent organization representing the interests of the environmental health profession. It offers a range of professional, educational, and membership services, as well as training courses, events, and publications. In January 2000 CIEH acquired the U.S.-based National Registry of Food Safety Professionals.
Publications, reports, or services: Offers HACCP training courses and numerous food safety publications, maintains a *Cryptosporidium* Information Resource Web site.

Chilled Food Association (CFA)
P.O. Box 14811
London, UK, NW10 9ZR
Email address: orion.kandh@easynet.co.uk
Web site: http://www.chilledfood.org/
Description: CFA's prime role is to promote and maintain standards of excellence in chilled food production and distribution. It accomplishes this by developing and maintaining common standards of safety and quality in the production and distribution of chilled prepared foods; representing the key interests of manufacturers of chilled prepared foods in their dealings with regulatory bodies and with other relevant groups; providing a common view and voice for the industry; and coordinating with organizations and other groups with related interests;
Publications, reports, or services: Food safety materials include: Guidelines for Good Hygienic Practice in the Manufacture of Chilled Foods, Guidelines for Microwaveable Products, Handwash Posters, Sous Vide Foods: Conclusions of an ECFF Botulinum Working Party.

Codex Alimentarius Commission
Secretariat of the Joint FAO/WHO Food Standards Programme
Viale delle Terme di Caracalla
00100 Rome, Italy
Telephone: +390657051 Fax: +390657054593
Email address: CODEX@FAO.Org
Web site: http://www.fao.org/waicent/faoinfo/economic/esn/codex/
Description: This commission is under the joint auspices of the Food and Agriculture Organization of the United Nations and the World Trade Association. Its purpose is to guide and promote the establishment of standards and requirements for food and food safety, to assist in their harmonization, and, in doing so, to facilitate international trade.
Publications, reports, or services: Publishes the Codex Alimentarius, an international standard for food products, which is recognized by more than 140 member nations and the World Trade Organization.

Conference for Food Protection
Web site: http://www.foodprotect.org
Description: The Conference for Food Protection is a nonprofit organization composed of representatives from regulatory agencies at all levels of government, the food industry, academia, and consumer organizations that work to improve food safety at the retail level by identifying problems, formulating recommendations, and developing and implementing practices that ensure food safety.

Consumer Alert
1001 Connecticut Ave. NW, Suite 1128
Washington, DC, 20036
Telephone: 202-467-5809 Fax: 202-467-5814
Email address: staff@consumeralert.org
Web site: http://www.consumeralert.org/
Description: Consumer Alert was founded in 1977 as a national, nonprofit, non-partisan, membership organization for people concerned about the excessive growth of government regulation at the national and state levels. As an independent consumer organization that supports the principles of sound science, consumer choice, and free-market competition, its mission is to represent average consumers as purchasers of goods and services in a dynamic and competitive marketplace.
Publications, reports, or services: Publishes monthly online newsletter—On the Plate, a newsletter to evaluate current policies and new proposals relating to food issues on the basis of sound science, risk assessment, and their impact on consumers. Submits testimony, formal comments, and petitions to regulatory agencies to help guide policy decisions that affect consumers. Food safety issues covered are pesticides, irradiation, and food biotechnology.

Consumer Information Center (CIC)
Department WWW
Pueblo, CO, 81009
Telephone: 888-8 PUEBLO
Fax: 719-948-9724
Email address: catalog.pueblo@gsa.gov
Web site: http://www.pueblo.gsa.gov/
Description: Since 1970 the Consumer Information Center has helped federal agencies and departments develop and distribute useful information to the public.
Publications, reports, or services: Has free food safety brochures that can be ordered.

Consumers Union (CU)
101 Truman Ave.
Yonkers, NY, 10703-1057
Telephone: 914-378-2000
Web site: http://www.consumersunion.org
Description: Consumers Union, publisher of Consumer Reports, is an independent, nonprofit testing and information organization serving only consumers. It is a comprehensive source for unbiased advice about products and services, health, and other consumer concerns. CU reports on current issues of concern to consumers, including many food safety issues.
Publications, reports, or services: Web site has issue papers, reports, and press releases on bovine growth hormone, food contaminants, genetically engineered food, mad cow disease, pesticides, risk assessment, and the food regulatory system.

Consumers Union, Food Quality Protection Act (FQPA) Project
New York, NY
Telephone: 914-378-2310
Email address: groted@consumer.org
Web site: http://www.ecologic-ipm.com/menu.html
Description: This Consumers Union project monitors the Food Quality Protection Act in a watchdog capacity to ensure the act brings about significant and sustained reductions in human exposure to pesticides, especially among vulnerable population groups like infants, children, and pregnant women.
Publications, reports, or services: Congressional documents, reports, and resources relating to the FQPA.

Council for Agricultural Science and Technology (CAST)
4420 West Lincoln Way
Ames, IA, 50014-3447
Telephone: 515-292-2125 Fax: 515-292-4512
Email address: cast@cast-science.org
Web site: http://www.cast-science.org
Description: CAST is a nonprofit organization composed of 36 scientific societies and many individual, student, company, and associate society members. Its mission is to identify food and fiber, environmental, and other agricultural issues and to interpret related scientific research information for legislators, regulators, and the media for use in public policy decision making.
Publications, reports, or services: Briefing papers on topics related to food safety cover pesticides, foodborne pathogens, and irradiation.

Council for Biotechnology Information
P.O. Box 34380
Washington, DC 20034-0380
Telephone: 202-467-6565
Email address: cbi@whybiotech.com
Web site: http://www.whybiotech.com/
Description: The Council for Biotechnology Information is a coalition of the world's leading biotechnology companies created to provide information to the public about the potential benefits of the technology, based on the best available scientific research, published reports, and expert opinion.
Publications, reports, or services: Fact sheets on biotechnology regulations, frequently asked questions about biotechnology crops, events calendar.

Council of Hotel and Restaurant Trainers (CHART)
P.O. Box 211
Avon By The Sea, NJ, 07717
Telephone: 800-463-5918 Fax: 800-427-5436
Email address: charthq@aol.com
Web site: http://www.chart.org
Description: The Council of Hotel and Restaurant Trainers is composed of training and development professionals working in the food and lodging industries. It promotes effective training and development as an element of the hospitality industry and provides opportunities for growth in training management and program design through the sharing of ideas and networking among members. CHART participates in the establishment of curriculum standards in the hospitality industry.
Publications, reports, or services: Training, including food safety, for hospitality industry.

Culinary Institute of America (CIA)
433 Albany Post Rd.
Hyde Park, NY, 12538
Telephone: 914-452-9600
Web site: http://www.ciachef.edu/
Description: The institute offers associate's degree programs in culinary arts and baking and pastry arts; bachelor's degree programs in culinary arts management and baking and pastry arts management; as well as continuing education courses for food service professionals.
Publications, reports, or services: Offers continuing education in sanitation, sells training materials through its Food and Beverage Institute.

Dietary Managers Association (DMA)
406 Surrey Woods Dr.
St. Charles, IL, 60174
Telephone: 630-587-6336 Fax: 630-587-6308
Email address: Webmaster@dmaonline.org
Web site: http://www.dmaonline.org/
Description: Dietary Managers Association is a nonprofit association established in 1960 whose mission is to provide optimum nutritional care through food service management. DMA members work in hospitals, long-term care, schools, correctional facilities, and other non-commercial settings. The association provides career training and resources—continuing education and professional—and monitors industry trends and legislative issues.
Publications, reports, or services: Sponsors the Certified Food Protection Professional (CFPP) credential and training.

Educational Institute of the American Hotel & Motel Association
800 N. Magnolia Ave., Suite 1800
Orlando, FL, 32803
Telephone: 800-752-4567 Fax: 407-236-7848
Email address: info@ei-ahma.org
Web site: http://www.ei-ahma.org/ei1/index.htm
Description: The institute is the nonprofit educational foundation of the American Hotel & Motel Association. It provides industry-tested, research-driven training using videos, textbooks, courseware, seminars, multimedia CD-ROM programs, and self-paced learning courses on the Internet to reach all levels of personnel.
Publications, reports, or services: FastTrack series of retail food safety training videos, Food Safety the HACCP Way video, Quality Sanitation Management training guide.

Environmental Working Group (EWG)
1718 Connecticut Ave. NW, Suite 600
Washington, DC, 20009
Telephone: 202-667-6982 Fax: 202-232-3592
Email address: info@ewg.org
Web site: http://www.ewg.org
Description: Founded in 1993, EWG provides information and policy analysis to the general public, environmental organizations and other public interest groups, journalists, and policy makers. Food safety areas of special emphasis at EWG are the threat posed to infants and children by pesticides and other toxic chemicals, and drinking water contamination by pesticides and other pollutants.
Publications, reports, or services: All You Can Eat—a program that lets users input their diet and tells them how many and which pesticides likely came along for the ride. Web site has information on reducing consumption of pesticide residues and chemicals in drinking water.

European Food Information Council (EUFIC)
1, Place des Pyramides
Paris, France, 75001
Telephone: +33140204440 Fax: +33140204441
Email address: eufic@eufic.org
Web site: http://www.eufic.org
Description: The European Food Information Council is an independent, nonprofit organization based in Paris. It was established to provide health educators, opinion leaders, and the news media with science-based information on foods and food-related issues to inform consumers in the European Union about the nutritional quality and safety of foods.

Federal Trade Commission
600 Pennsylvania Ave. NW
Consumer Response Center, CRC-240
Washington, DC, 20580
Telephone: 877-FTC-HELP (382-4357)
Web site: http://www.ftc.gov/
Description: Enforces a variety of laws that protect consumers from unfair, deceptive, or fraudulent practices, including deceptive and unsubstantiated advertising. Food safety issues include labeling and false advertising.

Food & Water
389 Vermont Route #215
Walden, VT, 05873

Telephone: 800-EAT-SAFE
Email address: info@foodandwater.org
Web site: http://www.foodandwater.org/
Description: The main mission of this consumer group is to stop food irradiation.
Publications, reports, or services: Published the report, Meat Monopolies: Dirty Meat and the False Promises of Irradiation, and *Food Irradiation: An Activist Primer.*

Food Allergy Network (FAN)
10400 Eaton Place, Suite 107
Fairfax, VA, 22030-2208
Telephone: 703-691-3179 Fax: 703-691-2713
Email address: fan@worldWeb.net
Web site: http://www.foodallergy.org/
Description: The Food Allergy Network is a nonprofit organization established to increase public awareness about food allergy and anaphylaxis, to provide education, and to advance research on behalf of all of those affected by food allergies.
Publications, reports, or services: Produces Food Allergy News newsletter, food allergy cookbooks and videos, food product recall lists on their Web site and by email, background information and fact sheets on food allergies.

Food and Agriculture Organization
Food and Nutrition Division
Viale delle Terme di Caracalla
Rome, Italy, 00100
Telephone: +390657051 Fax: +390657053152
Email address: Food-Quality@FAO.org
Web site: http://www.fao.org/
Description: The Food and Agriculture Organization was founded in October 1945 as part of the United Nations with a mandate to raise levels of nutrition and standards of living, to improve agricultural productivity, and to better the condition of rural populations. Many FAO projects have a food safety component, especially on the topics of pesticides, drug residues, food additives, environmental contaminants, food biotechnology, and food safety risk assessment.
Publications, reports, or services: Reports and conference proceedings are on the Web site.

Food and Drug Law Institute (FDLI)
1000 Vermont Ave. NW, Suite 200
Washington, DC, 20005-4903
Telephone: 202-371-1420 Fax: 202-371-0649
Email address: comments@fdli.org
Web site: http://www.fdli.org/
Description: FDLI is a nonprofit educational organization dedicated to improving the understanding of the laws, regulations, and policies affecting the food and drug industry. FDLI is neutral and non-partisan, and it does not lobby or take a stand on any issue.
Publications, reports, or services: Produces books, periodicals, educational resources, and reference materials for professionals in the food, drug, cosmetics, medical device, biologics, and veterinary medical products areas.

Food Biotechnology Communications Network (FBCN)
1 Stone Road West
Fourth Floor NW
Guelph, Ontario, N1G 4Y2 Canada
Telephone: 877-FOOD-BIO
Fax: 519-826-3441
Email address: info@foodbiotech.org
Web site: http://www.foodbiotech.org
Description: The Food Biotechnology Communications Network is a Canadian source for balanced, science-based facts about food biotechnology and its impact on our food system. FBCN brings together all those interested in food biotechnology, from the farmer to the consumer. Formerly the Food Biotechnology Centre.
Publications, reports, or services: Offers a monthly fax newsletter, information about biotechnology foods approved in Canada, a regional network of experts, biotechnology items in the news, and the Information About Food Biotechnology kit.

Food Institute
Box 972, 28-12 Broadway
Fair Lawn, NJ, 07410
Telephone: 201-791-5570 Fax: 201-791-5222
Web site: http://www.foodinstitute.com/
Description: Founded in 1928, The Food Institute is a nonprofit information and reporting association. The membership of more than 2,200 companies in 50 states and in more than 40 foreign countries spans the entire food distribution system, from seed companies to grocery chains and all bases between. Members include growers, food processors, importers, exporters, brokers, wholesalers, supermarket chains, independent retailers, food industry suppliers, food service distributors, advertising and banking executives, government officials, and others.
Publications, reports, or services: Offers the Food Safety Issues newsletter to members.

Food Marketing Institute (FMI)
655 15th St. NW, Suite 700
Washington, DC, 20005
Telephone: 202-452-8444 Fax: 202-429-4519
Email address: fmi@fmi.org
Web site: http://www.fmi.org/
Description: The Food Marketing Institute is a nonprofit association for food retailers and wholesalers that conducts programs in research, education, industry relations, and public affairs on behalf of its 1,500 members and their subsidiaries in the United States and around the world.
Publications, reports, or services: FMI produces food safety training videos and posters for retail workers and managers; reports on food safety issues such as foodborne illness, irradiation, biotechnology, and pesticides; and consumer brochures on food preparation and storage.

Food Marketing Policy Center
Department of Agricultural and Resource Economics, University of Connecticut
U-21, 1376 Storrs Road
Storrs, CT, 06269-4021
Telephone: 860-486-1927
Fax: 860-486-2461
Email address: fmpc@canr.uconn.edu
Web site: http://vm.uconn.edu/~wwware/FMktC.html
Description: The Food Marketing Policy Center conducts research on food and agricultural marketing and related policy questions. The general intent is to provide information that can contribute to improved performance of the food production and marketing system. The Policy Center is primarily an economic research organization, yet it conducts interdisciplinary research when appropriate, and it communicates results to the public. Key users include farmer and consumer organizations, agribusiness firms, public agencies, state legislatures, and the U.S. Congress. The center serves as the core research group for Regional Research Project NE-165: Private Strategies, Public Policies, and Food System Performance.
Publications, reports, or services: Reports and issue papers on food safety include: Mandatory vs. Voluntary Approaches to Food Safety, The Economics of Food Safety, Modeling the Costs of Food Safety Regulation, Implementation of the WTO Agreement on the Application of Sanitary and Phytosanitary Measures: The First Two Years, and Improving Cost/Benefit Analysis for HACCP and Microbial Food Safety: An Economist's Overview.

Food Processors Institute (FPI)
1350 I St. NW
Washington, DC, 20005-3305
Telephone: 202-393-0890 Fax: 202-639-5941
Email address: fpi@nfpa-food.org
Web site: http://www.fpi-food.org/
Description: The Food Processors Institute is the nonprofit education provider for the National Food Processors Association. Established in 1973, FPI offers Better Process Control Schools; a core curriculum of workshops, seminars, materials, and text; Hazard Analysis Critical Control Point (HACCP) training; and other industry training.
Publications, reports, or services: Numerous books, videos, and software for the food industry.

Food Research Institute
Department of Food Microbiology and Toxicology, University of Wisconsin-Madison
1925 Willow Dr.
Madison, WI, 53706
Telephone: 608-263-7777 Fax: 608-263-1114
Web site: http://www.wisc.edu/fri/
Description: The mission of the Food Research Institute is to provide a leadership role in identifying and addressing food safety issues to meet community, industry, and government needs; interact with industry, regulators, academia, and consumers on food safety issues; provide accurate, useful information and expertise; and deliver quality education and training in food safety.
Publications, reports, or services: Web site contains technical briefings on current food safety topics.

Food Safeguards Council
1925 North Lynn St., Suite 725
Arlington, VA, 22209
Telephone: 703-276-8444 Fax: 703-276-8447
Email address: foodsafec@aol.com
Description: The Food Safeguards Council is a nonprofit organization founded in 1996 in an attempt to form an industry-supported base to encourage food safety and the use of scientific methods to protect the public health. They have attempted to promote food irradiation and educate people about that process.

Food Safety Training and Education Alliance for Retail, Food Service, Vending, Institutions, and Regulators (FSTEA)
Web site: http://www.fstea.org
Description: Formed in 1998, FSTEA's mission is to reduce the risk of foodborne illness by coordinating efforts of government, industry, and educators to change behaviors of food workers, managers, and regulators through training and education based on current science as reflected in the Food Code. It's objectives include identifying competencies for food safety training, coordinating and sharing existing food safety training materials, promoting safe food preparation behaviors in food establishments, identifying languages/cultures where there is a need for food safety training, and promoting the development and delivery of multicultural programs.

Food Safety Research Information Office (FSRIO)
10301 Baltimore Ave.
National Agricultural Library
Beltsville, MD, 20705-2351
Email address: fsrio@nal.usd.gov
Web site: http://www.nal.usda.gov/fsrio
Description: The USDA's Food Safety Research Information Office is responsible for collecting government-funded and private food safety research information and making it accessible through the Web and by other means. Additionally, Internet links to other food safety resources are maintained.

Food Safety Consortium
University of Arkansas
110 Agriculture Building
Fayetteville, AR, 72701
Telephone: 501-575-5647 Fax: 501-575-7531
Email address: fsc@cavern.uark.edu.
Web site: http://www.uark.edu/depts/fsc/
Description: The Food Safety Consortium consists of researchers from the University of Arkansas, Iowa State University, and Kansas State University. The consortium was established by Congress in 1988 through a special USDA Cooperative State Research Service grant. The consortium's charge is to conduct extensive investigation into all areas of poultry, beef, and pork production and safety, from the farm to the consumer's table.
Publications, reports, or services: Web site has information about food safety—related research projects sponsored by the consortium, lists upcoming meetings and conferences, and links to other food safety sites.

Foodservice & Packaging Institute
1550 Wilson Blvd., Suite 701
Arlington, VA, 22209
Telephone: 703-527-7505 Fax: 703-527-7512
Email address: fpi@fpi.org
Web site: http://www.fpi.org/
Description: The Foodservice & Packaging Institute is the trade association for manufacturers, suppliers, and distributors of food service disposable products. FPI's mission is to promote the sanitation, safety, functional, economic, and environmental benefits of food service disposables.
Publications, reports, or services: Offers Take Aim at Sanitation video, conducts sanitation studies demonstrating the sanitary advantages of food service disposables.

Food Temperature Indicator Association (FTIA)
5470-B Oakbrook Parkway
Norcross, GA, 30093
Telephone: 770-441-1443 Fax: 770-441-3258
Description: Formed in 1999, the Food Temperature Indicator Association is a nonprofit organization for temperature indicator manufacturers, distributors, and allied industries associated with cooking temperatures and food safety. FTIA links the government, industry, and the consumer in advocating good food safety practices and proper usage of the variety of available food temperature indicators.

Gastroenteric Disease Center
The Pennsylvania State University
115 Henning Building
University Park, PA, 16802
Telephone: 814-863-2630 Fax: 814-863-6140
Web site: http://ecoli.cas.psu.edu
Description: Located in the Department of Veterinary Science at Penn State, the center serves as a laboratory and reference center for diagnosing cultures from outside sources. The Web site has extensive links to information about *E. coli* outbreaks, laboratory methods, legislation, animal health, and journals.
Publications, reports, or services: Repository of *E. coli* strains, information on *E. coli* detecting test kits.

George Washington University Center for Career Education
2029 K St. NW, Suite 600
Washington, DC, 20006
Telephone: 202-973-1150 Fax: 202-973-1165
Email address: cce@www.gwu.edu
Web site: http://www.gwu.edu/~cce/programs/
Description: Offers a professional advancement program in food studies for those pursuing a career in food and food-related businesses, including government regulators, trade association executives, food service professionals, and owners and managers of food-related businesses. Courses include food regulation and policy, food safety, food writing, food trends, and consumer advocacy in food safety.

Government Accountability Project (GAP)
1402 Third Ave., Suite 1215
Seattle, WA, 98101
Telephone: 206-292-2850
Email address: gap@whistleblower.org
Web site: http://www.whistleblower.org/
Description: The mission of the Government Accountability Project is to protect the public interest and promote government and corporate accountability by advancing occupational free speech, defending whistleblowers, and empowering citizen activists. It also advises public agencies and legislative bodies about management policies and practices that help government deal more effectively with substantive information and concerns, while protecting the jobs and identities of those who provide this critical information. GAP's Safe Food Campaign focuses on inspection issues in meat and poultry processing plants and government reform of the food safety system.
Publications, reports, or services: Reports, press releases, and white papers on food safety inspection.

Greenpeace
702 H Street NW
Washington, DC 20001
Telephone: 800-326-0959
Web site: http://www.greenpeace.org/
Description: Greenpeace's involvement with food safety consists mainly of their stance against genetically engineered foods.
Publications, reports, or services: Maintains on the Web site the True Food Shopping List: How to Avoid Genetically Engineered Food, a list that categorizes thousands of companies' brand-name food products based on their policies towards genetically engineered ingredients.

Grocery Manufacturers of America (GMA)
1010 Wisconsin Ave. NW, Ninth Floor
Washington, DC, 20007
Telephone: 202-337-9400 Fax: 202-337-4508
Email address: info@gmabrands.com
Web site: http://www.gmabrands.com/
Description: GMA is the trade association of food, beverage, and consumer product companies. The organization applies legal, scientific, and political expertise from its member companies to food safety, nutrition, and public policy issues affecting the industry.
Publications, reports, or services: Press releases, testimony, and background papers on biotechnology, food safety, irradiation, and food safety regulation.

The Groundwater Foundation
P.O. Box 22558
Lincoln, NE, 68542-2558
Telephone: 800-858-4844 Fax: 402-434-2742
Email address: info@groundwater.org
Web site: http://www.groundwater.org/
Description: The Groundwater Foundation is a nonprofit organization dedicated to informing the public about groundwater. Through programs and publications it shows the benefits everyone receives from groundwater and the very real risks to groundwater. The foundation strives to make learning about groundwater fun and understandable for kids and adultsalike.
Publications, reports, or services: Community action guides, workshop guides, children's videos and games, books, and brochures on groundwater. Web site has a page for kids.

Ground Water Protection Council (GWPC)
827 N.W. 63rd, Suite 103
Oklahoma City, OK, 73116
Telephone: 405-516-4972 Fax: 405-516-4973
Web site: http://www.site.net/
Description: The Ground Water Protection Council (GWPC) is a nonprofit organization whose members consist of state and federal groundwater agencies, industry representatives, environmentalists, and concerned citizens, all of whom come together within the GWPC organization to mutually work towards the protection of the nation's groundwater supplies. The purpose of the GWPC is to promote and ensure the use of best manage-

ment practices and fair but effective laws regarding comprehensive groundwater protection.

Publications, reports, or services: Web site has on online newsletter, reports, information on technology and legislation. There is also a home page for source water protection.

Institute of Food Research
Norwich Research Park
Colney, Norwich, UK, NR4 7UA
Telephone: +4401603255000 Fax: +4401603507723
Web site: http://www.ifrn.bbsrc.ac.uk/

Description: The institute's mission is to carry out independent, basic, strategic research on food safety, quality, nutrition, and health problems. In addition to research, the institute is involved in food safety and science education.

Publications, reports, or services: Publishes Science Briefs designed for journalists on food science and food safety topics to give an introduction to "science in progress"; and Food Science Information Sheets for use by school students, teachers, and the public, which also include food safety topics.

Institute of Food Science and Technology (IFST)
5 Cambridge Ct.
210 Shepherd's Bush Road
London, UK, W6 7NJ
Telephone: +4401716036316 Fax: +4401716029936
Email address: ifst@easynet.co.uk
Web site: http://www.ifst.org/

Description: IFST is an independent incorporated professional organization of food scientists and technologists who work to promote a wider understanding of food science and technology and its contribution to society and the well-being of consumers. The institute serves the public interest by furthering the application of science and technology in all aspects of the supply of safe, wholesome, nutritious, and attractive food, both nationally and internationally.

Publications, reports, or services: The Web site has numerous food safety papers on topics such as AIDS and the food handler, BSE, *Listeria* and other pathogens, risk assessment, irradiation, food allergens, home food safety, and more.

Institute of Food Technologists (IFT)
221 N. LaSalle St., Suite 300
Chicago, IL, 60601-1291
Telephone: 312-782-8424 Fax: 312-782-8348
Email address: info@ift.org
Web site: http://www.ift.org/

Description: Founded in 1939, the Institute of Food Technologists is a nonprofit scientific society with 28,000 members working in food science, food technology, and related professions in industry, academia, and government. The main mission of IFT is to advance the science and technology of food through the exchange of knowledge.

Publications, reports, or services: Publishes numerous backgrounders, statements, and testimonies on topics such as policy and regulation of food safety in the United States, BSE, food additives, food biotechnology, pesticides, and irradiation. IFT operates a national network of more than 70 university-based scientists trained to deliver the scientific perspective on food issues to the news media. IFT is also heavily involved in student education, offering awards, scholarships, and fellowships.

International Association for Food Protection
6200 Aurora Ave., Suite 200W
Des Moines, IA, 50322-2863
Telephone: 800-369-6337 Fax: 515-276-8655
Web site: http://www.foodprotection.org

Description: Formerly known as the International Association of Milk, Food and Environmental Sanitarians, the association's mission is to provide food safety professionals worldwide with a forum to exchange information on protecting the food supply. The association provides members with information on rapidly changing technologies, innovations and regulations, the latest findings in research, and contacts outside of their individual areas of expertise. Members work in all areas of food protection—industry, government, and academia.

Publications, reports, or services: Publishes two journals—Journal of Food Protection and Dairy, Food and Environmental Sanitation, and develops other food safety materials for sanitarians and consumers.

International Association of Culinary Professionals (IACP)
304 West Liberty St., Suite 201
Louisville, KY, 40202
Telephone: 502-581-9786 Fax: 502-589-3602
Email address: iacp@hqtrs.com
Web site: http://www.iacp-online.org/

Description: IACP is a worldwide society of professionals working in the many diverse facets of the culinary industry. The association provides continuing education and professional development for its members, as well as unique networking and special promotional opportunities.

Publications, reports, or services: Offers the Certified Culinary Professional program, which includes knowledge of food safety; provides tuition credit and cash scholarships annually to persons pursuing or furthering careers in the culinary arts.

International Bottled Water Association (IBWA)
1700 Diagonal Road, Suite 650
Alexandria, VA, 22314
Telephone: 703-683-5213 Fax: 703-683-4074
Web site: http://www.bottledwater.org/
Description: Founded in 1958, the International Bottled Water Association is the trade association representing the bottled water industry. IBWA plays an active role at all levels of state and federal government assisting in the development of stringent regulations for bottled water to ensure the greatest safety possible and high quality of bottled water products. IBWA has supported the U.S. Food and Drug Administration and state regulators/legislators in the development of strict regulations that will help guarantee bottled water's quality.

Publications, reports, or services: IBWA Model Code for bottled water, consumer and industry publications, Web site has FAQs and regulatory information.

International Commission on Microbiological Specifications for Foods (ICMSF)
Email address: John.Pitt@foodscience.afisc.csiro.au
Web site: http://www.dfst.csiro.au/icmsf.htm
Description: The International Commission on Microbiological Specifications for Foods is a nonprofit, scientific advisory body established in 1962 and is under the auspices of the International Union of Microbiological Societies (IUMS). Its primary goal is to provide timely, science-based guidance to government and industry on appraising and controlling the microbiological safety of foods. The main objectives of ICMSF have been to provide the scientific basis for microbiological criteria and to promote principles for their establishment and application, and to overcome the difficulties caused by nations' varying microbiological standards and analytical methods. Currently, emphasis is being given to the safety of foods in international commerce, the application of HACCP, and new quality assurance systems that incorporate science-based risk assessment to provide cost-effective control of food safety.

International Consultative Group on Food Irradiation (ICGFI)
Food and Environmental Protection Section, Joint FAO/IAEA Division of Nuclear Techniques in Food and Agriculture, International Atomic Energy Agency
Wagramerstrasse 5, P.O. Box 100
A-1400 Vienna, Austria
Telephone: 4312600 ext. 21638 or 21639 Fax: 43126007
Email address: Official.Mail@iaea.org
Web site: http://www.iaea.org/icgfi/
Description: In 1982 the directors general of FAO, IAEA, and WHO invited member states to consider forming a consultative group to focus on international cooperation in food irradiation. It was conceived as an independent body composed of government-designated experts. The functions of ICGFI are to evaluate global developments in the field of food irradiation, provide a focal point of advice on the application of food irradiation, and furnish information on the wholesomeness of irradiated food.

Publications, reports, or services: Maintains a database of which foods have been cleared for irradiation in which countries and a database of authorized food irradiation facilities around the world, publishes documents on the safety, legislation, and practical applications of food irradiation.

International Dairy-Deli-Bakery Association (IDDBA)
P.O. Box 5528
Madison, WI, 53705-0528
Telephone: 608-238-7908 Fax: 608-238-6330
Email address: Education@iddba.org
Web site: http://www.iddanet.org/
Description: IDDBA is a trade association that brings together retailers, manufacturers, brokers, distributors, and interested industry professionals who are united in providing safe, high-quality dairy, deli, and bakery products to the consumer.

Publications, reports, or services: Offers a variety of training programs that cover, among other topics, food safety and sanitation, such as the Be Safe, Not Sorry training kit for dairy-deli-bakery workers.

International Flight Catering Association (IFCA)
Surrey Place, Mill Ln., Godalming,
Surrey, UK, GU7 1EY
Telephone: +4401483419449
Fax: +4401483419780
Email address: mail@ifcanet.com
Web site: http://www.ifcanet.com/
Description: IFCA is a trade association for airlines, caterers, and those who supply products and equipment to airlines. It offers food safety and sanitation training and publishes food safety training materials for the in-flight catering industry.
Publications, reports, or services: HACCP booklets, Flight Catering Guide, A Travel Guide to Food Safety for Cabin Crew.

International Food Information Council Foundation (IFIC)
1100 Connecticut Ave. NW, Suite 430
Washington, DC, 20036
Email address: foodinfo@ific.health.org
Web site: http://ificinfo.health.org/
Description: Founded in 1985, the International Food Information Council is a nonprofit organization whose mission is to communicate science-based information on food safety and nutrition to health and nutrition professionals, educators, government officials, journalists, and others providing information to consumers. IFIC bridges the gap between science and communications by collecting and disseminating scientific information on food safety, nutrition, and health and by working with an extensive roster of scientific experts to help translate research into understandable and useful information for opinion leaders and, ultimately, consumers.
Publications, reports, or services: Publishes numerous documents for professionals, media, educators, and consumers on food irradiation, food biotechnology, foodborne illness, food additives, pesticide residues, and food allergies.

International Food Safety Council
Telephone: 312-715-1010 ext. 345
Web site: http://www.foodsafetycouncil.org/
Description: Organized in 1993 by the National Restaurant Association Educational Foundation, the council is a restaurant and food service industry coalition committed to education about safe food preparation and handling. The council's mission is to heighten the awareness of the importance of food safety education worldwide.
Publications, reports, or services: The council sponsors a variety of programs, including National Food Safety Education Month each September for which it prepares food safety training and promotional materials. Publishes Best Practices: Professional's Guide to Food Safety and Sanitation, a quarterly publication.

International Food Service Executives Association (IFSEA)
1100 S. State Road 7, Suite 103
Margate, FL, 33068
Telephone: 954-977-0767 Fax: 954-977-0874
Email address: hq@ifsea.org
Web site: http://www.ifsea.org/
Description: Organized in 1901, the International Food Service Executives Association is the food service industry's trade association for management-level professionals in all aspects of the food service and hospitality industry.
Publications, reports, or services: Offers National Food Manager Certification and HACCP training. Has scholarships for students.

International Fresh-Cut Produce Association
1600 Duke St., Suite 440
Alexandria, VA, 22314-3400
Telephone: 703-299-6282 Fax: 703-299-6288
Email address: fresh-cuts@fresh-cuts.org
Web site: http://www.fresh-cuts.org/
Description: The International Fresh-Cut Produce Association advances the industry by supporting its members with technical information, representation, and knowledge to provide convenient, safe, and wholesome food.
Publications, reports, or services: Publishes food safety and HACCP guides for fresh-cut produce, offers educational and technical seminars on food safety issues.

International HACCP Alliance
Texas A&M University
120 Rosenthal Center
College Station, TX, 77843-2259
Telephone: 409-862-3643 Fax: 409-862-3075
Email address: kharris@ifse.tamu.edu
Web site: http://haccpalliance.org
Description: The International HACCP Alliance was formed to provide a uniform program to assure safer meat and poultry products. The alliance is comprised of interested industry associations and is affiliated with several federal agencies, universities, and professional societies. Members de-

velop and disseminate standardized training materials for the meat and poultry industry.

Publications, reports, or services: Provides HACCP and other food safety information for the meat and poultry industry, offers training and videoconferences on food safety, develops approved training curricula.

International Inflight Food Service Association (IFSA)
304 West Liberty St., Suite 201
Louisville, KY, 40202
Telephone: 502-583-3783 Fax: 502-589-3602
Email address: ifsa@hqtrs.com
Web site: http://www.ifsanet.com
Description: Part of IFSA's mission is to develop and promote uniform standards of quality, sanitation, and safety within the in-flight food service industry.
Publications, reports, or services: Offers HACCP workshops for the in-flight food industry.

International Life Sciences Institute (ILSI)
1126 Sixteenth St. NW, Suite 300
Washington, DC, 20036
Telephone: 202-659-0074 Fax: 202-659-3859
Email address: ilsi@ilsi.org
Web site: http://www.ilsi.org
Description: The International Life Sciences Institute is a worldwide foundation that is making a difference in public health by advancing the understanding of scientific issues related to nutrition, food safety, toxicology, and the environment. By bringing together scientists from academia, government, industry, and the public sector, ILSI seeks a balanced approach to solving problems with broad implications for the well-being of the general public.
Publications, reports, or services: Exposure to Contaminants in Drinking Water: Estimating Uptake Through the Skin and by Inhalation, Safety of Water Disinfection: Balancing Chemical and Microbial Risks, Water Quality in Latin America: Balancing the Microbial and Chemical Risks in Drinking Water Disinfection, Microwave Ovens, Food Biotechnology: An Introduction, A Simple Guide to Understanding and Applying the Hazard Analysis Critical Control Point (HACCP) Concept, Food Allergy and Other Adverse Reactions to Food.

International Packaged Ice Association (IPIA)
P.O. Box 1199
Tampa, FL, 33601
Telephone: 800-742-0267 Fax: 813-251-2783
Email address: jane@packagedice.com
Web site: http://www.packagedice.com/
Description: The Packaged Ice Association is an international trade association representing manufacturers and distributors of packaged ice and manufacturers of ice-making equipment and supplies. PIA provides its members with educational information and sponsors meetings, publications, and seminars to update members on the most efficient, cost-effective ways to operate both large and small ice businesses.
Publications, reports, or services: Ice-The Forgotten Food video on ice food safety, A Guide to the Sanitation of Packaged Ice, and Ice News bimonthly publication.

International Sprout Growers Association (ISGA)
P.O. Box 2214
Amherst, MA, 01004-2214
Telephone: 413-253-8965
Email address: sprout1221@aol.com
Web site: http://www.isga-sprouts.org/
Description: As the professional association for sprout growers, ISGA promotes the sprout industry by encouraging the exchange of information among sprout growers and commercial suppliers. It is active in educating and informing members about important issues impacting the sprout industry, especially food safety.
Publications, reports, or services: Web site has full-text HACCP checklist for sprout growers, offers seminars and workshops on sprout safety.

Interstate Shellfish Sanitation Conference (ISSC)
115 Atrium Way, Suite 117
Columbia, SC, 29223-6382
Telephone: 803-788-7559 Fax: 803-788-7576
Email address: info@issc.org
Web site: http://www.issc.org/
Description: The Interstate Shellfish Sanitation Conference was formed in 1982 to foster and promote shellfish sanitation through the cooperation of state and federal control agencies, the shellfish industry, and the academic community. To achieve this purpose the ISSC adopts uniform procedures, incorporated into an Interstate Shellfish Sanitation Program, and implemented by all

shellfish control agencies; gives state shellfish programs current and comprehensive sanitation guidelines to regulate the harvesting, processing, and shipping of shellfish; provides a forum for shellfish control agencies, the shellfish industry, and the academic community to resolve major issues concerning shellfish sanitation; and informs all interested parties of recent developments in shellfish sanitation and other major issues of concern through the use of news media, publications, regional and national meetings, the Internet, and by working closely with academic institutions and trade associations.

Publications, reports, or services: Web site has documents for industry and shellfish education FAQs for consumers.

Joint Institute for Food Safety and Applied Nutrition (JIFSAN)
0220 Symons Hall
College Park, MD, 20742
Telephone: 301-405-8382 Fax: 301-405-8390
Web site: http://www.jifsan.umd.edu/
Description: Established in 1996, the institute is a jointly administered, multidisciplinary research and education program and includes research components from the FDA Centers for Food Safety and Applied Nutrition (CFSAN) and Veterinary Medicine (CVM) and the University of Maryland. The institute fosters the missions of FDA and the university through the creation of partnerships to increase the quantity and quality of research that will provide the basis for sound public health policy. It promotes food safety, human nutrition, and animal health and production through an integrated academic and regulatory science program that includes multidisciplinary research, outreach and educational programs, and policy studies.

Publications, reports, or services: Home of the Food Safety Risk Assessment Clearinghouse, offers food safety research internships and seminars on food safety topics.

Joint Institute for Food Safety Research (JIFSR)
Description: The mission of the Joint Institute for Food Safety Research is to efficiently coordinate all federal food safety research, including that with the private sector and academia, and to foster effective translation of research results into practice along the farm-to-table continuum. The ultimate goal of JIFSR is to coordinate food safety research, such that the incidence of foodborne illness is reduced to the greatest extent feasible. Leadership of the institute is shared between DHHS and USDA.

Mothers & Others
40 W. 20th St.
New York, NY, 10011-4211
Telephone: 212-242-0010
Email address: Mothers@mothers.org
Web site: http://www.mothers.org
Description: Mothers & Others, a national nonprofit education organization, works to promote consumer choices that are safe and ecologically sustainable for this generation and the next. By providing strategies that can reduce individual and community consumption of natural resources, and by mobilizing consumers to seek sustainable choices, it aims to effect lasting protection of public health and the environment. In the food safety realm, this group involves itself with pesticide residue and food biotechnology issues.

Publications, reports, or services: Organizes campaigns against genetically engineered foods and other "non-green" products and practices.

Mothers for Natural Law
P.O. Box 1177
Fairfield, IA, 52556
Telephone: 515-472-2809
Email address: mothers@fairfield.com
Web site: http://www.safe-food.org/
Description: Mothers for Natural Law is an organization formed to fight the genetic engineering of food. It campaigns to ban genetically engineered foods and to require mandatory labeling. Activities include a national public awareness campaign on the dangers of genetically engineered foods, finding genetically natural sources of ingredients for food manufacturers and producers, promoting a certification procedure for a "non-GE" label, and working to keep genetic engineering out of developing nations and out of the organic market.

Publications, reports, or services: Operates Consumer Right to Know Hotline: 877-REAL-FOOD, provides lists of non-GE foods for food manufacturers and consumers.

National Agricultural Biotechnology Council (NABC)
419 Boyce Thompson Institute
Tower Road
Ithaca, NY, 14853
Telephone: 607-254-4856

Email address: NABC@cornell.edu
Web site: http://www.cals.cornell.edu/extension/nabc/
Description: NABC provides an open forum to discuss agricultural biotechnology issues and encourage the ethical, safe, efficacious, and equitable development of the products and processes of agricultural biotechnology. Founded in 1988 by the Boyce Thompson Institute in collaboration with Cornell University, Iowa State University, and the University of California-Davis, the council is composed of senior management of the major nonprofit agricultural biotechnology research and/or teaching institutions in Canada and the United States.
Publications, reports, or services: Holds annual meetings and issues reports on agricultural biotechnology topics.

National Alliance for Food Safety (NAFS)
University of Arkansas
205 Agriculture Building
Fayetteville, AR, 72701
Telephone: 501-575-4446 Fax: 501-575-7273
Email address: nafs@cavern.uark.edu
Web site: http://www.uark.edu/depts/nafs/
Description: Formed in 1998, the National Alliance for Food Safety is composed of universities, government agencies, industry, and consumer groups who engage in major planning and coordination of activities in food safety research, education, and outreach. NAFS provides the overall framework, creating a partnership among universities and the federal government to identify needed research and education strategies with the aim towards better streamlining and allocation of the nation's limited food safety research and education resources.
Publications, reports, or services: Provides opportunities for collaboration among scientists engaged in all aspects of food safety research.

National Association of Catering Executives (NACE)
5565 Sterrett Place, Suite 328
Columbia, MD, 21044
Telephone: 410-997-9055 Fax: 410-997-8834
Web site: http://www.nace.net/
Description: The mission of NACE is to assist caterers in achieving career success by raising the level of education and professionalism of the catering industry.
Publications, reports, or services: Offers the Certified Professional Catering Executive certification, which includes knowledge of food safety.

National Association of College & University Food Services (NACUFS)
1405 S. Harrison Rd., Manly Miles Building, Suite 305
Michigan State University
East Lansing, MI, 48824-5242
Telephone: 517-332-2494 Fax: 517-332-8144
Email address: Webmaster@nacufs.org
Web site: http://www.nacufs.org
Description: The National Association of College & University Food Services is the trade association for food service professionals at more than 600 institutions of higher education in the United States, Canada, and abroad. Founded in 1958, NACUFS provides members with a full range of educational programs, publications, management services, and networking opportunities.
Publications, reports, or services: Training videos in personal hygiene, liability, sanitation; food service equipment database; grants to college sophomores, juniors, and seniors majoring in a food service field or employed by a college or university dining service; summer internships for food service management; job bulletin board.

National Association of County Health Officials (NACCHO)
1100 17th St., Second Floor
Washington, DC, 20036
Telephone: 202-783-5550 Fax: 202-783-1583
Web site: http://www.naccho.org
Description: NACCHO is a nonprofit membership organization serving all of the nearly 3,000 local health departments nationwide in cities, counties, townships, and districts. NACCHO provides education, information, research, and technical assistance to local health departments and facilitates partnerships among local, state, and federal agencies to promote and strengthen public health.
Publications, reports, or services: Works with health departments to strengthen their food protection and water quality programs,

National Association of State Departments of Agriculture (NASDA)
1156 15th St. NW, Suite 1020
Washington, DC, 20005
Telephone: 202-296-9680
Email address: nasda@patriot.net

Web site: http://www.nasda.org/nasda/nasda/index1.htm

Description: The association's mission is to support and promote the American agriculture industry, while protecting consumers and the environment, through the development, implementation, and communication of sound public policy and programs. NASDA's members are the executive heads (commissioners, secretaries, and directors) of the departments of agriculture in the 50 states and four territories. Members are involved in food safety legislation and policy matters.

Publications, reports, or services: Issues policy statements and backgrounders on animal health, biotechnology, food regulations, and pesticides.

National Automatic Merchandising Association (NAMA)

20 N. Wacker Dr., Suite 3500
Chicago, IL, 60606-3102
Telephone: 312-346-0370 Fax: 312-704-4140
Web site: http://www.vending.org/

Description: The National Automatic Merchandising Association is the national trade association of the food and refreshment vending and contract food service management industry.

Publications, reports, or services: Provides food safety training materials for vending machine operators.

National Cattlemen's Beef Association (NCBA)

1301 Pennsylvania Ave. NW, Suite 300
Washington, DC, 20004
Telephone: 202-347-0228 Fax: 202-638-0607
Email address: cows@beef.org
Web site: http://www.beef.org/

Description: Initiated in 1898, the National Cattlemen's Beef Association is the marketing organization and trade association for America's cattle farmers and ranchers. With offices in Denver, Chicago, and Washington, NCBA is a consumer-focused, producer-directed organization representing the nation's food and fiber industry. NCBA works to achieve the vision: "A dynamic and profitable beef industry, which concentrates resources around a unified plan, consistently meets global consumer needs and increases demand."

Publications, reports, or services: Web site has many consumer food safety documents and an Ask a Food-Safety Expert email address.

National Center for Food and Agricultural Policy (NCFAP)

1616 P St. NW, First Floor
Washington, DC, 20036
Telephone: 202-328-5048 Fax: 202-328-5133
Email address: stovall@ncfap.org
Web site: http://www.ncfap.org/

Description: The National Center for Food and Agricultural Policy is a nonprofit, nongovernmental organization whose purpose is to provide objective research and educational information on policy issues relating to U.S. and global agricultural policy issues.

Publications, reports, or services: Web site has sections on food safety and sanitary and phytosanitary (SPS) issues and pesticide use.

National Center for Food Safety & Technology (NCFST)

Illinois Institute of Technology
6502 South Archer Rd.
Summit-Argo, IL, 60501-9998
Telephone: 708-563-1576 Fax: 708-563-1873
Web site: http://www.iit.edu/~ncfs/

Description: NCFST is a unique consortium organized to address the complex issues raised by emerging food technologies. It is a place where academia, industry, and government pool their resources and work together to achieve the ultimate goal—ensuring the continued safety and quality of the nation's food supply. NCFST goals are to better understand the science and engineering behind food safety; conduct research promoting the safety and quality of the U.S. food supply; and conduct research needed to answer regulatory questions related to food safety. Staffing at NCFST includes food scientists from Illinois Institute of Technology, University of Illinois in Urbana-Champaign, 50 food companies, and the Food and Drug Administration.

Publications, reports, or services: Offers courses on food safety and microbiology, graduate research assistant positions are available, unique opportunities to apply theoretical research to pilot programs.

National Center for Toxicological Research

3900 NCTR Road
Jefferson, AR 72079
Web site: http://www.fda.gov/nctr/

Description: As part of the U.S. Food and Drug Administration, the National Center for Toxicological Research conducts peer-reviewed scientific research that supports and anticipates the FDA's current and future regulatory needs. Program initiatives include food safety, bioterrorism, biotechnology, and antimicrobial resistance.

Publications, reports, or services: The center's Science Internship Program is designed for science and mathematics students enrolled full-time in undergraduate or graduate schools located in the NCTR commuting area.

National Council for Science and the Environment (NCSE)

(Formerly the Committee for the National Institute for the Environment)
1725 K St. NW, Suite 212
Washington, DC, 20006-1401
Telephone: 202-530-5810 Fax: 202-628-4311
Email address: cnie@cnie.org
Web site: http://www.cnie.org/

Description: NCSE is a nonprofit organization dedicated to information dissemination by providing free, educational, non-advocacy resources such as daily news, congressional reports and briefings, laws and treaties, and educational resources.

Publications, reports, or services: NCSE makes available online in full-text Congressional Research Service reports that are prepared for the U.S. Congress. Some of these reports are on food safety topics.

National Drinking Water Clearinghouse

West Virginia University
P.O. Box 6064
Morgantown, WV, 26506-6064
Telephone: 800-624-8301 Fax: 304-293-3161
Email address: Webmaster@mail.estd.wvu.edu
Web site: http://www.estd.wvu.edu/ndwc/DiscussionFrame.html

Description: Intended for communities with fewer than 10,000 people and those who work with them, the National Drinking Water Clearinghouse (NDWC) assists small communities by collecting, developing, and providing timely information relevant to drinking water issues. The NDWC's technical assistants are available to answer questions related to drinking water.

Publications, reports, or services: NDWC maintains databases containing information on groundwater protection, water system design, water treatment processes, water conservation, alternative technologies and equipment manufacturers, drinking water regulations, water quality, and finance. The Web site has technical briefs and other drinking water–related information.

National Drinking Water Advisory Council

401 M St. SW
Washington, DC, 20460-0003
Telephone: 202-260-5543 Fax: 202-260-4383
Web site: http://www.epa.gov/safewater/ndwac/council.html

Description: The council, comprising members of the general public, state and local agencies, and private groups concerned with safe drinking water, serves in an advisory role to the EPA on everything that the agency does relating to drinking water. Twelve working groups concentrate on various issues related to water safety.

National Environmental Health Association (NEHA)

720 South Colorado Blvd.
South Tower, Suite 970
Denver, CO, 80246-1925
Telephone: 303-756-9090 Fax: 303-691-9490
Email address: staff@neha.org
Web site: http://www.neha.org/

Description: The mission of the National Environmental Health Association is "to advance the environmental health and protection professional for the purpose of providing a healthful environment for all."

Publications, reports, or services: NEHA offers the Registered Environmental Health Specialist/Registered Sanitarian (REHS/RS) and the Certified Food Safety Professional (CFSP) credentials. Supports the food safety professional through its food safety publications and annual meeting, offers undergraduate- and graduate-level scholarships.

National Fisheries Institute (NFI)

1901 N. Fort Myer Dr., Suite 700
Arlington, VA,
Telephone: 703-524-8880
Web site: http://www.nfi.org/

Description: NFI advocates the interests of the fish and seafood industry in Congress and before regulatory agencies. This includes firms operating fishing vessels and aquaculture facilities; those who buy, sell, process, pack, import, export, and distribute fish and seafood; and operators of retail stores and restaurants.

Publications, reports, or services: NFI sponsors HACCP workshops, offers seafood safety information for consumers on their Web site; science and technology staff provides technical information on food safety issues for industry.

National Food Safety and Toxicology Center
Food Safety and Toxicology Building, Room 165
East Lansing, MI, 48824-1302
Telephone: 517-432-3100
Email address: argeleri@msu.edu
Web site: http://foodsafe.msu.edu/
Description: The mission of the National Food Safety and Toxicology Center is to conduct research that will increase understanding of chemical and microbial hazards in foods, and to use this knowledge to develop a safer food supply, well-founded public policy, and a greater public understanding of food safety issues. The central concept underlying these goals is risk analysis involving the identification, assessment, management, and communication of risk.
Publications, reports, or services: Sponsors food safety training courses and research.

National Food Service Management Institute (NFSMI)
P.O. Drawer 188
University of Mississippi
University, MS, 38677-0188
Telephone: 800-321-3054 Fax: 800-321-3061
Email address: nfsmi@olemiss.edu
Web site: http://www.nfsmi.org/
Description: The mission of NFSMI is to provide information and services that promote the continuous improvement of child nutrition programs—school lunch, school breakfast, summer feeding, child and adult care, and Nutrition Education and Training (NET).
Publications, reports, or services: NFSMI provides food safety curricula and information, conducts applied research, and offers food safety training and education.

National Food Processors Association (NFPA)
1350 I St. NW, Suite 300
Washington, DC, 20005
Telephone: 202-639-5900 Fax: 202-639-5932
Email address: nfpa@nfpa-food.org
Web site:
For industry http://www.nfpa-food.org/.
For consumers http://safefood.org/
Description: NFPA is the voice of the food processing industry on scientific and public policy issues involving food safety, nutrition, technical and regulatory matters, and consumer affairs. It translates food science and technical knowledge into public policy strategies and communications programs, and offers food science and technical expertise to members.
Publications, reports, or services: Updates on policy and regulatory issues affecting the food industry, maintains the consumer food safety Web site.

National Grocers Association
1825 Samuel Morse Dr.
Reston, VA, 20190-5317
Telephone: 703-437-5300 Fax: 703-437-7768
Email address: info@NationalGrocers.org
Web site: http://www.nationalgrocers.org/
Description: The National Grocers Association is the national trade association representing retail and wholesale grocers that comprise the independent sector of the food distribution industry. The Grocers Research and Education Foundation, a nonprofit organization formed by NGA in 1992, serves the industry through industry research and educational programs.
Publications, reports, or services: Under the Grocers Research and Education Foundation, the National Grocers Association has established a food safety education program that includes classroom training, certification, and educational tools that assist employees in practicing proper food safety and sanitation. Scholarships are available.

National Institute for Animal Agriculture (NIAA)
1910 Lyda Ave.
Bowling Green, KY, 42104
Telephone: 270-782-9798 Fax: 270-782-0188
Email address: NIAA@animalagriculture.org
Web site: http://www.animalagriculture.org
Description: Formerly known as the Livestock Conservation Institute, NIAA is a nonprofit, consensus-building organization whose members influence the direction of research, product development, and regulations related to safe food animal production. Its mission is to unify organizations, allied industries, government agencies, researchers, and individuals interested in cooperatively addressing animal health, animal welfare, and food safety issues as they affect animal agriculture in North America.
Publications, reports, or services: Publishes materials related to animal health.

National Institute for Science, Law and Public Policy (NISLAPP)
1424 16th St. NW, Suite 105
Washington, DC, 20036

Telephone: 202-462-8800 Fax: 202-265-656
Email address: NISLAPP@swankin-turner.com
Web site: http://www.swankin-turner.com/nislapp/
Description: Founded in 1978 as a nonprofit organization by attorneys, scientists, and public policy planners, the National Institute for Science, Law, and Public Policy's mission is to bridge the gap between the consumer's need for laws that protect health and safety and the inability of science to state with certainty the impact of emerging technologies. This uncertainty raises significant concerns that affect public policy creation. NISLAPP seeks to develop intelligent policy on the points at which science and law intersect by forging dialogue among government, industry, and the concerned public.
Publications, reports, or services: Maintains the NutraMancer City Web-site Project, which endeavors to inform the public about the effects of aspartame.

National Meat Association (NMA)
1970 Broadway, Suite 825
Oakland, CA, 94612
Telephone: 510-763-1533 Fax: 510-763-6186
Email address: nma@hooked.net
Web site: http://www.nmaonline.org/
Description: The National Meat Association is a nonprofit trade association for meatpackers and meat processors, as well as equipment manufacturers and suppliers who provide services to the meat industry. National Meat Association's mission is to advocate the interests of the meat industry in federal regulatory issues and national legislation that impacts the industry. NMA assists its members in meeting the public's expectation for safe food produced in a competitive market environment.
Publications, reports, or services: Web site offers the Virtual HACCP Yellow Pages, NMA Scholarship Foundation awards scholarships to undergraduate students who pursue a curriculum leading to a degree in animal, meat, or food science.

National Pest Control Association (NCPA)
8100 Oak St.
Dunn Loring, VA, 22027
Telephone: 703-573-8330 Fax: 703-573-4116
Web site: http://www.pestworld.org/
Description: Founded in 1933, NCPA represents the pest management industry, communicating the role of the industry as protector of food, health, property, and the environment. The association achieves its goals through education and advocacy at workshops, regional conferences, and national meetings. It also works on legislative and regulatory initiatives on the federal and state levels, the creation of verifiable training, the changing technologies used by the industry, and public and media relations.
Publications, reports, or services: Web site offers an online discussion forum about pests and has sections for media, homeowners, or professionals. Produces training materials for pest exterminators.

National Pork Producers Council (NPPC)
P.O. Box 10383
Des Moines, IA, 50306
Telephone: 515-223-2600 Fax: 515-223-2646
Email address: pork@nppc.org
Web site: http://www.nppc.org/
Description: As the trade association for the pork industry, NPPC serves as the single unified voice for the nation's pork producers on a wide range of industry and public policy issues. It addresses issues affecting pork from production to consumer demand.
Publications, reports, or services: NPPC offers food safety information for pork producers and for the general public on its Web site. The council also sponsors food safety research through its grant program.

National Registry of Food Safety Professionals (NRFSP)
1200 East Hillcrest St., Suite 300
Orlando, FL, 32803
Telephone: 407-228-0909 Fax: 407-894-7748
Email address: pti@proftesting.com
Web site: http://www.nrfsp.com/
Description: The National Registry of Food Safety Professionals, Inc., tracks certified food safety managers who have successfully completed the Food Safety Manager Certification Examination (FSMCE). The registry serves the food service industry, regulatory agencies, and academia.

National Restaurant Association (NRA)
1200 Seventeenth St. NW
Washington, DC, 20036-3097
Telephone: 202-331-5900
Email address: info@dineout.org
Web site: http://www.restaurant.org/
Description: The National Restaurant Association is the membership-based business association for the restaurant industry, with its main mission to represent, educate, and promote the restaurant

industry. Founded in 1923, NRA is the leading source for research and information on the restaurant industry.

Publications, reports, or services: Talk papers on topics of interest to restaurateurs, including foodborne illness, government affairs, trends in the food service industry. Food safety education is administered through the nonprofit arm, the National Restaurant Association Educational Foundation.

National Restaurant Association Educational Foundation
250 South Wacker Dr., Suite 1400
Chicago, IL, 60606
Fax: 312-715-0713
Email address: info@foodtrain.org
Web site: http://www.edfound.org/
Description: The National Restaurant Association Educational Foundation provides educational and training solutions that serve the needs of the entire restaurant and hospitality industry: corporations, associations, schools, independent operators, and trainers-both national and international.
Publications, reports, or services: Offers ServSafe certification, training, books, videos, CD-ROM, and even a database to find a class. Also offers a restaurant HACCP training program. Publishes Fork in the Road, a biannual publication that promotes careers in the restaurant industry to high school students around the country. Undergraduate and graduate scholarships are available.

National Rural Water Association
2915 S. 13th St.
Duncan, OK, 73533
Telephone: 580-252-0629 Fax: 580-255-4476
Email address: mail@nrwa.org
Web site: http://www.nrwa.org/
Description: The National Rural Water Association is a nonprofit federation of more than 45 state rural water associations, representing more than 19,000 water and wastewater utilities across America. It's mission it is to provide support services to these state associations to improve the quality of water services for rural Americans while protecting natural resources. Activities include a Wellhead Protection Program; Quality On Tap, a nationwide, grassroots public relations and awareness campaign for the drinking water industry; and *Rural Water Magazine*.
Publications, reports, or services: Web site has an Ask Mr. Faucet section where consumers can post questions, links to state associations, a list of educational institutions offering course work in water, wastewater, and related fields of study.

New England Fisheries Development Association
197 Eighth St. Suite 600a
Charlestown, MA, 02129
Telephone: 617-886-0793 Fax: 617-886-0173
Email address: Fishdev@aol.com
Web site: http://www.fishfacts.com/
Description: The New England Fisheries Development Association provides information on the seafood industry in New England. Areas of interest include detailed information on the various fish species native to New England as well as species commonly distributed in the region, food service information, nutritional information, fishing methods and cooking methods.
Publications, reports, or services: The publication Seafood and Health: Risk and Prevention of Seafood-Borne Illness is available full-text at Web site.

North American Association of Food Equipment Manufacturers (NAFEM)
401 N. Michigan Ave.
Chicago, IL, 60611
Telephone: 312-644-6610 Fax: 800-336-0019
Email address: info@nafem.com
Web site: http://www.nafem.org/
Description: The North American Association of Food Equipment Manufacturers represents manufacturers of commercial food service equipment and supplies. It provides education and expands communications throughout the global food service industry; represents and supports members in regulatory processes that affect the global industry, its markets, and their business operations; provides forums for exchanges of information among members, suppliers, and customers; and maintains liaisons with allied organizations to improve interface with the industry.
Publications, reports, or services: Offers Certified Foodservice Professional certification. Publications on cleaning and care of food service equipment.

North American Meat Processors Association
1920 Association Dr., Suite 400
Reston, VA, 20191-1547
Telephone: 888-427-5499 Fax: 703-758-8001
Email address: namp@ix.netcom.com
Web site: http://www.namp.com/

Description: The North American Meat Processors Association is a nonprofit trade association comprised of meat processing companies and associates who share a continuing commitment to provide their food service customers with safe and consistent meat, poultry, seafood, game, and other meat products.

Publications, reports, or services: Provides services and educational opportunities for the benefit of its membership.

NSF International
P.O. Box 130140
789 N. Dixboro Road
Ann Arbor, MI, 48113-0140
Telephone: 800-NSF-MARK Fax: 734-769-0109
Email address: info@nsf.org.
Web site: http://www.nsf.org/

Description: NSF International, formerly known as the National Sanitation Foundation, develops standards, product testing, and certification services in the areas of public health safety and protection of the environment. It is an independent, nonprofit organization.

Publications, reports, or services: NSF certifies drinking water treatment units, bottled water, packaged ice faucets, and other plumbing devices and offers training courses in HACCP and food safety.

Office of Continuing Professional Education
Cook College, Rutgers University
102 Ryders Ln.
New Brunswick, NJ, 08901-8591
Telephone: 732-932-9271 Fax: 732-932-1187
Email address: cookce@aesop.rutgers.edu
Web site: http://www.cook.rutgers.edu/~ocpe/

Description: The Office of Continuing Professional Education focuses on the areas of agricultural production and competitiveness; food science and engineering; nutrition, health, and safety; marine and coastal resources; natural resources and the environment; and human and community resource development. Instructors are drawn from Rutgers Cooperative Extension; university faculty and staff; private industry; and local, regional, and nationwide organizations.

Publications, reports, or services: Courses include Food Safety Microbiology, Learning the 7 HACCP Principles and Developing a HACCP Plan, Food Service HACCP and Food Safety, Pest Management and Food Product Safety, Aseptic Packaging and Processing, Predicting and Controlling the Shelf-life of Foods, Controlling Crystallization to Improve Food Product Quality, Food Engineering for both Engineers and Non-Engineers, and Introduction to Food Science: Principles and Recent Advances.

Office of Water Resource Center (OWRC)
US EPA, Ariel Rios Building
1200 Pennsylvania Ave. NW
Washington, DC, 20460
Telephone: 202-260-7786 Fax: 202-260-0386
Email address: center.water-resource@epa.gov
Web site: http://www.epa.gov/safewater/rescnter.html

Description: The Office of Water Resource Center is a contractor-operated facility that provides library services to the public and Environmental Protection Agency staff regarding Office of Water programs. The center catalogues and distributes documents published by the Office of Ground Water and Drinking Water, the Office of Science and Technology, and the Office of Wastewater Management. The OWRC is part of the EPA National Library Network.

Publications, reports, or services: Distributes many of the EPA water quality documents and has EPA water program information.

Ontario Agri-Food Education, Inc. (OAFE)
8560 Tremaine Rd., Box 460
Milton, ON, L9T 4Z1 Canada
Telephone: 905-878-1510 Fax: 905-878-0342
Email address: resource@oafe.org
Web site: http://www.oafe.org/

Description: OAFE builds awareness and understanding of the importance of the agriculture and food system by providing educational programs and resources for students and teachers.

Publications, reports, or services: Numerous teacher workshops and resources for children to provide an understanding of where our food comes from, including the secondary school–level video and teacher's guide, Food Safety Can Be Fun.

Partnership for Food Safety Education
Web site: http://www.fightbac.org/

Description: The Partnership for Food Safety Education is a public-private partnership created to reduce the incidence of foodborne illness by educating Americans about safe food handling practices. The partnership developed and promotes the FightBAC! campaign.

Publications, reports, or services: Produces numerous publications, games, toys, curricula, and other materials to promote safe food handling to children and adults.

Pesticide Action Network North America (PANNA)
49 Powell St., Suite 500
San Francisco, CA, 94102
Telephone: 415-981-1771 Fax: 415-981-1991
Email address: panna@panna.org
Web site: http://www.panna.org
Description: The Pesticide Action Network North America is a nonprofit citizen-based organization that advocates adoption of ecologically sound practices in place of pesticide use.
Publications, reports, or services: Publishes Pesticide Research Updates and Pesticide Action Network Updates Service. The PANNA Information Clearinghouse is an extensive collection of books, reports, articles, periodicals, videos, slides, photos, and other materials about pesticides and related issues.

Physicians and Scientists for Responsible Application of Science and Technology (PSRAST)
Telephone: +46322622966
Fax: +46322620944
Email address: info@psrast.org
Web site: http://www.psrast.org
Description: Founded in 1998, PSRAST aims to establish itself as an international, interdisciplinary body that evaluates applications of science and technology from a comprehensive long-term global perspective including systemic/holistic considerations. PSRAST works independently of business and political interests. This group currently focuses on food biotechnology issues and working toward a global moratorium on the release into the environment of genetically engineered (GE) organisms and on the use of genetically engineered foods.
Publications, reports, or services: Web site has extensive food biotechnology information.

Produce Marketing Association
1500 Casho Mill Rd.
P.O. Box 6036
Newark, DE, 19714-6036
Telephone: 302-738-7100 Fax: 302-731-2409
Email address: Webmaster@mail.pma.com
Web site: http://www.pma.com/
Description: The Produce Marketing Association, founded in 1949, is a nonprofit trade association serving more than 2,500 members who market fresh fruits, vegetables, and floral products worldwide. Its members are involved in the production, distribution, retail, and food service sectors of the industry.
Publications, reports, or services: Produces food safety training resources for retail produce workers.

Public Citizen
1600 20th St. NW
Washington, DC, 20009
Telephone: 800-289-3787
Email address: pcmail@citizen.org
Web site: http://www.citizen.org/
Description: Founded by Ralph Nader in 1971, Public Citizen is the consumer's eyes and ears in Washington. Public Citizen's agenda includes public health topics, the environment, and energy resources.
Publications, reports, or services: Issues press releases, testimony, and public statements about food irradiation and other food safety policies.

Regional Research Project NE-165
Email address: ne165@resecon.umass.edu
Web site: http://www.umass.edu/ne165/
Description: NE-165 researches the impacts of changes in strategies, technologies, consumer behavior, and policies on the economic performance of the food system, and on how private and public strategies influence improvement in food safety and other quality attributes. It has more than 100 members around the world, primarily from universities and government agencies, and a core research group at the Food Marketing Policy Center, Universities of Connecticut and Massachusetts.
Publications, reports, or services: Research areas include food safety and quality, HACCP, benefit/cost analysis of food safety policies, agricultural biotechnology, and risk assessment. Conferences organized by NE-165 include Strategy and Policy in the Food System: Emerging Issues, The Economics of Reducing Health Risk from Food, The Economics of HACCP: New Studies of Costs and Benefits, and Valuing the Health Benefits of Food Safety.

Safe Food Coalition
1424 16th St. NW, Suite 604
Washington, DC, 20036
Telephone: 202-387-6121 Fax: 202-265-7989

Web site: http://www.consumerfed.org/fpi
Description: The Safe Food Coalition, a group of consumer, public health, senior citizen, and labor organizations that have worked together since 1986 to improve the nation's food safety system, represents consumers in seeking more effective prevention of bacterial contamination. Led by the Consumer Federation of America, coalition members include the American Public Health Association, Center for Science in the Public Interest, Government Accountability Project, National Consumers League, National Environmental Trust, Public Citizen, Safe Tables Our Priority, United Food and Commercial Workers International Union, and U.S. Public Interest Research Group.
Publications, reports, or services: Provides testimony before Congress on food safety issues.

Safe Tables Our Priority (S.T.O.P.)
P.O. Box 46522
Chicago, IL, 60646-0522
Telephone: 312-957-0284 Fax: 312-427-2307
Email address: feedback@stop-usa.org
Web site: http://www.stop-usa.org/
Description: Safe Tables Our Priority is a nonprofit grassroots organization devoted to victim assistance, public education, and policy advocacy for safe food and public health. The organization was founded in 1993 by families and friends of people who became ill or died from exposure to *E. coli* 0157:H7 and other pathogenic bacteria in meat and poultry.
Publications, reports, or services: Web site has consumer food safety information, medical information on foodborne illness, victim's stories, and FAQs.

Soap and Detergent Association (SDA)
475 Park Ave. South
New York, NY, 10016
Telephone: 212-725-1262 Fax: 212-213-0685
Web site: http://www.sdahq.org/about/
Description: The Soap and Detergent Association is the national, nonprofit trade association representing manufacturers of household, industrial, and institutional cleaning products; the ingredients used in cleaning products; and finished packaging. Established in 1926, SDA addresses the human and environmental safety of cleaning products and their ingredients, the safe and effective use and disposal of cleaning products, and the contributions of cleaning products to personal and public health.
Publications, reports, or services: Publications on proper handwashing and cleaning; antibacterial resistance; dishwashers; and the history, manufacture, chemistry, and use of soaps and detergents.

Society for Foodservice Management
304 W. Liberty St., Suite 201
Louisville, KY, 40202
Telephone: 502-583-3783 Fax: 502-589-3602
Email address: hq@sfm-online.org
Web site: http://www.sfm-online.org/
Description: The Society for Foodservice Management is the national association for individuals employed in or providing services to the on-site food service industry. The society's principal role is to enhance the ability of members to achieve career and business objectives through relevant research, industry information, continuing educational programming, and member interaction in a supportive environment.
Publications, reports, or services: Publications relating to food service management, food service planning, catering, vending, or food service equipment.

U.S. Department of Commerce, National Oceanic and Atmospheric Administration (NOAA)
Seafood Inspection Program
1315 East-West Highway
Silver Spring, MD, 20910
Telephone: 800-422-2750 Fax: 301-713-1081
Web site: http://seafood.nmfs.noaa.gov/
Description: NOAA oversees fisheries management in the United States, and through the 1946 Agricultural Marketing Act, provides a voluntary inspection service to the industry. Through its fee-for-service Seafood Inspection Program, NOAA inspects and certifies fishing vessels, seafood processing plants, and retail facilities for federal sanitation standards.
Publications, reports, or services: Provides access to seafood regulations and sanitation standards documents, sponsors HACCP training.

U.S. Environmental Protection Agency (EPA), Office of Pesticide Programs
401 M St. SW
Washington, DC, 20460-0003
Telephone: 202-260-2090
Email address: public-access@epamail.epa.gov
Web site: http://www.epa.gov/pesticides/

Description: EPA is responsible for regulating all pesticide products sold or distributed in the United States and for establishing tolerances for pesticide residues in or on food commodities and animal feed. Its mission is to protect public health and the environment from the risks posed by pesticides and to promote safer means of pest control.

Publications, reports, or services: Web site has consumer information regarding pesticide residues in food, and a searchable list of pesticide tolerances.

U.S. Environmental Protection Agency (EPA), Office of Ground Water and Drinking Water
401 M St. SW
Washington, DC, 20460-0003
Telephone: 202-260-5543 Fax: 202-260-4383
Email address: OW-General@epamail.epa.gov
Web site: http://www.epa.gov/safewater/

Description: The Office of Ground Water and Drinking Water, together with states, tribes, and other partners, protects public health by ensuring safe drinking water and protecting groundwater so that all Americans have drinking water that is clean and safe to drink.

Publications, reports, or services: Publications such as Water on Tap: A Consumer's Guide to the Nation's Drinking Water, EPA's drinking water glossary, and information on the Safe Drinking Water Act are available on the Web site. Maintains the National Drinking Water Contaminant Occurrence Database and the Safe Drinking Water Information System. Spanish version of the site is at http://www.epa.gov/safewater/agua.html.

U.S. Food and Drug Administration (FDA), Office of Regulatory Affairs (ORA)
Web site: http://www.fda.gov/ora

Description: The Office of Regulatory Affairs is the lead office for all field activities of the Food and Drug Administration. This includes the Division of Federal-State Relations, Division of Import Operations, Office of Enforcement, and Office of Criminal Investigations.

Publications, reports, or services: Products include inspectional references such as manuals and other documents that provide procedures and guidance to FDA personnel for conducting their inspectional and investigational activities; science references related to ORA laboratories, laboratory procedures, and new techniques in applied science; and consumer information on how to access FDA resources. Maintains a listing of state health officials.

U.S. Food and Drug Administration (FDA), Center for Food Safety and Applied Nutrition (CFSAN)
200 C St. SW
Washington, DC, 20204
Web site: http://vm.cfsan.fda.gov

Description: This office of the FDA is responsible for approving new food additives, assessing compliance with food labeling laws, examining and analyzing food shipments from abroad, and establishing new regulations based on modern food safety techniques to improve seafood safety. The FDA regulates all non-meat and poultry food products.

Publications, reports, or services: Web site has food safety information for consumers, educators, and industry on just about every food safety topic imaginable.

U.S. Food and Drug Administration (FDA), Center for Veterinary Medicine (CVM)
7500 Standish Place
Rockville, MD, 20855
Email address: CVMHomeP@cvm.fda.gov
Web site: http://www.fda.gov/cvm/

Description: The Center for Veterinary Medicine regulates the manufacture and distribution of food additives and drugs that will be given to animals. These include animals from which human foods are derived, as well as food additives and drugs for pets. CVM is responsible for regulating drugs, devices, and food additives given to, or used on, more than 100 million pets, plus millions of poultry, cattle, swine, sheep, and minor animal species.

Publications, reports, or services: Web site includes sections on antimicrobial resistance and some biotechnology information.

U.S. House Committee on Agriculture
1301 Longworth House Office Building
Washington, DC, 20515
Telephone: 202-225-2171
Email address: agriculture@mail.house.gov
Web site: http://agriculture.house.gov/

Description: As part of the U.S. Congress, the House Committee on Agriculture covers subjects relating to agriculture, and as such is the main House committee involved in food safety, covering food safety inspection, pesticide regulation, and agricultural biotechnology.

Publications, reports, or services: Web site contains committee hearings, schedules, audio of hearings, reports, briefing papers, committee actions, and anything else that happens in Congress related to the committee's interests.

U.S. Poultry & Egg Association
1530 Cooledge Rd.
Tucker, GA, 30084-7303
Telephone: 770-493-9401 Fax: 770-493-9257
Email address: promo@poultryegg.org
Web site: http://www.poultryegg.org/
Description: The U.S. Poultry & Egg Association (formerly the Southeastern Poultry and Egg Association) is dedicated to the growth, progress, and welfare of the poultry industry and all of its individual and corporate interests. All segments of the industry are represented, from producers of eggs, turkeys, and broilers to the processors of those products and allied companies that serve the industry.
Publications, reports, or services: Offers HACCP training, industry and consumer information on Web site, and sponsors research and education in poultry technology through a research grants program.

U.S. Senate Agriculture, Nutrition, And Forestry Committee
United States Senate
Washington, DC, 20510
Web site: http://www.senate.gov/~agriculture/
Description: As part of the U.S. Congress, the Senate Committee on Agriculture, Nutrition, and Forestry overseas subjects relating to agriculture, and as such is the main Senate committee involved in food safety, covering food safety inspection, general food safety issues, and agricultural biotechnology.
Publications, reports, or services: Web site contains committee briefs, hearing schedules and reports, and new legislation.

Union of Concerned Scientists
2 Brattle Square
Cambridge, MA, 02238
Telephone: 617-547-5552
Email address: ucs@ucsusa.org
Web site: http://www.ucsusa.org/
Description: The Union of Concerned Scientists works on issues pivotal to change where expertise in science is particularly useful. Its scientists try to persuade the government to encourage innovative ways to grow plants and animals, protect the safety of food, and ensure that consumers and citizens can make choices about how food is produced. Working in coalition with the environmental community, progressive farmers, and other public interest organizations, they urge new policies, analyze agency actions, and engage the public in advocacy efforts to improve the interlinked systems of agriculture, food, and the environment.
Publications, reports, or services: Two of the union's major issues are agricultural biotechnology and antibiotic resistance.

United States Animal Health Association (USAHA)
P.O. Box K227
Richmond, VA, 23288
Telephone: 804-285-3210 Fax: 804-285-3367
Web site: http://www.usaha.org/
Description: Formed in 1897, the United States Animal Health Association is a national nonprofit organization that works with state and federal animal health officials, veterinarians, livestock producers, national livestock and poultry organizations, research scientists, the extension service, and seven foreign countries to control livestock diseases in the United States. USAHA works to eliminate animal diseases and serves as an advisor to the U.S. Department of Agriculture.
Publications, reports, or services: Reports on animal health, biotechnology, feed safety.

USDA Agricultural Research Service (ARS)
Email address: arsWeb@nal.usda.gov
Web site: http://www.ars.usda.gov/
Description: ARS conducts research to develop and transfer solutions to agricultural problems of high national priority and provides information access and dissemination to ensure high-quality, safe food and other agricultural products; assess the nutritional needs of Americans; sustain a competitive agricultural economy; enhance the natural resource base and the environment; and provide economic opportunities for rural citizens, communities, and society as a whole.
Publications, reports, or services: Web site has a Find the Expert section for locating ARS scientists, and information on research initiatives and national programs.

USDA Agricultural Marketing Service (AMS)
Web site: http://www.ams.usda.gov/
Description: AMS conducts a program to collect and analyze data about pesticide residue levels in

agricultural commodities. It also administers the Pesticide Record Keeping Program, which requires all certified private applicators of federally restricted-use pesticides to maintain a record of all applications. The records will be put into a database to help analyze agricultural pesticide use.

USDA Animal and Plant Health Inspection Service (APHIS)
12th and Independence Ave. SW
Washington, DC, 20250
Email address: Web-requests@aphis.usda.gov
Web site: http://www.aphis.usda.gov/
Description: APHIS provides leadership in ensuring the health and care of animals and plants, improving agricultural productivity and competitiveness, and contributing to the national economy and the public health. APHIS guards U.S. borders against foreign agricultural pests and diseases; monitors agricultural diseases and pests; facilitates agricultural exports through scientifically based sanitary and phytosanitary standards; protects animal health by fighting domestic animal diseases and making sure veterinary biologics are safe, pure, potent and effective; and ensures the safety of genetically engineered plants and other products of agricultural biotechnology.
Publications, reports, or services: Web site has pages for animal health, plant health, BSE, and agricultural biotechnology.

USDA Cooperative State Research, Education, and Extension Service (CSREES)
Washington, DC, 20250-0900
Telephone: 202-720-3029 Fax: 202-690-0289
Email address: csrees@reeusda.gov
Web site: http://www.reeusda.gov/
Description: The CSREES mission emphasizes partnerships with the public and private sectors to maximize the effectiveness of limited resources. CSREES programs increase and provide access to scientific knowledge; strengthen the capabilities of land-grant and other institutions in research, extension, and higher education; increase access to and use of improved communication and network systems; and promote informed decision making by producers, families, communities, and other customers. This includes improved agricultural and other economic enterprises; safer, cleaner water, food, and air; enhanced stewardship and management of natural resources; and a stable, secure, diverse, and affordable national food supply.
Publications, reports, or services: Administers grant programs: Biotechnology Risk Assessment Research Grants Program, Food Safety and Quality National Initiative Grants, and Food Safety Special Research Grant Program.

USDA Economic Research Service (ERS)
1800 M St. NW
Washington, DC 20036-5831
Telephone: 202-694-5050
Email address: service@econ.ag.gov
Web site: http://www.ers.usda.gov
Description: The Economic Research Service conducts research on costs to society of foodborne diseases and the benefits of programs and policies to improve the safety of the nation's food supply.
Publications, reports, or services: Web site contains full-text of recent reports and a Food Safety Briefing Room.

USDA/FDA Foodborne Illness Education Information Center
10301 Baltimore Ave.
National Agricultural Library
Beltsville, MD, 20705-2351
Telephone: 301-504-5719 Fax: 301-504-6409
Email address: foodborne@nal.usda.gov
Web site: http://www.nal.usda.gov/foodborne/
Description: The USDA/FDA Foodborne Illness Education Information Center provides information about foodborne illness prevention to educators, trainers, and organizations developing education and training materials for food workers and consumers. The center is part of an interagency agreement between the USDA Food Safety and Inspection Service and FDA. It is housed at the Food and Nutrition Information Center (FNIC) of the National Agricultural Library. USDA and FDA established the center as part of a national campaign to reduce the risk of foodborne illness and to increase knowledge of food-related risks from production through consumption.
Publications, reports, or services: Sponsors foodsafe, the electronic food safety discussion group; maintains the Foodborne Illness Educational Materials Database and HACCP Training Programs and Resources Database; and compiles the Food Safety Index.

USDA Food Safety and Inspection Service
Room1175 South Building
1400 Independence Ave. SW

Washington, DC, 20250
Email address: fsis.Webmaster@usda.gov
Web site: http://www.fsis.usda.gov/
Description: The Food Safety and Inspection Service is the agency of the U.S. Department of Agriculture responsible for ensuring that the nation's commercial supply of meat, poultry, and egg products is safe, wholesome, and correctly labeled and packaged. FSIS sets standards for food safety and inspects meat, poultry, and egg products produced domestically and imported. Inspectors also test for the presence of drug and chemical residues that violate federal law.
Publications, reports, or services: Operates the Meat and Poultry Hotline, Web site has food safety information for consumers and educators, as well as technical and inspection information for industry.

USDA Grain Inspection, Packers and Stockyards Administration
1400 Independence Ave. SW
Washington, DC, 20250
Email address: gipsa-Webmaster@gipsadc.usda.gov
Web site: http://www.usda.gov/gipsa/
Description: GIPSA's mission is to facilitate the marketing of livestock, poultry, meat, cereals, oilseeds, and related agricultural products and to promote fair and competitive trading practices for the overall benefit of consumers and American agriculture. GIPSA provides an aflatoxin testing service for corn, sorghum, wheat, and soybeans. Testing is also provided for rice, popcorn, corn meal, corn gluten meal, corn/soy blend, and other processed products governed by the Agricultural Marketing Act.

USDA Rural Utilities Service (RUS)
1400 Independence Ave, SW
Washington, DC, 20250
Email address: Webmaster@rurdev.usda.gov
Web site: http://www.usda.gov/rus/
Description: The Rural Utilities Service is the federal "point" agency for rural infrastructure assistance in electricity, water, and telecommunications. As a federal credit agency in the United States Department of Agriculture, RUS provides a leadership role in lending and technical guidance for the rural utilities industries.
Publications, reports, or services: Web site has information on water programs and a kid's page.

Water Quality Association
4151 Naperville Rd.
Lisle, IL, IL 60532-1088
Web site: http://www.wqa.org/
Description: The Water Quality Association is the international nonprofit association representing the manufacturers and sellers of water treatment equipment, expertise, and services for homes, farms, commercial, industrial, and small community water systems.
Publications, reports, or services: Web site contains much technical and consumer information on water quality, including a section on diagnosing water quality and an online glossary.

Water Quality Information Center (WQIC)
National Agricultural Library
10301 Baltimore Blvd.
Beltsville, MD, 20705-2351
Email address: wqic@nal.usda.gov
Web site: http://www.nal.usda.gov/wqic/
Description: The center was established in 1990 to support USDA's coordinated plan to address water quality concerns. Activities include collecting, organizing, and communicating the scientific findings, educational methodologies, and public policy issues related to water quality and agriculture.
Publications, reports, or services: The center's Web site includes reports, bibliographies, and databases relating to water quality.

World Health Organization (WHO)
Food Safety Programme, Department of Protection of the Human Environment, Cluster on Sustainable Development and Healthy Environments (FOS/PHE/SDE)
1211 Geneva, 27 Switzerland,
Email address: foodsafety@who.ch
Web site: http://www.who.int/fsf/
Description: Since its inception in 1948, the World Health Organization has been working towards the improvement of food safety. Its work involves technical cooperation with member states to strengthen national food safety programs. Activities include development of national food safety policies and infrastructures, food legislation and enforcement, promotion of food technologies of public health importance, education of consumers in food safety, food safety in the urban setting, promotion of food safety in tourism, epidemiological surveillance of foodborne diseases, and monitoring of contaminants.
Publications, reports, or services: Web site contains full-text of recent reports on a variety of global food safety issues.

World Health Organization (WHO) Regional Office for Europe—Food Programme
European Centre for Environment and Health
via Francesco Crispi
10 - Rome, Italy
Telephone: 3906487751 Fax: 39064877599
Email address: Webmaster@who.it
Web site: http://www.who.it/Ht/food_safety.htm
Description: The Food Safety Programme was re-established in mid 1998 and operates to ensure that information on food safety is properly collected and circulated to provide the basis for policy and monitoring and that health-oriented guidelines are constantly updated. As an international independent body it plays a public health advocacy role in the areas of food production, retailing, and global marketing.
Publications, reports, or services: Web site contains reports on chemical contamination, irradiation, genetically modified foods, links to European foodborne disease surveillance sites, and EU food legislation.

World Trade Organization (WTO)
Centre William Rappard
Rue de Lausanne 154
CH-1211 Geneva 21, Switzerland
Telephone: +41227395111
Email address: enquiries@wto.org
Web site: http://www.wto.org/
Description: In the food safety arena, the World Trade Organization is responsible for the Agreement on the Application of Sanitary and Phytosanitary Measures (SPS Agreement). The SPS Agreement sets out the basic rules for international food safety and animal and plant health standards. It allows countries to set their own standards. But it also says regulations must be based on science. They should be applied only to the extent necessary to protect human, animal, or plant life or health. And they should not arbitrarily or unjustifiably discriminate between countries where identical or similar conditions prevail.
Publications, reports, or services: Full-text availability of the SPS Agreement from Web site.

World Veterinary Association
Rosenlunds Allé 8
DK-2720 Vanlose, Denmark
Telephone: +4538710156 Fax: +4538710322
Email address: wva@ddd.dk
Web site: http://www.worldvet.org/
Description: The World Veterinary Association is a global nonpolitical, nonprofit association guarding veterinary interests in the world society. The association acts to apply the results of veterinary science to protect and improve animal welfare, animal health, human health, and the environment.

COOPERATIVE EXTENSION OFFICES

Alabama

http://www.aces.edu/dept/

Chinella G. Henderson
Alabama A&M University
1890 Extension Programs
P.O. Box 222
Normal, AL 35762
Telephone: 205-851-5710
Fax: 205-851-5840
Email: chenders@aceag.auburn.edu

Mary Williams Hurt
Alabama A&M University
1890 Extension Program
P.O. Box 190
Normal, AL 35762
Telephone:205-859-7373
Fax: 205-851-5840
Email: mhurt@aceag.auburn.edu

Jannie Jones-Carter
Alabama A&M University
1890 Extension Programs
P.O. Box 967
Normal, AL 35762-1327
Telephone: 205-851-5710
Fax: 205-851-5840
Email: aamjws01@asnaam.aamu.edu

Evelyn F. Crayton
Auburn University
Cooperative Extension Service
Duncan Hall
Auburn University, AL 36849- 5621
Telephone: 334-844-2224
Fax: 334-844-9650
Email: ecrayton@acesag.auburn.edu

Jean Olds Weese
Auburn University
Cooperative Extension Service

364 Spidle Hall
Auburn University, AL 36849
Telephone: 334-844-3269
Fax: 334-844-3268
Email: jweese@acesag.auburn.edu

Eunice A. Bonsi
Tuskegee University
Cooperative Extension Programs
200 Extension Building
Tuskegee, AL 36088
Telephone: 205-727-8808/8816
Fax: 205-727-8812
Email: ebonsi@acd.tusk.edu

Alaska

http://www.uaf.edu/coop-ext/

Kristy Long
University of Alaska
Alaska Cooperative Extension
P.O. Box 756180
Fairbanks, AK 99775-6180
Telephone: 907-474-7974
Fax: 907-474-6567
Email: ffkal@aurora.alaska.edu

Bret Luick
University of Alaska-Fairbanks
Alaska Cooperative Extension
P.O. Box 756180
Fairbanks, AK 99775-6180
Telephone: 907-474-6338
Fax: 907-474-7439
Email: ffbrl@aurora.alaska.edu

American Samoa

Carol S. Whitaker
ASCC Land Grant Program
Cooperative Extension Service
P.O. Box 5319
Pago, Pago, AS 96799
Telephone: 684-699-1394
Fax: 684-699-4595
Email: wit@elele.peacesat.hawaii.edu

Arizona

http://ag.arizona.edu/extension/

Sharon Hoelscher Day
University of Arizona
Cooperative Extension System
4341 E. Broadway
Phoenix, AZ 85040
Telephone: 602-470-8086 ext. 332
Fax: 602-470-8092
Email: shday@ag.arizona.edu

Ralph Price
University of Arizona
Department of Nutritional Sciences
Shantz Building, Room 309A
Tucson, AZ 85721
Telephone: 520-621-1728
Fax: 520-621-9446
Email: rprice@ag.arizona.edu

Arkansas

http://www.uaex.edu/

Pamela Brady
University of Arkansas
Cooperative Extension Service
P.O. Box 391
2301 South University Ave.
Little Rock, AR 72203
Telephone: 501-671-2108
Fax: 501-671-2294
Email: pbrady@uaex.edu

James H. Denton
University of Arkansas
Poultry Science Center POSC 0-114
Fayetteville, AR 72701
Telephone: 501-575-4952
Fax: 501-575-3026
Email: jdenton@comp.uark.edu

David Edmark
University of Arkansas
Agricultural Publications
110 Agricultural Building
Fayetteville, AR 72701
Telephone: 501-575-5647
Fax: 501-575-7531Email: dedmark@comp.uark.edu

Luke Howard
University of Arkansas
Department of Food Science
272 Young Ave.
Fayetteville, AR 72701
Telephone: 501-575-2978
Fax: 501-575-6936
Email: LUKEH@COMP.UARK.EDU

John Marcy
University of Arkansas POSC 0-114
Poultry Science Center
Fayetteville, AR 72701
Telephone: 501-575-2211
Fax: 501-575-3026
Email: jmarcy@comp.uark.edu

Dr. John Meister
University of Arkansas-Pine Bluff
1200 North University Dr.
P.O. Box 4913
Pine Bluff, AR 71611
Telephone: 870-543-8526
Email: Meister_J@vx4500.uapb.edu

California

http://danrcs.ucdavis.edu/uclinks/

Christine M. Bruhn
University of California
Center for Consumer Research
One Shields Avenue
Davis, CA 95616
Telephone: 530-752-2774
Fax: 530-752-3975
Email: cmbruhn@ucdavis.edu

Arthur L. Craigmill
University of California
Environmental Toxicology Extension
One Shields Avenue
Davis, CA 95616-8588
Telephone: 530-752-2936
Fax: 530-752-0903
Email: alcraigmill@ucdavis.edu

Linda J. Harris, Ph.D.
Specialist in Microbial Food Safety
University of California
Department of Food Science and Technology
One Shields Ave.
Davis, CA 95616-8598
Telephone: 530-754-9485
Fax: 530-752-4759
Email: ljharris@ucdavis.edu

Amy Block Joy
University of California
Cooperative Extension Service
1143 Meyer Hall
One Shields Avenue
Davis, CA 95616
Telephone: 530-752-7959
Fax: 530-752-8966
Email: danrarw@uccvma.ucop.edu

Bill Sischo, DVM, Ph.D.
University of California
Veterinary Medical Teaching and Research Center
18830 Road 112
Tulare, CA 93274
Telephone:209-688-1731 ext. 225

Carl Winter
University of California
Department of Food Science and Technology
One Shields Avenue
Davis, CA 95616-8598
Telephone: 530-752-5448
Fax: 530-752-3975
Email: ckwinter@ucdavis.edu

Colorado

http://www.colostate.edu/Depts/CoopExt/

Pat Kendall
Colorado State University
Department of Food Science and Human Nutrition
Fort Collins, CO 80523-1571
Telephone: 970-491-1945 Fax: 970-491-7252
Email: pkendall@lamar.colostate.edu or Colorado State University kendall@cahs.colostate.edu

Mary McPhail Gray
Cooperative Extension Service
1 Administration Building
Fort Collins, CO 80523-4040
Telephone: 970-491-6281
Fax: 970-491-6208
Email: mgray@coop.ext.colostate.edu

Connecticut

http://www.canr.uconn.edu/ces/

Kenneth N. Hall
University of Connecticut
Cooperative Extension Service
Department of Nutritional Sciences
Storrs, CT 06269-4017
Telephone: 860-486-1763
Fax: 860-486-3674
Email: khall@canr1.cag.uconn.edu

Diane Wright Hirsch
Extension Educator/Food Safety
University of Connecticut
Cooperative Extension System
305 Skiff St.
North Haven, CT 06473
Telephone: 203-407-3173
Fax: 203-407-3176
Email: dhirsch@canr.cag.uconn.edu

Carol J. Lammi-Keefe, Ph.D., R.D.
Professor and Department Head
University of Connecticut
Department of Nutritional Sciences
Storrs, CT 06269
Telephone: 860-486-5762
Fax: 860-486-3674
Email: clammi@canr.cag.uconn.edu

Yanyun Zhao, Ph.D.
University of Connecticut
Department of Nutritional Sciences
3624 Horsebarn Road Extension, U Box 17
Storrs, CT 06269-4017
Telephone: 860-486-6885
Fax: 860-486-3674
Email: yzhao@canr.uconn.edu

Delaware

http://bluehen.ags.udel.edu/deces/fnf/fnf-list.htm

Dr. William Daniels
Delaware State University
Cooperative Extension Service
1200 N. Dupont Highway
Dover, DE 19901
Telephone: 302-739-6944
Fax: 302-739-2014
Email: bdaniels@dsc.edu

Sue Snider
University of Delaware
Cooperative Extension Service
Department of Animal and Food Sciences
Newark, DE 19717-1303
Telephone: 302-831-2524
Fax: 302-831-2822
Email: sue.snider@mvs.udel.edu

District of Columbia

http://udc2.org/lfsmt/Lifesmart.html

Dolores Langford Bridgette
University of the District of Columbia
Cooperative Extension Service
4200 Connecticut Ave. NW
Washington, DC 20008
Telephone: 202-274-6932
Fax: 202-274-6930

Dr. Lillie Monroe-Lord
Director
University of the District of Columbia
Cooperative Extension Service
4200 Connecticut Ave. NW
Building 52, Suite 322
Washington, DC 20008
Telephone: 202-274-7125
Fax: 202-274-7130
Email: Lmonroe-Lord@ces.udc.com

Florida

http://www.ifas.ufl.edu/www/extension/ces.htm

Mabel Edlow
Florida A&M University
1890 Extension Programs
215 Perry Paige Building
Tallahassee, FL 32307
Telephone: 904-561-2095
Fax: 904-561-2151
Email: medlow@vm.cc.famu.edu

Robert P. Bates
University of Florida
Cooperative Extension Service
329 Food Science Building
P.O. Box 110370
Gainesville, FL 32611-0370
Telephone: 352-392-1991
Fax: 352-392-8594
Email: rpb@gnv.ifas.ufl.edu

Eddie Richey
University of Florida
College of Veterinary Medicine
Building 459, Room 224B
P.O. Box 110136
Gainesville, FL 32610-0136
Telephone: 352-392-8059
Fax: 352-392-8289
Email: erichey.vetmed1@mail.health.ufl.edu

Ronald Schmidt
University of Florida

Cooperative Extension Service
325 Food Science Building
Gainesville, FL 32611-0370
Telephone: 352-392-8003
Fax: 352-392-8594
Email: RSCHMIDT@gnv.ifas.ufl.edu

Charles A. Sims
University of Florida
Cooperative Extension Service
349 FSHN Building
Gainesville, FL 32611-0370
Telephone: 352-391-1991
Fax: 352-392-9467
Email: fos@gnv.ifas.ufl.edu

Georgia

http://www.fcs.uga.edu/outreach/coopex/fsp/

Carol Ann Johnson
Fort Valley State University
1890 Extension Programs
P.O. Box 4061
Fort Valley, GA 31030-3298
Telephone: 912-825-6298
Fax: 912-825-6299
Email: johnson0@mail.fvsc.peachnet.edu

Elizabeth Andress
University of Georgia
Cooperative Extension Service
208 Hoke Smith Annex
Athens, GA 30602-4356
Telephone: 706-542-3773
Fax: 706-542-1979
Email: eandress@uga.edu

Judy Harrison
University of Georgia
Cooperative Extension Service
Hoke Smith Annex
Athens, GA 30602-4356
Telephone: 706-542-3773
Fax: 706-542-1979
Email: judyh@uga.edu

Estes Reynolds
University of Georgia
Cooperative Extension Service
Food Science Building
Athens, GA 30602
Telephone: 706-542-2574
Fax: 706-542-9066
Email: ereynold@uga.edu

Guam

Janet C. Benavente
University of Guam
Colleges of Agriculture and Life Sciences
303 University Dr.
Mangilao, GU 96923
Telephone: 671-735-2026
Fax: 671-734-4222
Email: jbenaven@uog.edu

Hawaii

http://www2.ctahr.hawaii.edu/extout/extout.asp

Aurora S. Hodgson
University of Hawaii
Cooperative Extension Service
1920 Edmondson Road
Honolulu, HI 96822
Telephone: 808-956-6564
Fax: 808-956-8663
Email: hodgsona@hawaii.edu

Lynn Nakamura-Tengan
University of Hawaii, CTAHR
Maui Extension Office
310 Kaahumanu Ave., Bldg 214
Kahului, HI 96732
Telephone: 808-244-3242
Fax: 808-244-7089
Email: tenganl@avax.ctahr.hawaii.edu

Wayne T. Nishijima
University of Hawaii, CTAHR
Hilo Extension Office
875 Komohana St.
Hilo, HI 96822
Telephone: 808-959-9155
Fax: 808-959-3101
Email: waynen@hawaii.edu

Idaho

http://www.uidaho.edu/ag/extension/

Linda Kirk Fox
University of Idaho
CES School of Family and Consumer Science
Niccolls Building, Room 105A
Moscow, ID 83844-3183
Telephone: 208-885-6698 or 6546
Fax: 208-885-5751
Email: lfox@uidaho.edu

Sandra McCurdy
University of Idaho
School of Family/Consumer Science
Niccolls Building 103C
Moscow, ID 83844-3183
Telephone: 208-885-6972/6545
Fax: 208-885-5751
Email: smccurdy@uidaho.edu

Illinois

http://www.extension.uiuc.edu/

Robert Reber
University of Illinois, CES
Cooperative Extension Service
339 Bevier, 905 S. Goodwin Ave.
Urbana, IL 61801
Telephone: 217-244-2851
Fax: 217-244-2861
Email: r-reber@uiuc.edu

Indiana

http://www.ces.purdue.edu/

James V. Chambers
Professor of Food Science and Extension Food Scientist
Purdue University
1160 Food Science Building
West Lafayette, IN 47907-1160
Telephone: 765-494-8279
Fax: 765-494-7953
Email: chamberj@foodsci.purdue.edu

Richard Linton
Purdue University
Department of Food Science
1160 Smith Hall
West Lafayette, IN 47907-1160
Telephone: 765-494-6481
Fax: 765-494-7953
Email: lintonr@foodsci.purdue.edu

April Mason
Purdue University
Cooperative Extension Service
1264 Stone Hall
West Lafayette, IN 47907-1264
Telephone: 765-494-8539
Fax: 765-494-0674
Email: MASONA@CFS.PURDUE.EDU

Charles R. Santerre, Ph.D.
Purdue University
Department of Foods and Nutrition
1264 Stone Hall
West Lafayette, IN 47907-1264
Telephone: 765-496-3443
Fax: 765-494-0674
Email: santerre@cfs.purdue.edu

Iowa

http://www.exnet.iastate.edu/

Jim Huss
Iowa State University
Hotel, Restaurant & Institutional Management
9 MacKay Hall
Ames, IA 50011-1120
Telephone: 515-294-3527
Fax: 515-294-8551
Email: x1huss@exnet.iastate.edu

William S. LaGrange
Iowa State University
2312 Food Sciences Building
Ames, IA 50011
Telephone: 515-294-3156
Fax: 515-294-8181
Email: foodsci@exnet.iastate.edu

Patricia Redlinger
Iowa State University
1127 Human Nutrition Sciences Building
Ames, IA 50011-1120
Telephone: 515-294-1381
Fax: 515-294-6193
Email: x1redlin@exnet.iastate.edu

Jane Ann Stout
Iowa State University
Families Extension
128 MacKay Hall
Ames, IA 50011-1120
Telephone: 515-294-8063
Fax: 515-294-5924
Email: x1stout@exnet.iastate.edu

Kansas

http://www.oznet.ksu.edu/pr_fsaf/

Fadi Michael Aramouni
Kansas State University
Research and Extension Service
Call Hall
Manhattan, KS 66506
Telephone: 785-532-1668

Fax: 785-532-5681
Email: faramoun@oz.oznet.ksu.edu

Liz Boyle, Ph.D.
Associate Professor and Extension Specialist, Meats
Kansas State University
Department of Animal Sciences and Industry
251 Weber
Manhattan, KS 66506
Telephone: 785-532-1247
Fax: 785-532-7059
Email: lboyle@oz.oznet.ksu.edu

Karen Penner
Kansas State University
Research and Extension Service
Call Hall
Manhattan, KS 66506
Telephone: 785-532-1672
Fax: 785-532-5681
Email: kpenner@oz.oznet.ksu.edu

Kentucky

http://www.ca.uky.edu/coopext/

Sandra Bastin
University of Kentucky
Cooperative Extension Service
Room 234, Scovell Hall
Lexington, KY 40546-0064
Telephone: 606-257-1812
Fax: 606-257-7792
Email: sbastin@ca.uky.edu

Mary J. Fant
State Extension Specialist
Kentucky State University
Child, Youth, Family Development and Management
Cooperative Extension Program
400 E. Main St.
Frankfort, KY 40601
Telephone: 502-227-6955
Fax: 502-227-5933
Email: mfant@gwmail.kysu.edu

Janet Kurzynske
University of Kentucky
College of Agriculture
733 Red Mile Road
Lexington, KY 40504
Telephone: 606-255-8640
Fax: 606-258-2670
Email: jkurzyns@ca.uky.edu

William B. Mikel
Univeristy of Kentucky
College of Agriculture
206 W.P. Garrigus Building
Lexington, KY 40546-0215
Telephone: 606-257-7550
Fax: 606-257-5318
Email: wmikel@ca.uky.edu

Melissa Newman
University of Kentucky
College of Agriculture
204 W.P. Garrigus Building
Lexington, KY 40546-0215
Telephone: 606-257-5881
Fax: 606-257-5318
Email: mnewman@ca.uky.edu

Joe O'Leary
University of Kentucky
CES Food Safety/Quality Task Force
234 Scovell Hall
Lexington, KY 40546-0064
Telephone: 606-257-1812
Fax: 606-257-7792
Email: japplega@ca.uky.edu

Anthony J. Pescatore
University of Kentucky
Cooperative Extension Service
604 W.P. Garrigus Building
Lexington, KY 40546-02151
Telephone: 606-257-7529
Fax: 606-257-2534
Email: apescato@ca.uky.edu

Bonnie Tanner
University of Kentucky
Cooperative Extension Service
206 Scovell Hall
Lexington, KY 40546-0064
Telephone: 606-257-3887
Fax: 606-257-7565
Email: btanner@ca.uky.edu

Janet Tietyen
University of Kentucky
College of Agriculture
234 Scovell Hall
Lexington, KY 40546-0064
Telephone: 606-257-1812
Fax: 606-257-7792
Email: jtietyen@ca.uky.edu

Louisiana

http://www.agctr.lsu.edu/wwwac/lces.html

Michael W. Moody
Louisiana State University
Cooperative Extension Service
P.O. Box 25100
Baton Rouge, LA 70894-5100
Telephone: 504-388-2152
Fax: 504-388-2478
Email: mmoody@agctr.lsu.edu

Ruth Patrick
Louisiana State University
Cooperative Extension Service
P.O. Box 25100
Baton Rouge, LA 70894-5100
Telephone: 504-388-6701
Fax: 504-388-2478
Email: rpatrick@agctr.lsu.edu

Chiquita Briley
Assistant Specialist—Nutrition
Southern University
Cooperative Extension Service
P.O. Box 10010
Baton Rouge, LA 70813
Telephone: 225-771-3822
Fax: 225-771-2861
Email: cbriley@sus.edu

Maine

http://www.umext.maine.edu/

Mahmoud El-Begearmi
University of Maine
Cooperative Extension
5717 Corbett Hall, Room 303
Orono, ME 04469-5717
Telephone: 207-581-3449
Fax: 207-581-3212
Email: mahmoud@umce.umext.maine.edu

Maryland

http://www.agnr.umd.edu/CES/

Henry M. Brooks
University of Maryland
1890 Extension Programs
Eastern Shore
Princess Anne, MD 21853
Telephone: 410-651-6206
Fax: 410-651-6207
Email: sterling@umes.bitnet

Mark A. Kantor
University of Maryland
Nutrition and Food Science
3306 Marie Mount Hall
College Park, MD 20742-7521
Telephone: 301-405-1018
Fax: 301-314-9327
Email: mk4@umail.umd.edu

Gayle Mason-Jenkins
University of Maryland-Eastern Shore
Richard Henson Center, Room 2127
Princes Anne, MD 21583
Telephone: 410-651-1212
Fax: 410-651-6207
Email: gmjenkins@mail.umes.edu

Thomas E. Rippen
University of Maryland
Sea Grant Extension Program
30921 Martin Ct.
Princess Anne, MD 21853
Telephone: 410-651-6636
Fax: 410-651-7656
Email: terippen@mail.umes.edu

Massachusetts

http://www.umass.edu/umext/

Nancy Cohen
University of Massachusetts Extension
Department of Nutrition
202 Chenoweth
Amherst, MA 1003
Telephone: 413-545-0552
Fax: 413-545-1074
Email: cohen@nutrition.umass.edu

Rita Brennan Olson, M.S.
Project Manager
University of Massachusetts Extension
Nutrition Education Program
Department of Nutrition
202 Chenoweth, Box 31420
Amherst, MA 01003-14220
Telephone: 413-545-0552
Fax: 413-545-1074

Michigan

http://www.msue.msu.edu/

Leslie Bourquin
Michigan State University
Department of Food Science and Human Nutrition
139 G.M. Trout Building
East Lansing, MI 48824-1224
Telephone: 517-353-9664
Fax: 517-353-8963
Email: bourqui1@pilot.msu.edu

Micronesia

Vernice Yuji
Palau Community College
Cooperative Research and Extension
P.O. Box 9
Koror, PW 96940
Telephone: 680-488-2746
Fax: 680-488-3307
Email: vernicey@yahoo.com

Anita R. Suta
Palau Community College
Cooperative Research and Extension
P.O. Box 9
Koror, PW 96940
Telephone: 680-488-2746
Fax: 680-488-3307

Minnesota

http://www.extension.umn.edu/

Paul Addis
University of Minnesota Extension Service
135E Andrew Boss Lab Meat Sciences
1354 Eckles Ave.
St. Paul, MN 55108-1011
Telephone: 612-624-7704
Fax: 612-625-5272
Email: addis@maroon.tc.umn.edu

Joellen Feirtag
University of Minnesota Extension Service
136B ABLMS
1334 Eckles Ave.
St. Paul, MN 55108-6099
Telephone: 612-624-3629
Fax: 612-625-5272
Email: jfeirtag@che2.che.umn.edu

H. William Schafer
University of Minnesota Extension Service
265 Food Science and Nutrition Building
1334 Eckles Ave.
St. Paul, MN 55108-6099
Telephone: 612-624-4793
Fax: 612-625-5272
Email: wschafer@che2.che.umn.edu

Mississippi

http://ext.msstate.edu/

Orlendtha McGowan
Alcorn State University
1000 ASU Dr., No. 479
Lorman, MS 39096
Telephone: 662-877-6559
Fax: 662-877-6694

Melissa Mixon
Mississippi State University Extension Service
Box 9745
Mississippi State, MS 39762- 9745
Telephone: 662-325-3080
Fax: 601-325-8188
Email: melissam@humansci.msstate.edu

Missouri

http://outreach.missouri.edu/hes/food.htm

Carol Giesecke, Ph.D., R.D.
Food, Nutrition and Health Specialist
Lincoln University Cooperative Extension
Allen Hall, Room 303
P.O. Box 29
Jefferson City, MO 65102-0029
Telephone: 573-681-5592
Fax: 573-681-5546
Email: giesecke@lincolnu.edu

Dale Brigham, Ph.D., R.D.
University of Missouri Outreach and Extension
Nutritional Sciences Extension
Gwynn Hall, Room 308
Columbia, MO 65211
Telephone: 573-882-2334
Fax: 573-884-5449
Email: brighamd@missouri.edu

Douglas L. Holt
University of Missouri Outreach and Extension
Food Science and Human Nutrition
122 Eckles Hall
Columbia, MO 65211
Telephone: 573-882-0593
Fax: 573-882-1150
Email: holtd@.missouri.edu

Montana

http://extn.msu.montana.edu/

Lynn C. Paul
Montana State University
Extension Service
101 Romney Gym
Bozeman, MT 59717-3360
Telephone: 406-994-5702
Fax: 406-994-7300
Email: lpaul@montana.edu

Nebraska

http://www.ianr.unl.edu/ianr/coopext/

Dicky Dee Griffin
Great Plains Veterinary Education Center
P.O. Box 187
State Spur 18D
Clay Center, NE 68933-0187
Telephone: 402-762-4500
Fax: 402-762-4509
Email: dgriffin@gpvec.unl.edu

Julie A. Albrecht
University of Nebraska-Lincoln
Cooperative Extension Service
202 F Ruth Leverton Hall
Lincoln, NE 68583-0806
Telephone: 402-472-8884
Fax: 402-472-1587
Email: hnfm063@unlvm.unl.edu

Dennis E. Burson
University of Nebraska-Lincoln
A213 Animal Sciences
Box 830908
Lincoln, NE 86583-0908
Telephone: 402-472-6457
Fax: 402-472-6362
Email: dburson1@unl.edu

Nevada

http://www.nce.unr.edu/

Jamie Benedict
University of Nevada-Reno
Department of Nutrition/Mailstop 142
Reno, NV 89557-0132
Telephone: 702-784-6445
Fax: 702-784-6449
Email: benedict@scs.unr.edu

Carolyn Leontos
University of Nevada-Reno
Cooperative Extenstion Service
2345 Red Rock St., Suite 100
Las Vegas, NV 89102
Telephone: 702-222-3130
Fax: 702-222-3100
Email: cleontos@agnt1.ag.unr.edu

Mary Spoon
University of Nevada-Reno
Cooperative Extension Service
P.O. Box 11130
Reno, NV 89520
Telephone: 702-784-4848
Fax: 702-784-4881
Email: mspoon@agnt1.ag.unr.edu

New Hampshire

http://ceinfo.unh.edu/

Catherine Violette
University of New Hampshire
Cooperative Extension System
129 Main St., 219 Kendall Hall
Durham, NH 3824
Telephone: 603-862-2496
Fax: 603-862-3758
Email: catherine.violette@unh.edu

Charlene Baxter
University of New Hampshire
Cooperative Extension System
59 College Road, Taylor Hall
Durham, NH 03824-3587
Telephone: 603-862-2485
Fax: 603-862-1585
Email: charlene.baxter@unh.edu

New Jersey

http://www.rce.rutgers.edu/

Daryl Minch
Rutgers University
Cooperative Extension of Somerset County
310 Milltown Road
Bridgewater, NJ 08807
Telephone: 908-526-6295
Fax: 908-704-1821
Email: minch@rutgers.aesop.edu

Debra Palmer-Keenan
Rutgers University, Cook College
Department of Nutritional Sciences
26 Nichol Ave., Davison Hall

New Brunswick, NJ 089012882
Telephone: 732-932-9853
Fax: 732-932-6522
Email: keenan@aesop.rutgers.edu

Donald W. Schaffner, Ph.D.
Rutgers University
65 Dudley Road
New Brunswick, NJ 08901-8520
Telephone: 732-932-9611 x214
Fax: 732-932-9611 x263
Email: Schaffner@aesop.rutgers.edu

New Mexico

http://www.cahe.nmsu.edu/ces/

Martha Archuleta
New Mexico State University
Cooperative Extension Service
Box 30003, Department 3AE
Las Cruces, NM 88003
Telephone: 505-646-3516
Fax: 505/646-5263
Email: maarchul@nmsu.edu

New York

http://www.cce.cornell.edu/

Robert B. Gravani
Cornell University
Cornell Cooperative Extension
11 Stocking Hall
Ithaca, NY 14853
Telephone: 607-255-3262
Fax: 607-254-4868
Email: RBG2@cornell.edu

Olga Padilla-Zakour
Cornell University
Department of Food Science and Technology
New York State Agricultural Experiment Station
Geneva, NY 14456
Telephone: 315-787-2259
Fax: 315-787-2284
Email: olp1@cornell.edu

Donna Scott
Cornell University
Cornell Cooperative Extension
8 Stocking Hall
Ithaca, NY 14853-7201
Telephone: 607-255-7922
Fax: 607-254-4868
Email: dls9@cornell.edu

Christina Stark
Cornell University
Cornell Cooperative Extension
Martha Van Rensselaer Hall
Ithaca, NY 14853
Telephone: 607-255-2141
Fax: 607-255-0027
Email: cms11@cornell.edu

Randy W. Worobo
Cornell University
Department of Food Science and Technology
New York State Agricultural Experiment Station
Geneva, NY 14456
Telephone: 315-787-2279
Fax: 315-787-2284
Email: rww8@cornell.edu

North Carolina

http://www.ces.ncsu.edu/

Wilda F. Wade
North Carolina A and T State University
Cooperative Extension Program
P.O. Box 21928
Greensboro, NC 27420-1928
Telephone: 910-334-7660
Fax: 910-334-7265
Email: wadew@rhema.ncat.edu

Marilyn Corbin
North Carolina State University
Cooperative Extension Service
Box 7605
Raleigh, NC 27695-7605
Telephone: 919-515-2781
Fax: 919-515-3483
Email: mcorbin@amaroq.ces.ncsu.edu

Pat Curtis
North Carolina State University
Cooperative Extension Service
P.O. Box 7624
Raleigh, NC 27695-7624
Telephone: 919-515-2956
Fax: 919-515-7124
Email: pat_curtis@ncsu.edu

Angela Fraser
North Carolina State University
Cooperative Extension Service
Box 7605, NCSU
Raleigh, NC 27695-7605

Telephone: 919-515-9150
Fax: 919-515-2786
Email: angela_fraser@ncsu.edu

Carolyn Lackey
North Carolina State University
Cooperative Extension Service
Box 7605
Raleigh, NC 27695-7605
Telephone: 919-515-2770
Fax: 919-515-3483
Email: carolyn_lackey@ncsu.edu

John E. Rushing
North Carolina State University
Cooperative Extension Service
Department of Food Science
Box 7624
Raleigh, NC 27695
Telephone: 919-515-2956
Fax: 919-515-7124
Email: John_Rushing@ncsu.edu

Brian W. Sheldon
North Carolina State University
Department of Poultry Science
234D Scott Hall
Box 7608
Raleigh, NC 27695-7608
Telephone: 919-515-5407
Fax: 919-515-7070
Email: brian_sheldon@ncsu.edu

Melissa C. Taylor
Food Safety Education and Communications Specialist
North Carolina State University
Department of Food Science
Cooperative Extension Service
Schaub Hall, Room 236B
Box 7624
Raleigh, NC 27695-7624
Telephone:919-513-2268
Fax: 919-515-7124
Email: foodsafety@ncsu.edu

Sandra Zaslow
North Carolina State University
Cooperative Extension Service
Box 7605
Raleigh, NC 27695-7605
Telephone: 919-515-9152
Fax: 919-515-3483
Email: sandra_zaslow@ncsu.edu

North Dakota

http://www.ext.nodak.edu/

Julie Garden-Robinson
North Dakota State University
Cooperative Extension Service
Food and Nutrition Department
351 EML Hall, Box 5059
Fargo, ND 58105-5059
Telephone: 701-231-7187
Fax: 701-231-8568
Email: jgardenr@ndsuext.nodak.edu

Northern Marianas

Floria P. James
Northern Marianas College
Cooperative Extension Service
P.O. Box 1250
Saipan, MP 96950
Telephone: 670-234-9023
Fax: 670-234-0054
Email: FloriaJ@nmcnet.edu

Ohio

http://www.ag.ohio-state.edu/~ohioline/lines/food.html

Lydia Medeiros
Ohio State University
Cooperative Extension Service
1787 Neil Ave., 315 Campbell Hall
Columbus, OH 43210-1295
Telephone: 614-292-2699
Fax: 614-/292-8880
Email: medeiros.1@osu.edu

Oklahoma

http://www.dasnr.okstate.edu/oces/

Barbara Brown
Oklahoma State University
Cooperative Extension Service
309 Home Economics Building
Stillwater, OK 74078-6111
Telephone: 405-744-6283
Fax: 405-744-3538
Email: bbrown@okstate.edu

Gerrit Cuperus
Oklahoma State University

Cooperative Extension Service
Department of Agricultural Economics
310 Agricultural Hall
Stillwater, OK 74078
Telephone: 405-744-6834
Fax: 405-744-8210
Email: bugs1@okstate.edu

Lynda Harriman
Oklahoma State University
Cooperative Extension Service
104 Home Economics
Stillwater, OK 74078-6111
Telephone: 405-744-6280
Fax: 405-744-7113
Email: lch@okstate.edu

Peter Michael Muriana
Oklahoma State University
109 Food and Agricultural Products Reseach and Technology Center
Stillwater, OK 74078
Telephone: 405-744-5563
Fax: 405-744-6313
Email: muriana@okstate.edu

Linda Murray
Oklahoma State University
Cooperative Extension Service
230 W. Okmulgee St., Suite B
Muskogee, OK 74401
Telephone: 918-687-2466
Fax: 918-687-2484
Email: lmurray@dasnr.okstate.edu

Oregon

http://osu.orst.edu/extension/

Carolyn A. Raab
Oregon State University
Extension Home Economics
161 Milam Hall
Corvallis, OR 97331-5106
Telephone: 541-737-1019
Fax: 541-737-0999
Email: raabc@orst.edu

Ellen Schuster
Oregon State University
Extension Home Economics
161 Milam Hall
Corvallis, OR 97331-5106
Telephone: 541-737-1017
Fax: 541-737-0999
Email: schustee@orst.edu

Pennsylvania

http://www.extension.psu.edu/

J. Lynne Brown
Pennsylvania State University
Department of Food Science
205A Borland Lab
University Park, PA 16802
Telephone: 814-863-3973
Fax: 814-863-6132
Email: f9a@psu.edu

Catherine Nettles Cutter, Ph.D.
Assistant Professor and Food Safety Extension Specialist—Muscle Foods
Pennsylvania State University
Department of Food Science
111 Borland Lab
University Park, PA 16802
Telephone: 814-865-8862 or lab. 814-863-1804
Fax: 814-863-6132
Email: cnc3@psu.edu

Hassan Gourama
Pennsylvania State University
Pennsylvania State Cooperative Extension
Tulpehocken Road
P.O. Box 7009
Reading, PA 19610-6009
Telephone: 610-396-6121
Fax: 610-396-6024
Email: hxg7@psu.edu

Stephen Knabel
Pennsylvania State University
Pennsylvania State Cooperative Extension
116 Borland Lab
University Park, PA 16802
Telephone: 814-863-1372
Fax: 863-863-6132
Email: sjk9@psu.edu

Luke LaBorde
Pennsylvania State University
Pennsylvania State Cooperative Extension
119 Borland Lab
University Park, PA 16802
Telephone: 814-863-2298Fax: 814-863-6132
Email: lfl5@psu.edu

Dana McElroy
Pennsylvania State University
Department of Food Science

106 Borland Lab
University Park, PA 16802
Telephone: 814-865-0640
Fax: 814/863-6132
Email: dmm39@psu.edu

Puerto Rico

http://sea.upr.clu.edu/

Vilma Gonzalez
University of Puerto Rico
Cooperative Extension Service
Building C, College Station
P.O. Box 5000
Mayaquez, PR 681
Telephone: 787-832-4040 ext. 306
Fax: 809-832-4220
Email: R_Justiniano@seam.upr.clu.edu

Ann Macpherson-Sanchez, Ed.D
Foods and Nutrition Specialist
University of Puerto Rico
Agricultural Extension Service
Mayaguez, PR 00681
Telephone: 787-832-4040 ext. 3066
Fax: 787-265-4130

Rhode Island

http://www.edc.uri.edu/

Marjorie Caldwell
University of Rhode Island
Cooperative Extension Service
530 Liberty Ln.
West Kingston, RI 2852
Telephone: 401-874-2254
Fax: 401-792-2994
Email: mcald@uriacc.uri.edu

Martha S. Patnoad
University of Rhode Island
Cooperative Extension Service
East Alumni Ave.
Kingston, RI 02881-0804
Telephone: 401-874-2960
Fax: 401-874-4017

Lori Pivarnik
University of Rhode Island
Cooperative Extension Service
530 Liberty Ln.
West Kingston, RI 2892
Telephone: 401-874-2972
Fax: 401-874-2994
Email: pivarnik@uriacc.uri.edu

South Carolina

http://virtual.clemson.edu/groups/extension/

Elizabeth H. Hoyle
Clemson University
Cooperative Extension Service
243 Poole Agricultural Center, Box 340315
Clemson, SC 29634-0315
Telephone: 864-656-5713
Fax: 864-656-5723
Email: lhoyle@clemson.edu

John Surak
Clemson University
Cooperative Extension Service
220 Poole Agricultural Center, Box 340371
Clemson, SC 29634-0371
Telephone: 864-656-2786
Fax: 864-656-0331
Email: jsurak@clemson.edu

South Dakota

http://www.abs.sdstate.edu/CES/

Carol Pitts
South Dakota State University
Cooperative Extension Service
NHE 239, Box 2275A
Brookings, SD 57007-0295
Telephone:605-688-6233
Fax: 605-688-6360
Email: pitts.carol@ces.sdstate.edu

Tennessee

http://www.utextension.utk.edu/

Thelma S. Sanders-Hunter
Tennessee State University
Cooperative Extension Service
3500 John Adam Merritt Blvd.
Nashville, TN 37209-1561
Telephone: 615-963-5547
Fax: 615-963-5884
Email: thunter01@picard.tnstate.edu

Janie L. Burney, Ph.D., R.D
University of Tennessee
Food, Nutrition and Health
Tennessee Agricultural Extension Service

P.O. Box 1071, 119 Morgan Hall
Knoxville, TN 37901-1071
Telephone: 423-974-7402
Fax: 423-974-7448
Email: jlburney@.utk.edu

John C. Campbell
University of Tennessee
Cooperative Extension Service
P.O. Box 415
Columbia, TN 38402-0415
Telephone: 615-388-9557
Fax: 615-380-2594

Dr. Michael P. Davidson
Associate Professor
University of Tennessee
Food Science and Technology
P.O. Box 1071, 201 McLeod Building
Knoxville, TN 37901-1071
Telephone: 423-974-7334
Fax: 423-974-7332
Email: pmdavidson@utk.edu

Bill Morris
University of Tennessee
Tennessee Agricultural Extension Service
P.O. Box 1071
Knoxville, TN 37901-1071
Telephone: 423-974-7334
Fax: 423-974-7332
Email: bmorris@utk.edu

Texas

http://agpublications.tamu.edu/

Linda Williams-Willis
Prairie View A & M University
Cooperative Extension Program
P.O. Box 3059
Prairie View, TX 77446
Telephone: 409-857-3829
Fax: 409-857-2004
Email: lw-willis@tamu.edu

Peggy Van Laanen
Texas A & M University
Texas Agricultural Extension Service
Department of Animal Science
352 Kleberg Center
College Station, TX 77843-2471
Telephone: 409-845-6379
Fax: 409-847-9225
Email: p-vanlaanen@tamu.edu

Anne Michelle Ledoux
Texas A & M University
Texas Agricultural Extension Service
Food Protection Management Program
352 Kleberg Center
College Station, TX 77843-2471
Telephone: 409-845-6379
Fax: 409-847-9225
Email: a-ledoux@tamu.edu

Utah

http://www.ext.usu.edu/food/

Charlotte Brennand
Utah State University
Cooperative Extension Service
Nutrition and Food Science
Logan, UT 84322-8700
Telephone: 435-797-2116
Fax: 435-797-2379
Email: foodsafe@cc.usu.edu

Vermont

http://ctr.uvm.edu/ext/nfsh/

Karen Schneider, CFCS
UVM Extension Specialist, Food Safety
University of Vermont
1 Scale Ave., Unit 55
Rutland, VT 05701
Telephone: 802-773-3349
Fax: 802-775-4840
Email: karen.schneider@uvm.edu or
karens@sover.net

Dale Steen
UVM Extension Specialist, Nutrition and Food Safety
University of Vermont
2176 Portland St., Suite 3
St. Johnsbury, VT 05819-8802
Telephone: 802-748-8177 ext. 29
Fax: 802-748-1955
Email: dale.steen@uvm.edu

Virgin Islands

http://rps.uvi.edu/CES/

Alice V. Henry
University of the Virgin Islands
Cooperative Extension Service
RR#2, Box 10,000, Kingshill St.

Croix, VI 850
Telephone: 340-692-4092
Fax: 340-692-4085
Email: alice.henry@uvi.edu

Virginia

http://www.ext.vt.edu/

Richard F. Booker
Virginia State University
Cooperative Extension Service
P.O. Box 9081
Petersburg, VA 23806
Telephone: 804-524-5871
Fax: 804-524-5967
Email: rbooker@vtvm1.cc.vt.edu

Anthony G. Hankins
Virginia State University
1890 Extension Programs
P.O. Box 9081
Petersburg, VA 23806
Telephone: 804-524-5962
Fax: 804-524-5967
Email: ex735@vtvm1.cc.vt.edu

Cameron Hackney
Virginia Polytechnic Institute and State University
Cooperative Extension Service
Food Science and Technology
Blacksburg, VA 24061-0418
Telephone: 540-231-5247
Fax: 540-231-9293
Email: hackneyc@vt.edu

Norman G. Marriott
Virginia Polytechnic Institute and State University
Cooperative Extension Service
Food Science and Technology
Blacksburg, VA 24061-0418
Telephone: 540-231-7640
Fax: 540-231-9293
Email: marriott@vt.edu

Tim Roberts, Ph.D, R.D.
Virginia Polytechnic Institute and State University
Department of Nutrition, Foods and Exercise
252 Wallace Hall
Blacksburg, VA 24061-0430
Telephone: 540-231-3464
Fax: 540-231-3916
Email: robertst@vt.edu

Susan S. Sumner
Virginia Polytechnic Institute and State University
Food Science and Technology 0418
Blacksburg, VA 24060
Telephone: 540-231-5280
Fax: 540-231-9293
Email: sumners@vt.edu

Brian Yaun
Virginia Polytechnic Institute and State University
Cooperative Extension Service
Food Science and Technology 0418
Blacksburg, VA 24061
Telephone: 540-231-8697
Fax: 540-231-9293
Email: byaun@vt.edu

Washington

http://ext.wsu.edu/

Richard Dougherty
Washington State University
Food Science and Human Nutrition
Pullman, WA 99164-6376
Telephone: 509-335-0972
Fax: 509-335-4815
Email: dougherty@wsu.edu

Virginia Val Hillers
Washington State University
Cooperative Extension Service
Food Science and Human Nutrition
Pullman, WA 99164-6376
Telephone: 509-335-2970
Fax: 509-335-4815
Email: hillersv@wsu.edu

West Virginia

http://www.wvu.edu/~exten/

Guendoline Brown
West Virginia University
Cooperative Extension Service
605 Knapp Hall
P.O. Box 6031
Morgantown, WV 26506-6031
Telephone: 304-293-2694
Fax: 304-293-7599
Email: gbrown2@wvu.edu

Wisconsin

http://www1.uwex.edu/

Dennis R. Buege
University of Wisconsin-Madison
Cooperative Extension
280 Muscle Biology Lab
1805 Linden Dr.
Madison, WI 53706
Telephone: 608-262-0555
Fax: 608-265-3110
Email: drbuege@facstaff.wisc.edu

Barbara Ingham
University of Wisconsin-Madison
Department of Food Science
1605 Linden Dr.
Madison, WI 53706-1565
Telephone: 608-263-7383
Fax: 608-262-6872
Email: bhingham@facstaff.wisc.edu

Steve Ingham
University of Wisconsin-Madison
Department of Food Science
1605 Linden Dr.
Madison, WI 53706-1565
Telephone: 608-265-4801
Email: scingham@facstaff.wisc.edu

Thomas Zinnen
University of Wisconsin-Madison
Cooperative Extension
1710 University Ave.
Madison, WI 53706
Telephone: 608-265-2420
Email: zinnen@macc.wisc.edu

Wyoming

http://www.uwyo.edu/ag/CES/ceshome.htm

Suzanne Pelican, M.S., R.D.
Food and Nutrition Extension Specialist
University of Wyoming
Department of Family and Consumer Sciences
Box 3354
Laramie, WY 82071-3354
Telephone: 307-766-5177
Fax: 307-766-3379
Email: pelican@uwyo.edu

FOOD AND DRUG ADMINISTRATION (FDA) PUBLIC AFFAIRS SPECIALISTS

FDA's public affairs specialists (PAS) can respond to consumer questions about the agency, its authorities, activities, and the products it regulates. The Public Affairs Specialists have publications, posters, teacher kits, press releases, and background papers on all kinds of FDA-related topics. The FDA maintains this list on their Web site at: http://www.fda.gov/ora/fed_state/DFSR_Activities/dfsr_pas.html.

Northeast Region

New England District Office
Serves Connecticut, Maine, Massachusetts, New Hampshire, Rhode Island, and Vermont
Paula Fairfield (ext. 184)
pfairfield@ora.fda.gov
Joseph Raulinaitis (ext. 186)
jraulina@ora.fda.gov
Susan Small (ext. 185)
ssmall@ora.fda.gov
Food and Drug Administration
One Montvale Ave.
Stoneham, MA 02180
Telephone: 781-279-1675
Fax: 781-279-1687

New York District Office
Serves New York City, Long Island (Nassau and Suffolk Counties), Westchester County, and Rockland County
Dicia Granville (ext. 5043)
dgranvil@ora.fda.gov
Vincent Zuberko (ext. 5755)
vzuberko@ora.fda.gov
Food and Drug Administration
850 Third Ave.
Brooklyn, NY 11232
Telephone: 718-340-7000
Fax: 718-340-7057

Central Region

New Jersey District Office
Serves all of New Jersey
Joan G. Lytle
jlytle@ora.fda.gov
Food and Drug Administration
Waterview Corporate Center
10 Waterview Blvd., 3rd Floor
Parisippany, NJ 07054
Telephone: 973-331-2926
Fax: 973-331-2969

Philadelphia District Office
Serves Delaware and Pennsylvania
Anitra D. Brown-Reed
abrown2@ora.fda.gov
Food and Drug Administration
2nd and Chestnut Sts.
Room 900, U.S. Customhouse
Philadelphia, PA 19106
Telephone: 215-597-4390
Fax: 215-597-6649

Baltimore District Office
Serves Maryland, Virginia, West Virginia, and Washington, D.C.
Jeanni Prego
jprego@ora.fda.gov
Food and Drug Administration
900 Madison Ave.
Baltimore, MD 21201
Telephone: 410-962-3731
Fax: 410-962-2307

Cincinnati District Office
Serves Kentucky and Ohio
Marilyn Zipkes
mzipkes@ora.fda.gov
Food and Drug Administration
6751 Steger Dr.
Cincinnati, OH 45237-3097
Telephone: 513-679-2700 ext. 110
Fax: 513-684-2905

Brunswick Resident Inspection Post
Serves Kentucky and Ohio
Ruth Weisheit
rweishei@ora.fda.gov
Food and Drug Administration
3820 Center Road
P.O. Box 838
Brunswick, OH 44212
Telephone: 330-273-1038
Fax: 330-225-7477

Chicago District Office
Serves the State of Illinois
Darlene Bailey
dbailey@ora.fda.gov
Kim Phillips
kphillip@ora.fda.gov
Food and Drug Administration
300 S. Riverside Plaza
Suite 550-South
Chicago, IL 60606
Telephone: 312-353-5863 (ext. 187)
Fax: 312-886-3280

Detroit District Office
Serves all of Michigan
Evelyn DeNike
edenike@ora.fda.gov
Linda Kettleson
lkettles@ora.fda.gov
Food and Drug Administration
1560 E. Jefferson Ave.
Detroit, MI 48207
Telephone: 313-226-6158 ext. 149
Fax: 313-226-3076

Indianapolis Resident Inspection Post
Serves all of Indiana
Janet LeClair (ext. 13)
jleclair@ora.fda.gov
Carol Gallagher (ext. 31)
cgallagh@ora.fda.gov
Food and Drug Administration
Resident Inspection Post
101 W. Ohio St.
Indianapolis, IN 46204
Telephone: 317-226-6500
Fax: 317-226-6506

Minneapolis District Office
Serves Minnesota, North Dakota, and South Dakota
Donald W. Aird
daird@ora.fda.gov
Food and Drug Administration
240 Hennepin Ave.
Minneapolis, MN 55401
Telephone: 612-334-4100 ext. 129
Fax: 612-334-4134

Milwaukee Resident Inspection Post
Serves all of Wisconsin
Steve Davis (ext. 19)
sdavis@ora.fda.gov
Kathy Rozewicz (ext. 20)
krozewic@ora.fda.gov
Food and Drug Administration

Resident Inspection Post
2675 N. Mayfair Road, Suite 200
Milwaukee, WI 53226-1305
Telephone: 414-771-7167
Fax: 414-771-7512

Southeast Region

San Juan District Office
Serves Puerto Rico and the Virgin Islands
Nilda Villegas
nvillega@ora.fda.gov
Ruth Marcano
rmarcano@ora.fda.gov
Food and Drug Administration
Puerta de Tierra Station
San Juan, PR 00906-3223
Telephone: 787-729-6852
Fax: 787-729-6847

Atlanta District Office
Serves Georgia, North Carolina, and South Carolina
JoAnn Pittman
jpittman@ora.fda.gov
Food and Drug Administration
60 Eighth St. NE
Atlanta, GA 30309
Telephone: 404-347-4001 ext. 5340
Fax: 404-347-1912

Raleigh Resident Inspection Post
Serves the State of North Carolina
Mary C. Lewis
mlewis@ora.fda.gov
Food and Drug Administration
310 New Bern Ave.
P.O. Box 25730
Raleigh, NC 27611
Telephone: 919-856-4456 ext. 17
Fax: 919-856-4776

Florida District Office
Serves Northern Florida
Lynne C. Issacs (ext. 202)
lisaacs@ora.fda.gov
Faye Bronner (ext. 203)
fbronner@ora.fda.gov
Frank Goodwin (ext. 221)
fgoodwin@ora.fda.gov
Food and Drug Administration
555 Winderley Place, Suite 200
Maitland, FL 32751
Telephone: 407-475-4700
Fax: 407-475-4768

Miami Resident Inspection Post
Serves South Florida including Miami, Palm Beach, and Fort Myers
Estela Niella-Brown
ebrown1@ora.fda.gov
Food and Drug Administration
6601 N.W. 25th St.
P.O. Box 59-2256
Miami, FL 33159-2256
Telephone: 305-526-2800 ext. 937
Fax: 305-526-2693

Nashville District Office
Serves Alabama and Tennessee
Sandra Baxter (ext. 122)
sbaxter@ora.fda.gov
Mancia Davis (ext. 147)
mdavis1@ora.fda.gov
Food and Drug Administration
297 Plus Park Blvd.
Nashville, TN 37217
Telephone: 615-781-5372
Fax: 615-781-5383

New Orleans District Office
Serves Louisiana and Mississippi
Darlene Tollestrup
dtollest@ora.fda.gov
Food and Drug Administration
4298 Elysian Fields Ave.
New Orleans, LA 70122
Telephone: 225-589-2420 ext. 121
Fax: 504-589-6360

Southwest Region

Dallas District Office
Serves Dallas, Fort Worth, and all of Oklahoma
Maria Velasco
mvelasco@ora.fda.gov
Helen Monda
hmonda@ora.fda.gov
Food and Drug Administration
3310 Live Oak St.
Dallas, TX 75204
Telephone: 214-655-5315 ext. 303
Fax: 214-655-5331

Houston Resident Inspection Post
Serves Houston Metro area and Eastern Texas (Beaumont, Galveston) and all of Arkansas
Sheryl Lunnon-Baylor
sbaylor@ora.fda.gov

Food and Drug AdministrationResident Inspection Post
1445 N. Loop West, Suite 420
Houston, TX 77008
Telephone: 713-802-9095 ext. 15
Fax: 713-802-0906

San Antonio Resident Inspection Post
Serves South Central Texas including Amarillo, Lubbock, Waco, Austin, San Antonio, El Paso, Laredo, Hidalgo, and Brownsville
Vacant
Food and Drug Administration
Resident Inspection Post
10127 Morocco, Suite 119
San Antonio, TX 78216
Telephone: 210-308-4531
Fax: 210-308-4548

Kansas City District Office
Serves all of Kansas and Nebraska including Kansas City, Missouri Metro area, Omaha, Council Bluff, and the Iowa Metro area
Tywanna Paul
tpaul@ora.fda.gov
Food and Drug Administration
11630 W. 80th St.
Lenexa, KS 66214
Telephone: 913-752-2141
Fax: 913-752-2111

St. Louis Branch Office
Serves St. Louis, Missouri, and all of Iowa
Mary-Margaret Richardson
mrichard@ora.fda.gov
Food and Drug Administration
12 Sunnen Dr., Suite 122
St. Louis, MO 63143
Telephone: 314-645-1167 ext. 123
Fax: 314-645-2969

Denver District Office
Serves all of Colorado, New Mexico, Utah, and Wyoming
Virlie Walker (303-236-3018)
vwalker@ora.fda.gov
Devin Koontz (303-236-3020)
dkoontz@ora.fda.gov
Food and Drug Administration
Denver Federal Center
Building 20, Room B-1121
6th Ave. and Kipling
Denver, CO 80225-0087
Fax: 303-236-3551

Pacific Region

San Francisco District Office
Serves Northern California including Fresno, Sacramento, San Jose, Guam, and Stockton. Also serves Nevada and the Pacific Rim territories such as Guam
Janet McDonald (510-337-6845)
jmcdonal@ora.fda.gov
Mary Ellen Taylor (510-337-6888)
mtaylor1@ora.fda.gov
Food and Drug Administration
1431 Harbor Bay Parkway
Alameda, CA 94502-7070
Fax: 510-337-6708

Los Angeles District Office
Serves Southern California including Calexico, Canoga Irvine, Los Angeles, San Diego, San Ysidro, Santa Barbara, Rancho Cucamonga, and Terminal Island
Laurel Eu (714-798-7609)
leu@ora.fda.gov
Rosario Quintanilla Vior (714-798-7607)
rqvior@ora.fda.gov
Food and Drug Administration
19900 MacArthur Blvd., Suite 300
Irvine, CA 92715-2445
Fax: 714-798-7715

Phoenix Resident Inspection Post
Serves all of Arizona
Gilbert V. Meza
gmeza@ora.fda.gov
Food and Drug Administration
Resident Inspection Post
4605 E. Elwood St., Suite 402
Phoenix, AZ 85040-1948
Telephone: 480-829-7396 ext. 225
Fax: 480-829-7677

Seattle District Office
Serves all of Washington State and Alaska
Susan Hutchcroft
shutchr@ora.fda.gov
Food and Drug Administration
22201 23rd Dr. SE
Bothell, WA 98021-4421
Telephone: 425-483-4953
Fax: 425-483-4996

Portland Resident Inspection Post
Serves Oregon, Idaho, and Montana
Alan Bennett
abennett@ora.fda.gov

Food and Drug Administration
Resident Inspection Post
9780 S.W. Nimbus Ave.
Beaverton, OR 97008-7163
Telephone: 503-671-9332 ext. 22
Fax: 503-671-9445

HOTLINES

Non-Food Company Hotlines

Alliance for Food and Fiber National Food Safety Hotline
Telephone: 800-266-0200 Fax: 310-446-1896
Description: Callers can access information on food safety topics related to agriculture at this educational clearinghouse to inform the public and the media on the issues of food safety and crop protection that impact the production, processing, and distribution of food and fiber products.
Web site: http://www.foodsafetyalliance.org/

American Academy of Allergy and Immunology
Telephone: 800-822-2762
Description: Brochures, physician referral

Ball Home Canning Hotline
Telephone: 800-240-3340
Description: Order their "How To" canning guides, ask questions about canning, or request recipes.

Butterball Turkey Talk-Line
Telephone: 800-323-4848 (English and Spanish) 800-TDD-3848 (hearing impaired)
Description: Information on recipes and food safety during the November/December holiday season.
Web site: http://www.butterball.com/

Consumer Right to Know Hotline
Telephone: 877-REAL-FOOD
Description: Sponsored by the Mothers for Natural Law, a group that campaigns to ban genetically engineered foods and to require mandatory labeling.
Web site: http://www.safe-food.org/

FDA Food Information Line
Telephone: 888-SAFEFOOD
Description: Information Specialists and recorded announcements offer consumers information on food safety, food additives, and dietary supplements.
Web site: http://vm.cfsan.fda.gov/

Food Biotechnology Communications Network
Telephone: 877-food-bio (366-3246)
Description: Information specialists at this information line answer questions on food biotechnology from the general public. Their mandate is to have a forum for the public to ask questions and have them addressed in a balanced way.
Web site: http://www.foodbiotech.org/

Food Safety and Technology Hotline
Telephone: 800-752-2751
Description: Mainly for Ohio residents, but will also take calls from others. Sponsored by Ohio State University.

International Bottled Water Association
Telephone: 800-WATER11
Description: Consumer information on the safety of bottled water.
Web site: http://www.bottledwater.org/

National Antimicrobial Information Network (NAIN)
Telephone: 800-447-6349 Fax: 541-737-0761
Description: NAIN responds to information requests about antimicrobial products-sanitizers, disinfectants, and sterilants-by phone or mail. A cooperative effort of Oregon State University and the U.S. EPA
Email address: nain@ace.orst.edu
Web site: http://ace.orst.edu/info/nain/

National Drinking Water Clearinghouse (NDWC)
Telephone: 800-624-8301
Description: The NDWC's technical assistants are available to answer questions related to drinking water. Some common topics include regulatory questions about specific requirements small drinking water systems must meet; financing questions, such as where communities might find funds to upgrade or build new water systems; and technical questions, such as what treatment processes alleviate specific water quality problems.
Web site: http://www.estd.wvu.edu/ndwc/DiscussionFrame.html

National Lead Information Center
Telephone: 800-424-LEAD 800-532-3394
Description: To receive a general information packet, to order other documents, or for detailed information or questions, you may call the Center's clearinghouse and speak with a specialist.
Email address: leadctr@epamail.epa.gov
Web site: http://www.epa.gov/opptintr/lead/nlic.htm

National Pesticide Telecommunications Network
Telephone: 800-858-7378 Fax: 541-737-0761
Description: NPTN is a cooperative effort of Oregon State University and the U.S. EPA offerring information on pesticides.
Email address: nptn@ace.orst.edu
Web site: http://nptn.orst.edu/

Safe Drinking Water Hotline
Telephone: 800-426-4791
Description: From the U.S. Environmental Protection Agency, Office of Ground Water and Drinking Water. Consumers may pose questions online at the Web site, via email, or on the phone
Email address: hotline-sdwa@epamail.epa.gov
Web site: http://www.epa.gov/safewater/drinklink.html

Safe Tables Our Priority (S.T.O.P.)
Telephone: 800-350-STOP Fax: 312-427-2307
Description: To provide information and improve services to those made ill by food. S.T.O.P. provides information and support to victims and their families through our hotline (800-350-STOP) and information clearinghouse, and promotes proper diagnostic and treatment practices in the medical community.
Email address: feedback@stop-usa.org
Web site: http://www.stop-usa.org/

USDA Meat and Poultry Hotline
Telephone: 800-535-4555
Description: Information specialists answer food safety questions about meat and poultry products.
Web site: http://www.fsis.usda.gov

Food Company Hotlines

Armour-Swift-Eckrich
Telephone: 800-325-7424
Description: Armour, Butterball, Swift Premium, Eckrich, Healthy Choice.
Web site: http://www.freshpork.com/

Banquet
Telephone: 800-722-1344
Description: Banquet foods.
Web site: http://www.conagra.com/

Beech-Nut
Telephone: 800-BEECH-NUT, 800-BEBITOS for Spanish
Description: Beech-Nut baby food products.
Web site: http://www.Beech-nut.com

Bob Evans Farm, Inc.
Telephone: 800-272-7675
Description: For food safety information on Bob Evans Farm products sold in stores and Bob Evans restaurants.

Campbell Soup Company
Telephone: 800-257-8443
Description: Prego, Pepperidge Farm, Pace, Franco-American, Swansons, Campbell Soups.
Web site: http://www.campbellsoup.com

Coca-Cola Company
Telephone: 800-438-2653
Description: All Coca-Cola beverages, Sprite, Surge, Barq's Root Beer, Minute Maid, Mr. Pibb, Fresca, Nestea Ice Tea, Fanta, Powerade, Dasani, Lift, Citra, Mellow Yellow.
Web site: http://www.thecocacolacompany.com/

Dole Consumer Center
Telephone: 800-232-8800
Description: Dole products.
Web site: http://www.dole.com

Eckrich Products
Telephone: 800-325-7424
Description: Eckrich products.

Empire Kosher Customer Service Hotline
Telephone: 800-EMPIRE4
Description: Empire kosher products.
Web site: http://www.empirekosher.com/

Fiesta Nut Candy Company
Telephone: 800-645-3296
Description: Fiesta nut and candy products.
Web site: http://fiestanut.com

Fleischmann's
Telephone: 800-227-6202
Description: Fleischmann's products.
Web site: http://breadworld.com

Frito-Lay
Telephone: 800-352-4477.
Ask for operator 100.
Description: Fritos, Lays, Ruffles, Doritos, Cheetos, 3Ds, Tostitos, Rold Gold, Sun Chips, Cracker Jacks, Grandma's, Santitas.
Web site: http://www.fritolay.com

General Mills Consumer Response Center
Telephone: 800-328-6787
Description: Betty Crocker, Yoplait, Gold Medal, Nature Valley, Lloyd's, Farmhouse, Colombo.
Web site: http://www.generalmills.com

Gerber
Telephone: 800-443-7237 (800-4-GERBER)
Description: Gerber baby food products.
Web site: http://www.gerber.com

Gorton's Fish Consumer Services
Telephone: 800-222-6846
Description: Gorton's fish products.
Web site: http://www.gortons.com/

Healthy Choice Consumer Affairs
Telephone: 800-323-9980
Description: Healthy Choice products.
Web site: http://www.healthychoice.com/

Heinz USA Consumer Affairs Department
Telephone: 800-USA-BABY
Description: For Heinz baby food products only.
Web site: http://www.heinz.com/

Hershey's Consumer Relations
Telephone: 800-468-1714
Description: Hershey's products.
Web site: http://www.hersheys.com

Hillshire Farm and Kahn's Consumer Affairs
Telephone: 800-543-4465
Description: Hillshire Farm, Kahn's products.

Hormel Foods
Telephone: 800-523-4635
Description: Hormel products, Dinty Moore, Mary Kitchen, Spam, Stagg, Herb-ox, Black Label, Old Smokehouse, Mrs. Paterson's, Quick Meal, Marrakesh Express, Peloponnese, Patak's, Herdez, House of Tsang, Chi-Chi's.
Web site: Hormel.com or spam.com

Kraft-General Foods Consumer Resource Center
Telephone: 800-431-1001
Description: Post cereals, Toblerone, Jell-o, Calument, Minute, Baker's, Stove Top, Cracker Barrel, Shake N Bake, Velveeta, Sure-Jel, Certo, Dream Whip, Good Seasons, Knudson, Country Time, Crystal Light, Kool-aid, Tang, Breakstone's, Bull's Eye, Miracle Whip, Breyers, Oscar Mayer, Digiorno, Capri, Seven Seas, Claussen, Cool Whip, Tombstone.
Web site: http://www.Kraftfoods.com

Kroger Product Line
Telephone: 800-632-6900
Description: Kroger private label foods.

LaChoy Foodservice
Telephone: 800-633-0112
Description: LaChoy products.
Web site: http://www.lachoyfoodservice.com/

Land O'Lakes
Telephone: 800-328-4155
Description: Land O'Lake products.
Web site: http://landolakes.com/

Louis Rich
Telephone: 800-722-1421
Description: Louis Rich products.
Web site: http://www.Kraftfoods.com

McCormick/Schilling Spices
Telephone: 800-632-5847
Description: McCormick products, Old Bay, Golden Dipt, Produce Partners, Schilling.
Web site: http://www.McCormick.com

Minute Maid Company
Telephone: 888-884-8952
Description: Minute Maid juices, Hi-C, Kapo, Cappy, Andifruit, Bacardi Mixers, Five Alive, Southern Sun, Bright and Early. Also speak Spanish.
Web site: http://www.minutemaid.com

Nabisco Consumer Affairs
Telephone: 800-8NABNET

Description: Nabisco products, Grey Poupon, Knox, Peek Freans.
Web site: http://www.nabisco.com/

Nestle USA Consumer Services Center
Telephone: 800-637-8539 800-452-1971
Description: Nestle products,Stouffer's, Carnation, Libby's, Ortega, Taster's Choice, Toll House, Juicy Juice.
Web site: http://www.nestle.com

Nutra-Sweet
Telephone: 800-321-7254
Description: Nutra-Sweet products.
Web site: http://www.equal.com

Omaha Steaks International
Telephone: 800-228-9872
Description: Omaha Steak products.
Web site: http://www.omahasteaks.com

Pepsi Cola Consumer Relations
Telephone: 800-433-2652
Description: Pepsi beverages.
Web site: http://www.pepsi.com

Pillsbury Company
Telephone: 800-767-4466
Description: Pillsbury products, Häagen-Dazs, Green Giant, Old El Paso, Totino's, Jeno's, Progresso, Martha White, Hungry Jack.
Web site: http://www.Pillsbury.com

Proctor & Gamble Consumer Relations
Telephone: 800-543-7276
Description: Pringles (800-568-4035), Crisco (800-543-7276), Folgers (800-937-9745), Jif (800-283-8915), Sunny Delight (800-395-5849).
Web site: http://www.pg.com

Tropicana
Telephone: 800-237-7799
Description: Tropicana products.
Web site: http://www.tropicana.com/

STATE DEPARTMENTS OF HEALTH AND/OR AGRICULTURE

State and local health and/or agriculture departments are responsible for the inspecting and licensing of grocery stores, restaurants, and other institutions that serve or sell food. In some states these duties are shared between the department of health and the department of agriculture; in other states one of the two agencies may have complete jurisdiction. To report a suspected foodborne illness or potential food safety violation in a food store or restaurant, call the state or county department where the facility is located. These are also the offices to contact for obtaining a license and for information on regulations to produce a food product or open a food establishment. This list is adapted from a Food and Drug Administration's list available on the Internet at: http://www.fda.gov/ora/fed_state/directorytable.htm. State offices are also responsible for the animal health, manufactured foods, milk processing, meat processing, and pesticides.

Alabama State Department of Public Health
Bureau of Environmental Services
Division of Food, Milk and Lodging
334-206-5375
http://www.alapubhealth.org/environmental/overview.htm

Alaska State Department of Environmental Conservation
Division of Environmental Health
Environmental Sanitation/Food Safety Program
907-451-2110
http://www.state.ak.us/dec/deh/sanitat/homesan.htm

American Samoa Department of Health
Division of Preventive and Environmental Health
011 684-633-4606

Arizona State Department of Health Services
Bureau of Epidemiology and Disease Control
Office of Environmental Health
Food Safety and Environmental Services
602-230-5917
http://www.hs.state.az.us/edc/oeh/fsandes.htm

Arkansas State Department of Health
Bureau of Environmental Health Services

Division of Environmental Health Protection
Food Protection Services
501-661-2171
http://health.state.ar.us/services/services_eh1_all.html

California State Department of Health Services
Division of Food, Drug and Radiation Safety
Food and Drug Branch
Food Safety Section
916-445-2263
http://www.dhs.cahwnet.gov/org/ps/fdb/

Colorado State Department of Public Health and Environment
Division of Consumer Protection
303-692-3620
http://www.cdphe2.state.co.us/cp/

Connecticut State Department of Public Health
Bureau of Regulatory Services
Environmental Health Division
Food Protection Program
860-509-7297
http://www.state.ct.us/dph/junk/food_protectiontext.htm

Delaware State Department of Health and Social Services
Division of Public Health
Health Systems Protection Branch
Office of Food Protection
302-739-38410

District of Columbia Department of Health
Environmental Health Administration
Food Protection Branch
202-727-7250
http://www.dchealth.com/eha/services.htm

Florida State Department of Agriculture and Consumer Services
Division of Food Safety
850-488-0295
http://doacs.state.fl.us/~fs/

Florida Department of Business and Professional Regulation
Division of Hotels and Restaurants
850-488-1133
http://www.state.fl.us/dbpr/html/hr/

Florida Department of Health
http://www.doh.state.fl.us/

Georgia State Department of Human Resources
Division of Public Health
Environmental Health Section
404-657-6534
http://www.ph.dhr.state.ga.us/publications/foodservice/index.shtml

Guam Department of Public Health and Social Services
Division of Environmental Health
671-735-7210
http://www.gov.gu/pubhealth/envh.html

Hawaii State Department of Health
Environmental Health Administration
Environmental Health Services Division
Sanitation Branch/Food Services
808-586-8000
http://www.hawaii.gov/health/eh/index.html

Idaho State Department of Health and Welfare
Bureau of Environmental Health and Safety
Food Protection Program
208-334-5938
http://www.state.id.us/dhw/hwgd_www/FoodSafety/index.htm

Illinois State Department of Public Health
Office of Health Protection
Division of Food, Drugs and Dairies
Food Section
217-782-7532
http://www.idph.state.il.us/about/fdd/fddintro.htm

Indiana State Department of Health
Assistant Commissioner for Consumer Regulatory Services
Food Protection
317-233-7467

Iowa State Department of Inspections and Appeals
Division of Inspections
515-281-7114

Kansas State Department of Health and Environment
Division of Health

Bureau of Environmental Health Services
85-296-5599
http://www.kdhe.state.ks.us/fpch/index.html

Kentucky Cabinet for Health Services
Department for Public Health
Division of Public Health Protection and Safety
Food Safety/Cosmetics Branch
502-564-7181

Louisiana State Department of Health and Hospitals
Division of Environmental Health Services
Retail Food Program
225-763-5553
http://www.dhh.state.la.us/OPH/ehs/default.htm

Maine State Department of Agriculture
Food and Rural Resources
Division of Quality Assurance and Regulations
Food Program
207-287-3841
For retail food stores. http://janus.state.me.us/agriculture/quality/homepage.htm

Maine State Department of Human Services
Bureau of Health
Division of Health Engineering
207-287-5672
For restaurants and other food service establishments. http://janus.state.me.us/dhs/eng/index.htm

Maryland State Department of Health and Mental Hygiene
Community and Public Health Administration
Division of Food Control
410-767-8440
http://www.dhmh.state.md.us/cpha/

Massachusetts Executive Office of Human Services
State Department of Public Health
Bureau of Health Quality Management
Food Protection Program
617-983-6700
http://www.state.ma.us/dph/fpp/fpp.htm

Michigan State Department of Agriculture
Food and Dairy Division
517-373-1060
http://www.mda.state.mi.us/food/index.html

Minnesota State Health Department
Division of Environmental Health
651-215-0731
For restaurants and other food service establishments.
http://www.health.state.mn.us/divs/dpc/food/foodsafe.htm

Minnesota State Department of Agriculture
Dairy and Food Division
651-296-2627
For retail food stores.
http://www.mda.state.mn.us/foodsafe.htm

Mississippi State Board of Health
Bureau of Environmental Health
General Environmental Services
601-576-7690
http://www.msdh.state.ms.us/sanitation/index.htm

Missouri State Department of Health
Division of Environmental Health and Communicable Disease Prevention
Section for Environmental Public Health
573-751-6095

Montana State Department of Public Health and Human Services
Health Policy and Services Division
Food and Consumer Safety Section
406-444-5309
http://www.dphhs.state.mt.us/hpsd/pubheal/healsafe/fcss/index.htm

Nebraska State Department of Agriculture
Bureau of Dairies and Foods
402-471-25360
http://www.agr.state.ne.us/division/daf/food.htm

Commonwealth of The North Mariana Islands Department of Public Health
Division of Public Health
670-234-8950

Nevada State Department of Human Resources
Health Division
Bureau of Health Protection Services
702-687-4750
http://www.state.nv.us/health/bhps/

New Hampshire State Department of Health and Human Services
Bureau of Food Protection
Food Sanitation Section
603-271-4673

New Jersey State Department of Health and Senior Services
Division of Epidemiological/Environmental/Occupational Health
Consumer and Environmental Health Services
Food and Milk Program
609-588-3123
http://www.state.nj.us/health/eoh/foodWeb/

New Mexico State Department of Environment
Food Program
505-827-2855
http://www.nmenv.state.nm.us/

New York State Department of Health
Bureau of Community Sanitation and Food Protection
518-402-7600
For restaurants and other food service establishments.
http://www.health.state.ny.us/nysdoh/environ/bcsfp.htm

New York State Department of Agriculture and Markets
Division of Food Safety and Inspection
518-457-4492
For retail food stores.

New York City Department of Health
Environmental Health Services
Bureau of Inspections
212-676-1600
http://www.ci.nyc.ny.us/html/doh/html/inspect/insp.html

North Carolina State Department of Agriculture
Food and Drug Protection Division
919-733-7366
For retail food stores.
http://www.agr.state.nc.us/fooddrug/FDRPROG.HTM

North Carolina State Department of Health and Human Services
Division of Environmental Health
919-733-2870
For restaurants and other food service establishments.
http://www.deh.enr.state.nc.us/ehs/ehs.htm

North Dakota State Department of Health
Administrative Services Section
Division of Food and Lodging
701-328-6150 or 800-472-2927
http://www.health.state.nd.us/ndhd/admin/food/

Ohio State Department of Health
Division of Quality Assurance
Bureau of Local Health Services
614-466-0061
For restaurants and other food service establishments. http://www.odh.state.oh.us/directory/directory-f.htm

Ohio State Department of Agriculture
Division of Food Safety
614-728-6250
For retail food stores.
http://www.state.oh.us/agr/FoodSafetyDiv.html

Oklahoma State Department of Health
Deputy Commissioner for Special Health Services
Environmental Health Services
405-271-5217

Oregon State Department of Human Resources
Food Protection Program
503-731-4012
For restaurants and other food service establishments.
http://www.ohd.hr.state.or.us/esc/food/welcome.htm

Oregon State Department of Agriculture
Food Safety Division
503-986-4720
For retail food stores.
http://www.oda.state.or.us/Food_Safety/FSDINFO.html

Pennsylvania State Department of Agriculture
Bureau of Food Safety and Laboratory Services
717-787-4315

http://www.state.pa.us/PA_Exec/Agriculture/bureaus/food_safety/index.html

Puerto Rico Department of Health
Environmental Health Secretariat
Food Hygiene Division
787-274-7810

Rhode Island State Department of Health
Division of Environmental Health
Office of Food Protection
401-222-2750
http://www.health.state.ri.us/yhd08.htm

South Carolina State Department of Health and Environmental Control
Health Services
Bureau of Environmental Health
803-935-7945
http://www.state.sc.us/dhec/envhlth/hseh.htm

South Dakota State Health Department
Office of Health Protection
605-773-3364
For restaurants and other food service establishments.
http://www.state.sd.us/doh/Protect/

South Dakota State Department of Agriculture
State Department of Commerce and Regulations
Commercial Inspection and Regulation
605-773-3697
For retail food stores.
http://www.state.sd.us/dcr/inspection/SIP.htm

Tennessee State Department of Health
Division of General and Environmental Health
615-741-7206
For restaurants and other food service establishments.

Tennessee State Department of Agriculture
Regulatory Services Division
800-628-2631
For retail food stores.
http://www.state.tn.us/agriculture/regulate/regulate.html

Texas State Department of Health
Environmental and Consumer Health
Bureau of Food and Drug Safety
Retail Foods Division
512-719-0232
http://www.tdh.state.tx.us/bfds/bfds-hom.htm

Trust Territory of the Pacific Department of Health Services
691-320-2619/2609

Utah State Department of Health
Division of Epidemiology and Laboratory Services
Bureau of Food Safety and Environmental Health
801-538-6856
http://hlunix.ex.state.ut.us/els/envsvc/foodsafety/

Vermont State Department of Health
Environmental Health Division
802-863-7220

Virgin Islands Department of Health
Division of Environmental Health
809-774-6880

Virginia State Department of Health
Office of Environmental Health Services
Division of Food/Environmental Services
804-786-1750
For restaurants and other food service establishments.
http://www.vdh.state.va.us/oehs/food/food.htm

Virginia State Department of Agriculture and Consumer Services
Division of Consumer Protection
Office of Dairy and Foods
804-786-8899
For retail food stores.
http://www.vdacs.state.va.us/index.html

Washington State Department of Health
Environmental Health Programs
Office of Community Environmental Health
360-236-3050
http://www.doh.wa.gov/ehp/

West Virginia State Department of Health and Human Resources
Bureau for Public Health
Environmental Health Services
304-558-2981
http://www.wvdhhr.org/bph/enviro.htm

Wisconsin State Department of Agriculture
Trade and Consumer Protection
Division of Food Safety
608-224-4700
For retail food stores.
http://datcp.state.wi.us/fsafety/

Wisconsin State Department of Health and Family Services
Environmental Sanitation Section
608-266-8294
For restaurants and other food service establishments.
http://www.dhfs.state.wi.us/reg_licens/PH Sanitarians.htm

Wyoming State Department of Agriculture
Consumer Health Services Section
307-777-6587
http://wyagric.state.wy.us/CHS/foodsafe/foodsafe.html.

STATE MEAT INSPECTION PROGRAMS

To obtain information about individual State Meat Inspection Programs, contact the following state officials:

Alabama
Director
Meat and Poultry Inspection
Richard Beard Building
P.O. Box 3336
Montgomery, AL 36109-0336
334-240-7210

Alaska
State Veterinarian
Division of Environmental Health
500 S. Alaska, Suite A
Palmer, AK 99645
907-745-3236

Arizona
State Veterinarian
Arizona Dept. of Agriculture
Meat and Poultry Inspection Branch
1688 W. Adams, Room 333
Phoenix, AZ 85007
602-542-4971

California
(Custom Exempt Only)
Chief
Department of Food and Agriculture
Meat and Poultry Inspection Branch
1220 N St., Room A-126
Sacramento, CA 95814
916-654-0504

Delaware
Administrator
Delaware Department of Agriculture
2320 S. DuPont Highway
Dover, DE 19901
302-739-4811

Georgia
Director
Meat Inspection Division
Georgia Department of Agriculture
19 Martin Luther King Jr. Dr.
Room 108
Capitol Square
Atlanta, GA 30334
404-656-3673

Illinois
Bureau Chief
Illinois Department of Agriculture
State Fairgrounds
P.O. Box 19281
Springfield, IL 62794-9281
217-782-6684

Indiana
Director
Division of Meat and Poultry
Indiana State Board of Animal Health
805 Beachview Dr., Suite 50
Indianapolis, IN 46224-7785
317-227-0359

Iowa
Bureau Chief
Iowa Department of Agrculture and Land Stewardship
Wallace Building
Des Moines, IA 50319
515-281-5597

Kansas
Program Director
Meat and Poultry Inspection
Kansas Department of Agriculture

Division of Inspections
901 S Kansas Ave., 7th Floor
Topeka, KS 66612
785-296-3511

Louisiana
Program Manager
Louisiana Department of Agriculture and Forestry
P.O. Box 1951
Baton Rouge, LA 70821
504-922-1358

Minnesota
Director
Food Insepction Division
Minnesota Department of Agriculture
90 West Plato Blvd.
St. Paul, MN 55107
612-296-2629

Mississippi
Director
Meat Inspection Division
Mississippi Department of Agriculture
P.O. Box 1609
Jackson, MS 39201-1609
601-354-1193

Montana
Administrator
Meat, Milk, and Egg Inspection Division
Montanta Department of Livestock
P.O. Box 202001
Helena, MT 59620-2001
406-444-5202

New Mexico
Supervisor of Meat Inspection
New Mexico Livestock Board
7013 Central Ave., NE
Albuquerque, NM 87108-2049
505-841-4000

New York
(Custom Exempt Only)
Supervisor
Food Safety and Compliance Unit
New York Department of Agriculture
1 Winners Circle
Albany, NY 12235
518-457-2840

North Carolina
State Director
Meat and Poultry Inspection Service
North Carolina Department of Agriculture
P.O. Box 27647
Raleigh, NC 27611
919-733-4136

Ohio
Chief
Division of Meat Inspection
Ohio Department of Agriculture
8995 E. Main St., 2nd Floor
Reynoldsburg, OH 43068
614-728-6260

Oklahoma
Director
Meat Inspection Program
Coordinator
Animal Industry Services
Oklahoma Department of Agriculture
2800 N. Lincoln Blvd.
Oklahoma City, OK 73105-4298
405-521-3741

South Carolina
Director
South Carolina Meat and Poultry Inspection Division
P.O. Box 102406
Columbia, SC 29224
803-788-8747

South Dakota
State Veterinarian and Administrator
South Dakota Animal Industry Board
411 S. Fort St.
Pierre, SD 57501-4503
605-773-3321

Texas
Director
Meat Safety Assurance Division
Bureau of Food and Drug Safety
100 W. 49th St.
Austin, TX 78756
512-719-0205

Utah
Manager
Meat and Poultry Inspection Bureau
Utah Department of Agriculture

350 N. Redwood Road
Salt Lake City, UT 84116-6500
801-538-7117

Vermont
Director
Vermont Department of Agriculture
Meat Inspection Service
116 State St.
Drawer 20
Montpelier, VT 05620-2901
802-828-2426

Virginia
Program Manager
Office of Meat and Poultry Service
Virginia Department of Agriculture and Consumer Services
Washington Building
1100 Bank St., Suite 614
Richmond, VA 23219
804-786-4569

West Virginia
Director
West Virginia Department of Agriculture
Meat and Poultry Inspection Division
1900 Kanawha Blvd., E
State Capitol Building
Charleston, WV 25305-0179
304-558-2206

Wisconsin
Director
Meat Safety Inspection Bureau
Wisconsin Department of Agriculture
Trade and Consumer Protection
P.O. Box 8911
Madison, WI 53708-8911
608-224-4725

Wyoming
Director
Consumer Health Services
Wyoming Department of Agriculture
2219 Carey Ave.
Cheyenne, WY 82002-0100
307-777-7321

Glossary

Acute. An immediate (i.e., within hours or days), usually short-lived adverse health effect.

Adulterated. When a food contains a bacteria, contaminate, or other ingredient considered illegal.

Aerobic. Needs oxygen to grow.

Aflatoxin. Toxin produced by the mold *Aspergillus flavus* that contaminates grains and nuts.

Anaerobic. Grows in the absence of oxygen.

Antibiotic. Substance usually produced by microorganisms that can kill or inhibit the growth of other microorganisms.

Antibiotic resistance. The ability of some microorganisms to resist the effects of antibiotics.

Antibiotic resistance marker (ARM) gene. A gene inserted into genetically modified organisms that lets genetic engineers know the gene modification was successful.

Antitoxin. Substance that can neutralize a specific toxin.

Assize. A law regulating price, measure, weight, ingredients, etc. for goods to be sold.

Bacillus thuringiensis (Bt). A naturally occurring bacterium present in soil that produces a toxin that is toxic to only certain insect larvae. Is used as a natural pesticide.

Bacteria (singular: bacterium). Living, one-celled organisms found everywhere in the environment. Bacteria can be carried by water, food, wind, insects, plants, animals, people, and soil. Some bacteria can cause foodborne illness, but others are helpful and are used to make yogurt, alcoholic beverages, and cheeses.

Biological hazard. Disease-causing microorganisms or toxins that are found in some plants and animals. Includes bacteria, viruses, parasites, protozoa, and fungi.

Biotechnology. A variety of techniques that use living organisms, or substances from them, to make or modify products; improve plants, animals, and microorganisms; or develop novel organisms for specific uses.

Botulism. Food poisoning from consuming food containing toxin produced by the bacteria *Clostridium botulinum*. The toxin attacks the central nervous system and can cause muscle weakness, paralysis, and death unless an antitoxin is administered.

Bovine somatotropin (BST, rBST, bST). A naturally occurring hormone in milk-producing cows that is given to cows to increase milk production. Also called bovine growth hormone (BGH, rBGH).

Bovine spongiform encephalopathy (BSE). Degenerative brain disease of cattle characterized by sponge-like development of brain tissue. The human form is called Creutzfeldt-Jakob disease (CJD).

Carcinogen. Any substance that causes cancer.

Chemical hazard. Substance such as pesticide residue and cleaning solution that can cause illness.

Chronic. An adverse health effect that is persistent or recurring and may develop over many years. Example: Accumulation of heavy metals in the liver from years of drinking contaminated water.

Cold pasteurization. Any process that doesn't use heat to reduce the level of pathogenic or spoilage organisms in a food product. Examples: irradiation, ultraviolet (UV) radiation.

Coliform. A group of related bacteria, common in the environment and the digestive tracts of humans and animals, whose presence in drinking water may indicate contamination by disease-causing microorganisms.

Contamination. Unintended presence of potentially harmful substances, including microorganisms, chemicals, or physical objects in food.

Creutzfeldt-Jakob disease (CJD). Degenerative brain disease of humans characterized by sponge-like development of brain tissue. Similar to bovine spongiform encephalopathy (BSE) or mad cow disease.

Critical control point (CCP). Step or procedure along the food preparation path at which a control, such as heating, can be applied to prevent, reduce, or eliminate a food safety hazard. *Example:* Washing hands prior to handling food.

Cross-contamination. Transfer of harmful microorganisms to food by hands, food-contact surfaces, sponges, cloth towels, and utensils. Cross-contamination also occurs when raw food touches or drips onto cooked or ready-to-eat foods.

Danger zone. The range of temperatures at which most bacteria multiply rapidly, between 40 and 140 degrees F.

Defect action levels. Levels of permissible filth or extraneous matter established by FDA for specific foods or products for which a zero tolerance would be unrealistic. Example: Staples in a sack of potatoes.

Disinfection by-products (DBPs). Chemicals that form when disinfectants such as chlorine react with plant matter and other naturally occurring materials in water. These by-products may pose health risks.

DNA fingerprinting. Bacteria replicate themselves by dividing in two. When a bacterium divides, the two daughter bacteria have the same genetic make-up as the parent bacterium. Even after many generations, bacteria descended from the same original parent will have virtually identical genetic material, or DNA. DNA "fingerprinting" by pulsed-field gel electrophoresis (PFGE) is a simple way of comparing genetic material that involves cutting up the DNA into pieces, then measuring the number and sizes of those pieces. The pieces are separated by a jelly-like substance (gel). The DNA that has been cut into pieces is placed at one end of the gel. A pulsing electric field applied across the gel drives the DNA pieces across the gel over a period of hours. The smallest pieces move more quickly, so the pieces are separated as distinct bands on the gel. This pattern of bands, which resembles a bar code, is the "fingerprint."

Emerging infectious diseases. Infectious diseases that were little-known or unknown but that have greatly increased in the last two decades and threaten to increase in occurrence and severity in the future. *Example: Listeria monocytogenes* because it has only recently been discovered.

Epidemiology. The study of the incidence and distribution of disease and/or toxic effects in a population.

Ergotism. Also called St. Anthony's Fire, a disease caused by the ingestion of ergot toxin produced by the mold *Claviceps purpurea,* which infects rye and other cereals.

Exposure. Contact between a person and a chemical. Exposures are calculated as the amount of chemical available for absorption by a person.

Facultative anaerobe. Bacteria that can grow with or without oxygen.

Fecal-oral route. When a microscopic amount of fecal material on the hands is transmitted to the digestive system by putting the hands in the mouth.

Foodborne illness. Sickness resulting from disease that is transmitted to humans by food or water containing harmful microorganisms. Also sometimes called food poisoning.

Foodborne infection. Foodborne illness caused when pathogenic microorganisms consumed in food multiply within the gastrointestinal tract and attack tissues. Examples: *Salmonella, Campylobacter.*

Foodborne intoxication. Foodborne illness caused when miroorganisms produce toxins within food or the gastrointestinal tract. Examples: *Clostridium, Staphylococcus.*

Foodborne outbreak. Two or more people experiencing the same foodborne illness after eating the same food.

Food chain. A sequence in which each species serves as a food source for the next bigger species. Food chains usually begin with small species that consume plant material and proceed to larger and larger carnivores. Example: Grasshopper eaten by snake eaten by bird eaten by fox.

FoodNet. A federal surveillance program to determine the frequency and severity of foodborne illness.

Food irradiation. Process of preserving food through exposure to radiation (rays of energy).

Food poisoning. General term that includes almost all forms of sickness resulting from eating contaminated food.

Fungi. Group of microorganisms that include molds and yeasts.

Fungicide. Type of pesticide used to kill fungi.

Gastroenteritis. Inflammation of the stomach lining and intestines, often caused by a foodborne infection.

Gastrointestinal tract. Path food takes during digestion, stretching from the mouth to the anus, including the pharynx, esophagus, stomach, and intestines.

Gene. A section of a DNA molecule that is responsible for the production of specific proteins; a unit of hereditary information.

Genetic modification. A technique where an individual gene can be copied and transferred to another living organism to alter its genetic make-up. Also referred to as genetic engineering, genetic manipulation, and gene technology.

Growth hormones. Natural or synthetic hormones given to animals to promote faster, more efficient growth and to make leaner cuts of meat.

Hazard. A biological, physical, or chemical substance that may cause a food to be unsafe for consumption.

Hazard Analysis and Critical Control Points (HACCP) system. A preventive approach to food safety that involves determining where the hazards are in the manufacture or preparation of a food, and then controlling those critical points to eliminate, prevent, or minimize hazards.

Hemolytic uremic syndrome (HUS). Condition where red blood cells are broken down faster than new ones can be made by the bone marrow. Often requires kidney dialysis and blood transfusions and can result in death. Has been associated with *E. coli* O157:H7 infection.

Immunocompromised. When an individual has an existing disease or weakened physical condition that makes him or her more susceptible to becoming ill from foodborne illness.

Infectious dose. The number of organisms required to cause foodborne illness.

Inorganic chemicals. Mineral-based compounds such as metals, nitrates, and asbestos.

Integrated pest management (IPM). The use of pest and environmental information in conjunction with available pest control technologies to prevent unacceptable levels of pest damage by the most economical means and with the least possible hazard to persons, property, and the environment.

Ionizing radiation. Rays of energy that move in short, fast wave patterns that can penetrate cells.

Kuru. A degenerative brain disease, similar to Creutzfeldt-Jacob disease, found in certain tribes in New Guinea and originally linked to cannibalism practiced by those tribes.

Mad cow disease. *See* bovine spongiform encephalopathy (BSE).

Maximum contaminant level (MCL). Maximum permissible level of a contaminant in water that is delivered to any user of a public water system.

Microbiology. The study of microorganisms.

Microorganism. A form of life that can be seen only with a microscope, including bacteria, viruses, molds, and yeast.

Minimally processed foods. Foods that are only lightly processed to maintain the highest eating quality.

Modified atmosphere packaging (MAP). Packaging foods in a reduced-oxygen environment to extend shelf life.

Mycotoxin. A toxin produced by a fungus.

No observable effect level (NOEL). The highest dose of a chemical given to laboratory animals that does not produce any observable adverse effect.

Non-ionizing radiation. Rays of energy that move in long, slow wave patterns that do not penetrate cells.

nvCJD. New variant CJD. First identified in 1996 as being associated with BSE.

Organic chemicals. Chemical molecules that contain carbon and other elements such as hydrogen. Organic contaminants of concern in drinking water include chlorohydrocarbons and pesticides.

Organoleptic. Using the sight, touch, and smell for inspection.

Parasite. An organism that grows and feeds on or within another organism (host), but offers no benefits to the host.

Pasteurization. Process used to destroy foodborne pathogens. Often refers to heating food to a high enough temperature to reduce most of the pathogenic and spoilage microorganisms to a safe level. Irradiation is sometimes referred to as cold pasteurization.

Pathogen. A bacterium, virus, or other microorganism that causes disease.

Pathogenic. Disease-producing.

Pathogenic bacteria. Bacteria that cause foodborne illness. As opposed to spoilage bacteria, which cause food to deteriorate and develop unpleasant odors, tastes, and textures. Spoilage bacteria do not necessarily cause human illness.

Pesticide. The EPA defines a pesticide as, "any substance or mixture of substances intended for preventing, destroying, repelling, or mitigating any pest, and any substance or mixture of substances intended for use as a plant regulator, defoliant or dessicant."

Pesticide residue. A film of pesticide left on the plant, food, soil, container, equipment, handler, etc. after application of a pesticide.

Physical hazard. Foreign particles such as glass or metal in foods.

Potentially hazardous food (PHF). Foods with a high moisture and protein content that are low in acid and thus are known to support the growth of microorganisms that can cause foodborne illness. Examples: meats, eggs, milk products.

Prion. Tiny protein particles thought to be responsible for spongiform encephalopathies such as BSE and CJD.

Pulsed-field gel electrophoresis (PFGE). A laboratory technique that generates a DNA fingerprint. *See* DNA fingerprinting.

PulseNet. A national electronic network of public health laboratories and the CDC that performs DNA fingerprinting on bacteria suspected of causing a foodborne outbreak.

Radiation dose. Quantity of radiation energy absorbed by food as it passes through the radiation field during processing.

Radura. Circular symbol that must appear on all irradiated foods in the United States unless the food is used as an ingredient in a processed food or is served in a restaurant.

Ready-to-eat foods. Food that is in a form that is edible without washing, cooking, or additional preparation by the food establishment or consumer, and that is reasonably expected to be consumed in that form. Examples: Raw fruits and vegetables, processed lunch meats.

Reference Dose (RfD). Level of a chemical that an individual could be exposed to on a daily basis for a lifetime with minimal probability of experiencing any adverse effect. While this term is used in the United States, internationally the term Acceptable Daily Intake (ADI) is used.

Residue. A minute amount of a drug, antibiotic, hormone, pesticide, insecticide, or other contaminant that remains in meat and poultry after slaughter, or on fruits and vegetables after harvesting.

Risk. An estimate of the likelihood of an occurrence.

Risk assessment. An evaluation of the health risk resulting from exposure to a hazard. It combines exposure with degree of toxicity to estimate risk.

Rodenticide. Poisonous substance used to kill rodents, especially rats and mice.

Spoilage bacteria. Microorganisms that cause food to look, smell, or feel rotten, but that do not cause human disease.

Spore. A stage in the life cycle of some bacteria similar to hibernation in which the cell dries up and becomes dormant. Spores can survive cooking, freezing, or other sanitizing measures. When the environment becomes more hospitable the spore can revive and produce new active cells.

Standards of identity. Requirements a food must meet to be called a specific type of food. Example: Cream cheese must contain 51 percent moisture and 33 percent fat to be called "cream cheese."

Sterilization. Reduction of all vegetative cells and dormant spores to a safe level. This is the process used to make canned food.

Substances generally recognized as safe (GRAS). Additives in use prior to January 1958 that were thought to be safe due to a substantial history of safe use were declared generally recognized as safe (GRAS) and exempted from the provisions in the Additives and Color Amendments of 1958 and 1960.

Tolerance. For pesticides, a legal limit established by EPA for the maximum amount of a pesticide residue that may be present in or on a food.

Total coliform. Bacteria that are used as indicators of fecal contaminants in drinking water.

Toxicity. The capacity of a substance to cause adverse health effects.

Toxicology. The study of poisoning and its treatment.

Toxin. A poisonous substance produced by microorganisms.

Ultrahigh temperature (UHT). Modern method of pasteurization using higher temperatures for shorter periods of time. Provides longer shelf life, and no refrigeration is necessary until package is opened.

Unique radiolytic products (URPs). Chemicals produced in food when it is irradiated that are different from chemicals produced during cooking.

Vacuum packaging. A form of packaging food that eliminates most of the air from a package. This increases the shelf life of products and reduces shrinking due to moisture loss.

Vegetative cell. Cell in an active metabolic state in which bacteria are growing and multiplying.

Virulence. The power of a bacterium or virus to cause disease.

Virus. Smallest and simplest of microorganisms, basically just a ball of genes wrapped in a protein shell. Examples: Norwalk virus, hepatitis A.

Volatile organics. Chemicals that, when in a liquid form, evaporate into the air.

Water activity (Aw). The amount of water in a food that is available for bacterial growth.

Waterborne disease. Illness caused by ingesting water contaminated with a bacterium, virus, or other microorganism. Examples: typhoid fever, cholera, cryptosporidiosis.

Zero tolerance. If there is a zero tolerance for a substance or organism, the presence of that substance or organism in a food is illegal. Example: If any *E. coli* O157:H7 bacteria are found in a product, that product is considered adulterated.

Index

Page references followed by "t" or "f" indicate that the information is located in a table or figure.

About the Author

CYNTHIA A. ROBERTS is a faculty member at the Department of Nutrition and Food Science, University of Maryland. She has been the Coordinator of the USDA/FDA Foodborne Illness Education Information Center since its creation in 1994. The center is located at the National Agricultural Library in Belstville, MD and is funded and supported as part of a partnership between the U.S. Department of Agriculture, the Food and Drug Administration, and the National Agricultural Library. In 1998 Ms. Roberts was a recipient of the Food and Drug Administration Commissioner's Special Citation for fostering the exchange of information about food safety education between public and private sector organizations.